DIAGNOSIS OF SPEECH AND LANGUAGE DISORDERS

Second Edition

DIAGNOSIS OF SPEECH AND LANGUAGE DISORDERS

Second Edition

James E. Nation, PhD
Department of Communication Sciences
Case Western Reserve University
Cleveland, Ohio

Dorothy M. Aram, PhD
Department of Pediatrics
Case Western Reserve University
Cleveland, Ohio

SINGULAR PUBLISHING GROUP, INC.
SAN DIEGO, CALIFORNIA

Singular Publishing Group, Inc.
4284 41st Street
San Diego, California 92105

© 1984 College-Hill Press, Inc.
© 1991 Singular Publishing Group, Inc.

Library of Congress Cataloging in Publication Data

Nation, James E.
  Diagnosis of speech and language disorders.
  Bibliography: p. 379
  Includes index.
  1. Speech, Disorders of— Diagnosis. 2. Language disorders— Diagnosis. I. Aram, Dorothy M. II. Title. [DNLM: 1. Language disorders— Diagnosis. 2. Speech disorders — Diagnosis. WM 475 N275d]

| RC423.N25 | 1983 | 616.85'5075 | 83-23133 |

ISBN 1-879105-05-5

Printed in the United States of America

For

The Nations, Compardos, and Arams

In Special Remembrance

Brian, Norma, Herb

Preface

Diagnosis of speech and language disorders is a professional skill. The basic goals of the diagnostician are to discover the patient's speech or language problem, understand the potential causes of the problem, and propose appropriate management recommendations. To accomplish these goals the speech–language pathologist must have a basic fund of knowledge concerning normal and disordered speech and language, organize this information into a conceptual framework for easy retrieval, and understand the methodology necessary for solving the speech and language problem. Therefore diagnosis is a far different skill from just learning a series of testing procedures applicable to specific speech and language disorders, that is, tests for articulation disorders, voice disorders, stuttering, language disorders, and so forth.

The study of speech and language disorders is a field of inquiry within the realm of the behavioral sciences. As a behavioral science, a logical approach to diagnosis is available—the method of science. Scientific methodology as adapted to the clinical process should be the diagnostician's major tool. This approach can demonstrate a more unified ordering of information to students. They can acquire knowledge within a conceptual framework, behavior can be studied within this framework, advances in knowledge can be made, and arbitrary distinctions such as that between scientist and clinician can be broken down. The scientific orientation to diagnosis allows students to pursue diagnosis as a problem-solving process with the goal of understanding the nature, extent, and consequences of speech and language disorders.

A fundamental purpose of the second edition of *Diagnosis of Speech and Language Disorders* continues to demonstrate how the method of science can be applied to the diagnostic process. We feel students need an organized framework for learning, recalling, and using information vital to the diagnostic process. Therefore our intent is to retain a conceptual framework for organizing the information needed by the diagnostician and a scientific methodology that demonstrates how this framework can be applied to the individual diagnosis.

The second edition retains its emphasis on teaching an approach to diagnosis, not specific content about speech and language disorders or tests used in the diagnostic process. Emphasis is placed on how knowledge is acquired and used and how we must continue to expand on the information we need rather than on the learning of specific content. Throughout the text we have embedded patient examples to assist students in thinking through their approach to diagnosis as problem solving.

Our approach to learning tests and other diagnostic procedures is to do this through a variety of case studies—here referred to as patient projects—chosen to represent the major types of speech and language disorders. These patient projects are introduced in chapter 4. One patient project, Katherine Compardo, is developed throughout all subsequent chapters to serve as an example demonstrating the diagnostic tasks under discussion. The remainder of the patients serve as projects for the students to learn and practice the tasks presented in the given chapter. A series of study questions are included at the conclusion of every chapter which are intended to direct the student to additional sources of information.

This second edition no longer presents the material in two parts. The first part of the earlier edition has been condensed into three chapters in the new edition and some of the material has been incorporated into other chapters. The second edition now contains 10 chapters. Chapter 1 introduces diagnosis as a professional activity, the goals of which are to determine the given speech and language disorder, to understand causal factors, and to propose patient management. To accomplish these goals the diagnostician must command a specialized fund of knowledge related to normal and disordered speech and language, a problem-solving skill, and patient concern. Chapter 2 develops our framework, referred to as the Speech and Language Processing Model, for providing an organizational schema for integrating the diagnostician's fund of knowledge, for hypothesizing cause–effect relationships, for designing and selecting tools, and for interpreting clinical data. Chapter 3 discusses the applicability of the scientific method to speech and language diagnosis and outlines a series of steps for diagnosis that parallel the steps of the scientific method. The remaining seven chapters each address one of these steps, demonstrating specifically and systematically how the steps of the scientific method can be applied to the diagnostic process. We demonstrate how students can retrieve information from their fund of knowledge and expand on it when attempting to define and delimit the clinical problem under consideration. We discuss how diagnostic hypotheses can be formulated, and we follow this with a discussion of the selection of tools to test these hypotheses. We then go on to discuss general and specific procedures for administering testing tools, how to analyze and synthesize the information obtained in order to make decisions as to whether a problem exists, and what should be done about it. We also consider report writing as a means of communicating the information obtained in the diagnosis, emphasizing that reports can also reflect the scientific method.

We believe the orientation presented in this book allows speech pathologists to approach diagnosis as an ongoing process of hypothesis formulation and testing, utilizing and expanding on the knowledge and theories we have about human communication and its disorders. This orientation should allow speech–language pathologists to feel more comfortable in approaching any diagnostic problem that may be presented. It should allow for flexibility and change rather than a static testing procedure approach, since the primary emphasis is placed on problem solving rather than on a series of tests for specific disorders.

Diagnosis of Speech and Language Disorders can serve as a textbook in courses at both the graduate and undergraduate levels. The student using this book should possess fundamental information in the areas of the normal human communication process, language acquisition and use, child growth and development, and various speech and language disorders and their causes.

A few editorial decisions taken by the authors are worth comment. We have chosen to refer to patients and diagnosticians alike by the generic use of "he," considering this to be a simple, unobtrusive means of dealing with different pronoun genders. We also have chosen the term, *patient*, to refer to the person being diagnosed, although we are quite aware of the issues surrounding the choice of the term *patient* versus *client*, which have continued to be debated in our profession, most recently for example by Brodnitz (1983) and Naylor (1983). We have included bibliographic information for tests and other diagnostic procedures in the Tool Retrieval Tables: Appendix III and, to avoid lengthy redundancy, have not reiterated this information in the references.

Finally, many people are involved in preparing a textbook. To each person who has assisted we offer our thanks. Special acknowledgment and appreciation is expressed to Maureen Wetherbee, who helped with the Tool Retrieval Tables, to Claire Svet, who within a very short deadline typed almost the entire manuscript, and to Meg Guncik, who also typed and tracked down endless details. A special thanks to Margaret Olson who, besides working on many details of this book, assisted Dr. Nation immeasurably while he chaired the Department of Communication Sciences, and to Alex Johnson who has always provided a great deal of communicative competence. Finally, thanks go to Edward F. Moore for his special contribution to Dr. Nation's emotional well-being during the later phases of this book's completion.

James E. Nation
Dorothy M. Aram

CONTENTS

Chapter 1

Diagnosis as a professional activity

THE DIAGNOSTICIAN'S JOB

Meg, aged 2½, is brought to a hospital-based speech and language clinic because her parents want to know why she has not yet begun to talk. Max is seen in a community agency because he has lost his previously developed high level of verbal ability following a recent stroke. Jonathan is referred to the school speech–language pathologist by his classroom teacher because of his hesitancy to talk in class. Each is consulting a speech–language pathologist for a diagnosis of a speech and language disorder. Each wants to know what kind of speech and language disorder is present? What caused it? What can be done about it?

To answer these questions the diagnostician's job necessitates meeting three goals: first he focuses on the presented speech and language behavior to determine if it is disordered. Second, he wants to understand how that behavior came to be, that is, to understand what causal factors may be related to the behavior. Third, he utilizes the information gathered to decide what, if anything, can be done to help the patient.

Determining the speech and language disorder

The first goal of diagnosis is to describe the patient's speech and language behavior with particular emphasis on areas of greatest variation. This phase can be relatively objective. Three perspectives are used in the description of the patient's speech and language behavior: (1) as a speech and language *variation*: (2) as a speech and language *disorder*; and (3) as a speech and language *problem*.

First the diagnostician describes the behavior of concern with close attention to variability from normal expectations within different linguistic and interpersonal contexts. After the speech and language variation has been described, the diagnostician's task is to judge if the observed variation is normal or disordered. He recognizes that speech and language behavior exhibit a range of acceptable variability. What he needs to determine is whether the given variation falls within or outside of this normal range. If the specific behavior departs far enough from what is accepted as normal, he then has identified a speech or language disorder. The diagnostician determines that a disorder exists by comparing the observed speech and language behavior to normative data and acceptability criteria. For example, 5-year-old Janet who only speaks in single-word utterances is clearly outside the range of normal syntactic expectancies.

Further, through a comparison of the obtained behavioral variation with the diagnostician's known standard, a statement regarding the severity of the disorder may also be achieved. Thus, all other factors being equal, 2-year-old Margaret, demonstrating a total spoken vocabulary of 10 words, would not be judged to have as severe a language disorder as 4-year-old Sandra demonstrating the same behavior. While it is recognized that there is a considerable range in the ages at which children acquire certain features of their language, the competent diagnostician can arrive at a judgment of severity (1) by comparing the obtained behavior to normative data, (2) by noting the pattern of deviation, and (3) by referring to his own knowledge of the sequence of normal acquisition when specific normative data is not available. Shriberg and Kwiatkowsi (1982) illustrate the use of this concept in their discussion of phonological disorders.

Finally, the diagnostician must judge whether the identified speech and language disorder constitutes a problem for the patient and/or other involved persons. Here the diagnostician must use his professional judgment in evaluating the patient's speech and language behavior. For example, Jim claims he is a stutterer; however, the diagnostician does not observe Jim's speech to be abnormally dysfluent. What appears "normal" from an observable viewpoint is not normal to the patient. Thus, even if Jim's behavior is not considered variant to the diagnostician, Jim may still have a speech "problem" because of his own perceptions and feelings about his speech. Similarly, 4-year-old Philip's sound variations may be judged as normal developmental variations by the diagnostician. If this evaluation is accepted by Philip's parents and significant others in his environment, these normal sound variations probably will not present a problem. However, if the parents or others do not regard the behavior as normal, a problem may exist. On the other hand, a foreign-born speaker of English may talk with a foreign accent, which, while at variance with standard English, may not present a problem for the speaker or his listeners. Similarly, a person judged by his listeners as having a strident voice quality may not consider his voice quality a problem.

The diagnostician may rely heavily on the patient's verbal report of his feelings and attitudes about his speech and language, but he also gains information from observing the effect of the speech and language variation on the patient and his listeners. The patient's verbal statement may or may not coincide with the diagnostician's observations, which again calls for professional judgment in evaluating whether a "real" speech and language problem exists. On identification of a speech and language disorder, the diagnostician has to place the behavior into a broader context if he is to determine whether a problem exists for his patient.

In determining the nature and extent of the speech and language disorder, then, the diagnostician does three things: He describes the particular speech and language variation; he evaluates if the variation constitutes a disorder and the severity of the disorder; and he judges if the disorder constitutes a problem for persons involved.

Understanding causal factors

The second goal of diagnosis is to understand the causal factors that account for the presenting speech and language disorder. What does gaining such an understanding do for the diagnostician? Identifying causal factors allows him to have a better understanding of the nature of the speech and language disorder, its severity, and the prognosis. It also raises considerations for patient management and serves as a guide to therapeutic intervention. For example, Robert's sibilant distortions may be caused by a malocclusion, an inability to hear or discriminate the appropriate sounds, a deviant model presented by his father, or a variety of other reasons. The approach to changing the distorted sounds would vary depending on the identified causal factors. The fact that Mr. Weiss' profound language problem resulted from a cerebrovascular accident (CVA) 5 years earlier has quite clear implications for prognosis. Learning that Barbara's hypernasality is due to lack of velopharyngeal closure raises the consideration of referral for surgical procedures. Innumerable examples can demonstrate that subsequent decisions and actions taken by the diagnostician rest on an understanding of causal factors.

When investigating causal factors, the diagnostician should not expect to identify a single cause for a given effect. Even in the physical sciences, one-to-one cause–effect relationships are difficult to demonstrate. When dealing with human behavior, the relationship between a cause and an effect is even more tenuous. Rather, the diagnostician looks at multiple causes and interactions among numerous potential causal factors. He is not attempting to identify *the cause* but rather to suggest *probable causal relationships.* In approaching his search for causal factors, the diagnostician views causation in two ways.

First, he may search for *historical causal factors,* that is, past events that may have contributed to the current disorder. In this case, he studies information about the patient's past history. Second, he investigates *contemporary causal factors,* that is, events that are currently operating to account for, or maintain the speech and language disorder.

Historical and contemporary factors may include *extrinsic* situations that presently contribute to the disorder, for example, limited language stimulation from the immediate environment. In addition, contemporary causal factors may be viewed as physical processing deviations that are *intrinsic* to the patient. For example, an auditory discrimination problem can be viewed as a contemporary causal factor contributing to or maintaining a patient's disordered speech. Conditions that originally occurred in the past but are currently operating, sometimes referred to as maintaining causes, may be viewed as both historical and contemporary. While it is desirable to have an understanding of both historical and contemporary causation, many times historical causation is unknown or speculative. The more immediate disruptions in processing are more available for evaluation, more readily understood, and often serve as the basis for remediation.

Although at times the diagnostician may not be able to arrive at definitive causal factors, it is our contention that an attempt toward understanding causation is an indispensable goal of a complete diagnosis. Thus, the second major goal of the diagnostician's job is to understand historical, contemporary, and multicausal factors that potentially contribute to or maintain the speech and language disorder.

Proposing patient management

The final goal of diagnosis is to determine patient management (Nation, 1982). The major reason for delineating speech and language disorders and understanding causal factors is to arrive at a plan of action for the patient. Before the diagnostician can proceed in making plans for patient management, he must first assess whether or not the speech and language disorder constitutes a problem for the patient.

After establishing that a disorder constitutes a problem, the diagnostician then develops a plan of action for him—patient management. This goal incorporates any further steps that are to be taken, including recommendations for speech and language therapy, educational placement, medical referrals, and psychological evaluations, among others. At times, no further plans are indicated. A consideration of patient management should include a statement of probable prognosis. Prognostic statements will weigh the nature and severity of the disorder, the causal factors, and the personal characteristics of the patient such as age, motivation, and intelligence and the likelihood that management alternatives will be carried out.

CHARACTERISTICS OF THE SPEECH–LANGUAGE DIAGNOSTICIAN

Meeting the goals of speech and language diagnosis requires the knowledge and specialized training of professionals whose specialty is communication disorders. The characteristics needed by a competent speech and language diagnostician include (1) a fund of knowledge relevant to speech and language disorders, (2) skill in applying this knowledge to solving clinical problems, and (3) an overriding concern for helping his patient understand and manage his speech or language problem. These three characteristics—a fund of knowledge, a problem-solving skill, and patient concern—are fundamental to the diagnostician's professional service.

A fund of knowledge

A profession is generally defined as a vocation based on specialized knowledge in some area of learning or science. A professional is seen as one who has a broad range of information from which he selectively draws to solve the problem at hand. His competence is judged on the basis of the range of information he possesses, his ability to see relationships among areas of information, and his skill in selectively applying this information base. The diagnostician in practice and the student in training confront a wide range of speech and language disorders stemming from many possible causes and requiring countless management decisions. One day it may be a 4-year-old nonverbal child and the next an adult with a laryngectomy. The diagnostician must be prepared to work with many different types of patients. Only rarely will he work in a setting that specializes in a narrowly defined disorder, for example, in an aphasia rehabilitation unit. Also, the diagnostician is not likely to remain in the same professional setting throughout his career. The professional speech and language diagnostician therefore needs a diverse fund of knowledge which will allow him to shift to differing patient populations.

While relevant information comes from our study of the communication sciences, other important information comes from diverse areas, including, among others, the biological and physical sciences, linguistics, psychology, sociology, medicine, and education. Because the study of disordered speech and language is multidisciplinary, one of the chief problems facing the diagnostician is drawing together all this information into an organizational framework that is readily usable for addressing clinical problems. Learning to become a diagnostician, therefore, is not simply a matter of learning a body of knowledge or course content. Developing a frame of reference for his fund of knowledge and making it readily applicable to clinical problems are equally, if not more, important. Two notable implications follow from this orientation.

First, an organizational framework for funds of knowledge should not be directed to specific "problem types." The professional diagnostician is not a preprogrammed technician with certain information for certain conditions. Rather the professional's approach toward organizing knowledge should be integrative and not simply segmented or departmentalized into knowledge about voice disorders, stuttering, aphasia, autism, and so forth. The diagnostician must arrive at a framework that is equally appropriate to whatever speech and language behavior his patients may present. Before he sees a new patient, the diagnostician often does not know what *problem type* to expect. Even when anticipating a certain pattern, he is often surprised to find that what he expected did not turn out to be the primary disorder. For example, a child with a cleft palate may not have significant difficulty in the production of speech, but may experience difficulty in language formulation or perhaps may even stutter. Therefore the diagnostician needs a superordinate view of speech and language processing and its disorders that allows him to shift gears flexibly and relate his fund of knowledge to whatever behavior occurs.

Second, our orientation implies that diagnoses are arrived at through application of this broad base of acquired knowledge. The diagnostic process stems from a culmination and integration of past experience and learning and may be viewed as the pinnacle of professional activity. Although a diagnostician may have his current information organized for application, it should be understood that his frame of reference must allow for continued acquisition of knowledge. The diagnostician must realize that his present knowledge does not necessarily represent reality accurately. Instead, it only represents his understanding of his experiences and the available information at any given time.

The diagnostician keeps in mind that much of what is "known" may be theoretical. Additional knowledge not only will be forthcoming and acquired, but current information may change over time. The professional is committed to developing broadly based knowledge, while at the same time realizing the incompleteness and tentativeness of the knowledge. It is vital that the diagnostician maintains an inquisitive, searching attitude toward knowledge acquisition that leads to a revitalization and a reevaluation of acquired information. He must keep current in his profession.

The primary funds of knowledge needed by the speech and language diagnostician concern speech and language acquired within an interdisciplinary framework. The diagnostician requires specialized knowledge of the following, each of which will be addressed further below:

1. Normal speech and language development and use;
2. Disorders of speech and language;
3. Causal factors that disrupt normal speech and language;
4. Various management alternatives.

Normal speech and language

In order to determine if speech and language is disordered the diagnostician must have a fundamental grounding in what is normal. We have identified four normative or normal content areas as prerequisites for speech and language diagnosis. (1) language as a rule-based system, (2) the normal speech and language user; (3) changes in speech and language use during a lifespan; and (4) communicative interaction. Within each area we briefly describe the needed information, the disciplines that provide the information, and the relevance of the information for the diagnostician.

• *Language as a rule-based system.* Language, an ordered, predictable system for communication, can be abstracted from individual speakers and studied as an idealized system. Such study aims to describe language in and of itself and to present the rules that account for the creation of permissible language sequences. Students of language typically subdivide the language system into levels or parameters:

1. *Phonology*, which concerns the description of sounds in a language and the rules for ordering sound sequences (e.g., Edwards & Shriberg, 1983).
2. *Syntax*, which generally concerns word order, inflectional endings, and functional words (e.g., Miller, 1981).

3. *Semantics,* which focuses on meaning of single words (lexicon) and between words (semantic relations; e.g., Leonard, 1976).

4. *Pragmatics,* which attempts to understand the functional use of language and modifications required by the communicative context (e.g., Gallagher & Prutting, 1983).

Linguistics has become the primary discipline devoted to the study of language as an idealized system. While writers have been intrigued with the study of language for hundreds of years, in the 1960s an outpouring of linguistic study and thought began with the advent of Chomsky's work (1957, 1965) in transformational–generative grammar. While differing approaches to the study of the language system have been presented, such as descriptive linguistics (Francis, 1958; Gleason, 1961), stratificational grammar (Lamb, 1966), and case grammar (Fillmore, 1968), certainly Chomsky's influence was a major force in accelerating the study of the structure of language.

With information for studying language as a rule-based system, the diagnostician is armed with an indispensable tool for clinical use. He may borrow the linguist's methods for describing, measuring, and understanding the language used by his patients. Through linguistic description the diagnostician may order, categorize, and see relationships among speech sounds, syntactic devices, semantic systems, and communicative interactions.

• **The normal speech and language user.** The diagnostician needs knowledge about normal speech and language processes if he is to understand speech and language disorders. The focus here is on the normal person's ability to receive, comprehend, integrate, formulate, and produce speech and language—the human as a processing system.

The diagnostician needs knowledge of the biological, physiologic, and psychological requisites for speech and language. He needs information about human anatomy, especially concentrating on those structures involving hearing, understanding, and speaking. He also needs information about the cognitive and psychological experience underlying and relating to speech and language. For example, when considering auditory reception, the diagnostician needs to know the anatomy and physiology of the hearing mechanism—its structure and function. He also has to understand the hearer's psychological response to sound and the role played by other psychological factors such as attention, motivation, and memory. He must relate cognitive development to auditory and language mechanisms and stages in development.

The biological sciences (including anatomy and physiology, neuroanatomy and neurophysiology, genetics, and embryology) have provided much information pertaining to the biological basis for speech and language. The speech and hearing sciences (speech perception, psychoacoustics, motor phonetics, etc.) have been central in accumulating and organizing pertinent anatomic and physiologic information as it relates to the study of speech reception and production. An understanding of the psychological dimensions of speech and language has been contributed to by a number of applied disciplines, including clinical neurology, psychology, and psychiatry. The study of speech and language as a system has resulted in the emergence of disciplines whose concern is with the normal speech and language user. Psycholinguistics "wedded" the study of psychology and language; neurolinguistics has come to refer to the interface between language behavior and its neuroanatomic basis; and bioacoustics has brought together the sciences of biology and acoustics.

Essentially the diagnostician's study of the normal speech and language user helps him understand why disorders do occur. For example, he may be able to relate an articulation disorder to a defective speech-producing mechanism as seen in a child with a cleft palate, or the language formulation disorder may be related to known left cerebral hemisphere damage. By understanding the relationship of <u>anatomic</u>, <u>physiologic</u>, and <u>psychological</u> factors to speech and language processing, the diagnostician can better determine the reasons for the speech and language symptoms presented by his client.

→ add to Dx mission tree

• ***Changes in speech and language development during life.*** It is not enough for the diagnostician to acquire knowledge about speech and language as mature and static systems. Speech and language emerge in childhood, achieve a relative plateau during adulthood, and undergo further changes in later life. Speech and language disorders are seen at all ages, and diagnosticians must have an understanding of how the process develops and varies at different ages if they are to make appropriate comparisons of patients suspected of having speech and language disorders.

Knowledge related to child language development prior to the 1960s has been summarized by McCarthy (1954), including commentaries and criticisms. These earlier studies were primarily biographic and analytic, measuring quantitatively what a child did at a certain age in such areas as vocabulary development, sound development, sentence structure, and length of response.

Beginning in the late 1950s but with greater emphasis toward the late 1960s and the 1970s, a tremendous accumulation of language acquisition data resulted, corresponding to the outgrowth of theories regarding language and communication. New knowledge about speech and language development has come from many disciplines, including psycholinguistics, cognitive psychology, education, and speech pathology.

Numerous theories of speech and language acquisition have been proposed, and the developmental sequence of various parameters of language have been described in detail (e.g., Brown, 1973a, 1973b; deVilliers & deVilliers, 1978; Menyuk, 1977; Miller & Chapman, 1981). Rather than striving for quantitative measures, the presumption is that each stage of development represents for the child his own rule-based system. In addition to the considerable attention now given to speech and language development per se, language acquisition is being more thoughtfully integrated with information about the child's physical, cognitive, and emotional development within an interpersonal context (e.g., Prutting, 1982b; Steckol & Leonard, 1981). A fund of knowledge that is growing quite rapidly because of our (interdisciplinary interest) in child growth and development is the information about language–cognitive relationships in the young child from birth to 2 years of age. This interest is leading to assessment and management principles and procedures with an eye toward
→ prevention of later language-learning disorders. Currently the information tends to be more theoretical than applicable to clinical situations (Stark, 1981). ← *support for mott program*

Knowledge of normal speech and language development provides the diagnostician with a yardstick against which to judge the rate, sequence, and characteristics of the speech and language behavior presented by young patients, a yardstick that has great variability. Theories of acquisition provide insight into how and why the observed speech and language behavior may be disordered and descriptions of sequential development offer guides for remediation (e.g., Bloom & Lahey, 1978; Ingram, 1976; Leonard, 1979; Miller, 1981; Mills, 1983; Prutting, 1979). Only by knowing what is expected in the way of speech and language during normal development can the diagnostician determine if a variation from normal constitutes a speech and language disorder (Aram & Nation, 1982).

At the other end of the development spectrum, the speech and language diagnostician must have knowledge of the speech and language changes that accompany the aging process. As the population includes an increasing number of elderly people, the speech and language pathologist is being called upon to evaluate growing numbers of persons in their 70s and

80s and beyond. He therefore must know what may be expected in these age groups in, for example, voice quality, rate of speech, or word retrieval, in order to differentiate normal changes from pathological symptoms evidenced in a range of neurological or psychiatric conditions commonly seen in the elderly. Further, he needs to have an appreciation of the more general biological, psychological, and social changes in later life to better understand his elderly patients' perspectives and problems. While information bearing on the elderly is included in long-established disciplines such as psychology, neurology, sociology, and biology, the field of gerontology has emerged to bring together these many facts of the study of the aging. Within speech-language pathology, the past 10 years also has seen an increased interest in studying speech and language changes in later life, especially as these relate to pathological conditions such as Alzheimer's disease and presbycusis (e.g., Bayles & Boone, 1982; Marshall, 1981; Oyer & Oyer, 1976; Ramig & Ringel, 1983; Walker, Hardiman, Hedrick, & Holbrook, 1981).

• ***Communicative interaction.*** Our field in recent years has come full circle from its early beginnings in "general speech," where interferences with ones' ability to speak with others was first recognized, to the present where communicative interactions have become a major focus of study, under umbrella terms of "pragmatics," "discourse analysis," and "conversational competence" (Prutting, 1983).

Communicative interaction through creative speech and language use is unique to the human being. Speech and language as the primary means of human interaction can be considered as fulfilling the human lifestyle. People talk to themselves and to one another to learn, impart information, control behavior, express anger, solve problems, fantasize, remember, reason, and persuade—the list is extensive and the categories are seldom mutually exclusive.

The study of theories of human communication, including communicative interaction, understandably is multidimensional and interdisciplinary (e.g., Littlejohn, 1983). Such diverse persons as business executives, psychologists, educators, actors, philosophers, and health practitioners, among others, have all addressed communicative interaction, especially the problematic aspects. Academic areas such as speech communication, psycholinguistics, sociology, psychiatry, social psychology, and other people-related fields have all made contributions.

Because of this diversity of interest, we are often left with a fragmented framework. Mortensen (1972) has indicated that there may be as many definitions of communication as there are research interests about it. In his work on communication as a study of human interaction, Mortensen (1972) sees human communication as made up of three interrelated systems—the *intrapersonal, interpersonal,* and *sociocultural.* Each of these systems shares essential components with the others within the overall human communication system.

Adapting Mortensen's views to speech and language disorders we believe most disorders stem from disruptions within the intrapersonal system, to us disruptions of speech and language processing. These disorders then can result in difficulties with interpersonal communicative interactions. Therefore the phonologic, syntactic, and semantic levels of language could be viewed as primarily intrapersonal whereas the pragmatic level is more specifically related to interpersonal and sociocultural systems of communication. While the majority of speech and language disorders probably originate within the intrapersonal system (that is, intrinsic speech and language processing breakdowns), some arise within the interpersonal system as has been hypothesized in the diagnosogenic view of stuttering (Johnson, 1942).

Need description + measurement of abnormality

Irrespective of the origin of speech and language breakdowns, understanding the impact of a speech and language disorder on communicative interaction is an integral part of a diagnostician's needed knowledge. For example, 42-year-old James who has an /s/ distortion may communicate effectively and be unconcerned about the distortion. If so, the diagnostician must question whether there is truly an interpersonal communication problem vs. or if the speech disorder is merely an intrapersonal variation about which James has no concern.

In still broader perspective the diagnostician must understand how the speech and language disorder affects the overall psychological adjustment his patients make to their intrapersonal, interpersonal, and sociocultural worlds. Since speech and language are used for so many purposes, disorders frequently have significant effects on many areas of development and adjustment. For example, in the young child with a language disorder we may see significant subsequent effects on learning (e.g., Aram, Ekelman, & Nation, in press; Aram & Nation, 1980). The child who has no language because he is deaf also demonstrates this point clearly.

It is only when he understands the overall communication process as it relates to a specific language community with its personal, social, and cultural expectations that the diagnostician can place speech and language disorders into their appropriate contexts.

Disorders of speech and language

While normal speech and language provide diagnosticians with a base for measuring and understanding disordered behavior, speech–language pathologists' unique area of expertise is their specialized knowledge about speech and language disorders. To fulfill the first purpose of diagnosis, determining the speech and language disorder, the diagnostician needs specific information about the symptoms and classifications used to describe speech and language disorders. When the behavior departs from normal expectations, the diagnostician has to know how to observe, describe, and measure what he hears and sees. While, for example, his internalized normal standard may signal that a particular voice quality is not normal, he should have information that allows him to say more than "the voice quality is not normal." His detailed knowledge of voice disorders allows him to provide additional description and measurement of the behavior presented. He may study the patient's voice range, listening for variations in quality as a function of pitch. He may have the patient attempt different manners of voice production and note the effects on voice quality under each condition. The diagnostician's prior exposure to voice disorders allows him to descriptively classify the voice quality characteristics. In addition, he may wish to employ instrumental aids to provide objective study of the vocal tone. Thus, what the diagnostician knows specifically about each speech and language disorder points the way for detailed analysis and description.

As specified by The American Speech–Language–Hearing Association (Asha, 1982) certification requirements, speech–language pathologists must have clinical training in four primary disorder areas. These areas are disorders of *voice, fluency, articulation,* and *language.* Students are required to gain academic information and clinical practicum in each of these areas, usually through one or more courses, independent study, and clinical experience in each area.

Because of the emphasis placed on each disorder area, relating the disorders to each other has typically received less attention. The diagnostician can be left with a disjointed view of speech and language disorders. Often the student and professional diagnostician function as if they have mutually exclusive funds of knowledge for each disorder area rather than examining the relationships between, for example, articulation and language disorders. While it is essential to have information about specific speech and language disorders, it is equally essential to relate these areas to each other since the patient may well present behaviors characteristic of more than a single disordered area, for example, the dysfluencies often seen in young language delayed children (Bloodstein, 1974; Hall, 1977; Merits-Patterson & Reed, 1981).

Similarly, the diagnostician does not have available to him an agreed upon system for classifying the majority of speech and language disorders presented. Classification of speech and language disorders has been approached from several perspectives, including those that address primarily etiology, behavioral description, clinical problem types, or processing. Etiologic classification systems have grouped disordered speech and language in terms of the presumed cause of the disorder, for example, cleft palate speech, developmental dysphasia, or psychosocial language delay. Behavioral description classification systems emerged in part as a reaction to the inadequacies in the use of etiologic classification systems. In such systems a phrase or paragraph often was used to describe a patient's speech and language strengths and limitations (e.g., Milisen, 1957). A clinical problem-type approach to classification has been reflected in many introductory texts in speech and language pathology. What usually results in problem-type classifications is a mixture of etiologic, behavioral, and processing terms with little internal consistency. For example, Erikson and Van Riper (1967) use the term "clinical type" and include within this classification the following disorders: stuttering, misarticulation, dysphonia, cerebral palsy, aphasia, postlaryngectomy, delayed language, and hearing loss. Finally, processing approaches to speech and language classification have attempted to relate observed speech and language behavior to presumed underlying processes. Processes specified in many such classification systems include phonation, resonation, articulation, prosody, and symbolization.

The development of processing classification systems for speech and language disorders has assisted the diagnostician in drawing better relationships between the behavioral disorders observed and disrupted speech and language processes. These systems went beyond describing the characteristics of the disorder; they provided insight into the basis of the behavioral disorder. Further, processing approaches to classification have aided speech–language pathologists in seeing commonalities and differences among disorder types and, to some degree, have helped counteract the entrenched practice of studying, diagnosing, and treating distinct disorder types.

Thus, the diagnostician needs extensive information about the various speech and language disorders. Equally important, however, is that his fund of knowledge include a system for classifying and drawing relationships among disorder types (Nation & Aram, 1977).

Causal factors

To arrive at the second goal of diagnosis, understanding causal factors, the diagnostician must possess information pertinent to general and specific causes of speech and language disorders. He needs to gain knowledge about the intrinsic and extrinsic (biological–environmental) factors that may potentially affect the development and use of speech and language. He is interested in those physical, psychological, emotional, and environmental factors that may have a direct or indirect effect on the patient's speech and language mechanisms and processes. For example, an amputated arm, although not directly needed for speech and language, may influence 6-year-old Bertheva's self-esteem, thus making her less outgoing and energized in attempting to communicate.

The diagnostician's fund of knowledge about causal factors should help him do the following:

1. Understand ways of categorizing causal factors that have a bearing on the speech and language disorder, information that helps him view and interpret various levels of causation;
2. Gain a complete understanding of historical causal factors to assist in establishing how the present disorder came to be;
3. Evaluate what interactions may have existed among multiple causal factors in the patient's history to produce the disorder;
4. Evaluate contemporary causal factors, as these are currently operating and may be more amenable to change;
5. Identify probable cause–effect relationships in order to plan appropriate patient management.

In order to answer questions regarding causation, the diagnostician uses many sources. He considers his knowledge of normal speech and language development and use, emphasizing factors and determinants that could disrupt the process. Specific study of disordered speech and language provides considerable data about causation. As well, information that bears on questions of causation comes from disciplines outside speech pathology, including medicine, child growth and development, anatomy and physiology, psychology and psychiatry, and many others. With relevant information coming from many fields of study, cataloging potential causal factors has become significantly difficult for the diagnostician.

Within speech and language pathology, diverse orientations to causation have coexisted. Different positions have been taken about the need to understand the causes of speech and language disorders. Probably the least emphasis is given to causation by those who profess to be interested in behavioral symptoms only. At the other end of the continuum are those whose orientation justifies working only with the "underlying" or "overriding" cause for the disordered behavior. In addition, settings in which speech–language pathologists train or work promote different approaches and biases to the study of causal factors. For example, a speech–language pathologist working with neurologists, may well come to view most disorders as neurologically based, while work in a psychiatric setting may well exaggerate the importance of psychogenic factors. Thus, the causal emphasis for almost any speech and language disorder can vary significantly from one professional to another.

These diverse orientations to causation have resulted in inconsistent and often confusing approaches to causal factors for speech and language disorders. Three persistent and, to us, dead-end practices have dominated much of the work in our field. We have already mentioned the etiological classification system, whereby disorder types were grouped in terms of presumed etiology. A second practice has involved open-ended listing or cataloging of the endless potential causes of disordered speech and language. A final, equally unsatisfying, approach has been to dichotomously classify causes as "functional" or "organic," failing to recognize that for something to function it must also exist as an organic structure, and thus in the final analysis all behavior is organically based.

These three persistent practices that have evolved around causation have resulted in a limited understanding of causal factors for speech and language disorders. They often lead the diagnostician toward a simplistic view of causation rather than a dynamic interactive view. Emphasis has been placed on finding a cause rather than discovering a cause–effect relationship. Diagnosticians often search the patient's history to see if it reveals a causal factor that is on the etiology "list." These diagnostic practices seem to arise because the diagnostician somehow feels obligated to tie a cause to a disorder or to label the disorder as functional or organic, but he does not feel the obligation to discover how and if the causal factor is important to management decisions that need to be made.

Lists and catalogs of etiologic factors have little explanatory power; they do not automatically reveal the interactions that existed between the causal factors and the speech and language disorder. Thus, it is of limited value in diagnosis to gather historical data of etiologic significance without considering how the causal factors interacted with speech and language processing to result in the disordered speech and language behavior. Multiple causation, chains of cause–effect relationships, time of occurrence, severity, and the direct–indirect nature of causation must be evaluated.

Fortunately, more professionals are rethinking causation in relationship to diagnosis and treatment of speech and language disorders. They are recognizing the presence of multiple causation and different levels of causal description. From this process, new schemata are being developed out of the old. Better insights into the complexities of causation for speech and language disorders are being sought (Nation & Aram, 1977).

Management alternatives

Finally, within his fund of knowledge the diagnostician needs expert knowledge of management approaches and alternatives. From his study of speech and language disorders he has acquired detailed and up-to-date information outlining remediation principles and procedures for various disorder types. His extensive course work and continuing education have equipped him with numerous therapy alternatives for working with language, articulation, phonology, fluency, and voice disorders. Beyond knowing how to remediate a range of speech and language disorders, he also needs to be knowledgeable in the availability and appropriateness of management alternatives which may involve other professionals or other alternatives not involving direct speech and language therapy. His information base in causal factors coupled with his expertise in speech and language disorders will point to management alternatives other than therapy. For example, understanding the relationship between articulation disorders and velopharyngeal incompetence directs referral to a prosthodontist, plastic surgeon, or possibly a craniofacial team—all potentially more appropriate management alternatives to direct speech therapy. Similarly, a child with verbal auditory agnosia may be more appropriately treated by a neurologist prior to or coincident with speech and language therapy (Nation, 1982).

Thus, the diagnostician must have specific knowledge regarding the range of management approaches needed for speech and language disorders. He must know when referrals are necessary to other professionals, what remedial programs (modes of therapy) are needed, and what effect the remedial program might have, that is, the skill of prognostication (Nation, 1982).

To make these decisions concerning patient management, the diagnostician needs both theoretical and practical knowledge. He needs generalized information about what procedures and functions other professionals provide if he is to determine if a particular referral is indicated and appropriate. Practically, the diagnostician needs to know specific names of professionals and agencies that provide services in his community and how to go about obtaining that service. For example, on a theoretical level, a diagnostician may know that any one of a number of professionals can provide child guidance or psychotherapy; practically, however, the diagnostician has to know who is likely to accept the patient within a reasonable period and at a manageable cost. In making recommendations for therapy programs, including speech and language therapy, the diagnostician must know the range of potential therapy alternatives and be aware of practical limitations in arranging for any of them. Finally, the diagnostician's data base in communicative interaction provides him with an intrapersonal, interpersonal, and sociocultural perspective from which to judge the importance of the disorder to both the patient and others.

Problem solving skill

The second characteristic fundamental to the professional diagnostician is skill in applying his fund of knowledge to solving clinical problems. The professional diagnostician does not arrive at clinical solutions purely by intuition; rather, he approaches clinical problems through a systematic, explicit methodology based on his reasoning and training as a behavioral scientist. As a behavioral scientist, the diagnostician states cause–effect hypotheses pertaining to each patient that he sees; he develops procedures for testing his clinical hypotheses; and he collects, analyzes, interprets, and generalizes from his clinical data.

The chief point to be made here is that diagnosis is something other than just testing or learning specified test procedures for a specific disorder. The diagnostician is a problem solver, a decision maker, not a technician or a "prescription filler." He carries with him a scientific methodology that allows him systematically to utilize his fund of knowledge in addressing the clinical problems presented to him. His scientific method organizes and guides his clinical work. While he may artfully employ procedures and relate to his patients, he has little use for "cookbook" approaches to diagnosis in which one routinely and invariably administers a set battery of tests for a given disorder. Rather, he approaches each diagnosis as a creative problem-solving activity that follows positively from a scientific methodology. Therefore, if confronted with symptomatology that does not fit a particular condition, he has a rational approach for studying the presented behavior. Similarly, he can readily assimilate new tests and testing procedures into his overall approach to diagnosis.

With the problem-solving methodology provided by his scientific orientation, the diagnostician is able to employ his professional judgment, discretion, and knowledge in tailor-making each diagnosis. He is better able to efficiently and competently evaluate each patient's unique speech and language disorder. As he continues to solve clinical questions with the scientific method, he learns more, he adds more information to his fund of knowledge, and his problem-solving abilities become more finely tuned.

Basic then to the development of a professional diagnostician is his utilization of a problem-solving methodology. A speech pathologist with a high level of knowledge but no approach to problem solving is not a diagnostician. Occasionally, we encounter very knowledgeable speech–language pathologists who have little ability to relate their knowledge to patient's problems. Because their knowledge is not available for clinical problem solving, these individuals, in our minds, are not diagnosticians.

Patient concern

The final characteristic essential to a speech and language diagnostician is professional commitment to serving the best interests of his patients. Whatever we do as diagnosticians, we must acknowledge the wants and needs of the person who comes to us. Unless the diagnostic process benefits the patient and addresses his needs, the activity becomes a sterile, academic exercise with little professional involvement. However, benefit to the patient does not necessarily imply direct speech and language therapy. The diagnostician should be accountable for helping his patient understand his disorder, its possible causes, and its prognosis as well as plan for appropriate future management of the problem when needed. Even if therapy or referral is not indicated, the diagnostician has added to his patient's understanding of and future orientation to his problem.

The diagnostician must know how and why the patient was motivated to seek help. Does he come of his own volition, in agreement with the recommendation of another, or is he brought passively or actively against his will by a dutiful parent or spouse? The reality is that diagnosticians sometimes see people who do not want to be seen; for example, the preadolescent stutterer who does not take responsibility for his stuttering or cannot admit to having a problem, or the aphasic who is so depressed about his total physical condition that he cannot accept the proddings of his spouse. These nonvoluntary patients should make us evaluate patient concern carefully. To whom are we responsible? Is it always the patient, or in some instances is it to an interested relative or professional?

Above all, the professional diagnostician must consider the patient as a person with feelings, needs, and abilities beyond just the speech and language problem. It is the patient who has the problem, not the problem that has the patient. The diagnostician is the patient's consultant in understanding that problem. His orientation should therefore be toward diagnosing a human being with a speech and language problem, not merely adding to his own sophistication and experience in recognizing and understanding disordered speech and language. If he has merely treated the patient as a "problem type" to which he administers x number of tests, the diagnostician has failed to see the patient as an individual and thereby neglects to meet an essential characteristic of his professional responsibility. Diagnosticians have not fulfilled their ethical contract with their patient if they have not addressed *his* questions and provided as best they can for *his* needs.

OTHER VIEWS OF DIAGNOSIS AND RELATED TERMS

We have now presented the particular viewpoint toward diagnosis and the diagnostician that is used in this book and expanded on in subsequent chapters. We do not wish to imply that all persons in speech–language pathology use the term "diagnosis" in the same sense as we do. Many writers have chosen other words to refer to the total activity we call diagnosis. Rather than assume that everyone means the same thing by these words we will discuss our understanding of these related terms.

A medical heritage

The term "diagnosis" has a medical orientation: to determine by physical examination and laboratory tests the nature of a disease or condition. The medical model generally implies that the symptoms and observable signs are not the underlying cause. Rather than deal with symptomatology, the focus in medicine generally has been an attempt to identify and treat the cause of a given condition. A number of writers in speech–language pathology use the word "diagnosis" in the medical sense and suggest that diagnosis should remain within the domain of the physician. Perkins writes:

Where assessment is the province of the speech pathologist, diagnosis is accomplished by the physician. The speech pathologist seeks to understand the disabilities that produce and maintain the speech disorder. The physician seeks the etiology of these disabilities. He seeks diseases and lesions that disable functions of the apparatus required for speech. The speech pathologist can often aid in this task.... Because the speech pathologist is interested in the biologic correlates of these skills, he may study them anatomically and physiologically. He may, if asked, be able to venture an informed opinion about the neurologic, laryngeal, respiratory, or orofacial condition of a speech-handicapped patient. But if he is not asked, he will be well advised to limit his contributions to diagnosis to a report of information about which he has special competence: speech behavior. To venture unsolicited observations about the physical status of a patient can be construed by a physician as a novice telling a professional about his own specialty. (Perkins, 1977, pp. 339–350)

Since the medical use of diagnosis focuses on underlying causation, other behavioral scientists also suggest that the term "diagnosis" is not appropriate for those who primarily want to describe and understand behavior (Palmer, 1970).

Despite these views, the term "diagnosis" has a long tradition in speech–language pathology. The primary diagnosis texts use the term "diagnosis," although not always supporting the causal implications the term implies (Darley, 1964; Darley & Spriestersbach, 1978; Emerick & Hatten, 1979; Peterson & Marquardt, 1981; Singh & Lynch, 1978). The activity engaged in is called diagnosis or diagnostics.

Aside from the tradition of common usage, we consider the term "diagnosis" to hold significant professional implications for speech–language pathologists. As specialists educated in describing and understanding speech and language disorders, their causes, and management procedures, we rightfully should be in the most knowledgeable position to diagnose speech and language disorders. While we do not presume to make medical diagnoses, it is our position that because of his professional knowledge the speech–language pathologist takes a major role in searching for and identifying probable causal factors. He should not be merely a passive recipient of medical diagnoses.

There are numerous instances in which speech–language pathologists as diagnosticians and physicians as diagnosticians work hand in hand to arrive at a determination of causal factors. In many of these situations the boundaries between the speech–language pathologist and physician are blurred—active cooperation rather than abrogation should be the role of each. For example, a speech–language pathologist may refer the patient to a physician for further evaluation that employs the use of more sophisticated cinemdiographic techniques. Or the speech–language pathologist may be in a position to both perform and evaluate the cineradiographhic studies as they relate to his patient's speech and language disorder.

Knowing how certain medical conditions affect speech and language keeps the diagnostician aware that there may be an undiagnosed medical condition requiring attention underlying the speech and language disorder. Therefore referrals are made to physicians with clear statements as to the diagnostician's suspicions about medical conditions. For example, if he saw a patient with a speech pattern characteristic of some form of dysarthria, he would certainly refer the patient to a neurologist, providing him with any information known about the relationship of the patient's speech pattern to certain neurologic diseases. Or, in the case of a hypernasal patient, if the examination of the velopharyngeal musculature along with the speech pattern led the diagnostician to suspect palatal paralysis or a submucous cleft of the palate, he would again refer to the appropriate physician with a clear statement of his suspicions of the underlying physical condition.

It is the diagnostician's professional responsibility to communicate causal concerns to the physician; however, he must refrain from discussing them as if he had made a medical diagnosis. His job is to understand the onset and development of a speech and language disorder: How it came to be, what caused it? Some of the causal factors are medical, some are psychological, some are emotional, and some are unknown. In doing his job, the diagnostician must know his professional boundaries and how to relate to and work with other specialists who interact with his. Speech–language pathologists make speech and language diagnoses—not medical diagnoses, psychological diagnoses, psychiatric diagnoses, educational diagnoses, dental diagnoses, or neurologic diagnoses—nor should these other specialists make speech and language diagnoses. Each specialty uses information from others to understand its own diagnostic concerns. Therefore to us there is a major difference between making a *medical diagnosis* (establishing the presence of and reasons for a condition, a disease, or other abnormality of structure and function in the individual) and making a *speech and language diagnosis* (analyzing, interpreting, and establishing causal relationships for observed speech and language disorders).

Comparison to similar terms

Numerous terms other than diagnosis have been used by writers in speech–language pathology to refer to the activity engaged in when determining the speech and language status of a given patient. Words such as *testing, examination, appraisal, evaluation,* and *assessment* exist in the literature and are sometimes used interchangeably. While these words are often introduced within a textbook with little discussion as to their implication, we would like to point out some distinctions and make explicit our use of *diagnosis* as it relates to these terms.

Testing

While testing can refer to a form of data collection or one aspect of a more complete diagnosis, the term has come to suggest the routine administration of a test or battery of tests. Frequently the connotation is that few selective decisions have been made prior to testing and that this activity results in a test score with little or no interpretation of the test performance. Often testing has been used in a pejorative sense, as when a diagnostician denies being a "test giver."

Testing as a form of data collection is, in our view, both a part of determining the patient's speech and language variation as well as understanding causal factors. Testing elicits data that allows the diagnostician to describe the presented speech and language variation and to some extent determine if it is disordered. Testing also aids in the understanding of causal factors, as when the results of audiometric testing reveal a hearing loss. Testing, to us, is the objective data-gathering part of diagnosis, allowing little role for the interpretive, evaluative aspects of a complete diagnosis. Thus, we see testing as a limited part of diagnosis, contributing primarily to the goal of describing the speech and language variation and at times to the goal of understanding causal factors.

Examination

The term "examination" similarly has come to imply a systematic, although sometimes perfunctory, inventory of a patient's behavior. As used by some writers, examination seems to carry a medical connotation. It often is used to refer to physical inspection of the peripheral speech mechanism, or to determine auditory functioning. Examination, like testing, accounts for only a limited part of the total concept of diagnosis. While an examination may reveal information relevant to a description of the speech and language variation, most often examination implies inspection of the physical person rather than his speech and language behavior per se. Such inspection provides information most directly pertinent to causal factors, particularly contemporary disruptions of speech and language processes. For example, an examination of tongue movement may reveal motor limitations contributing to faulty articulation.

Appraisal

As frequently used, appraisal also implies a certain routinization of activity. One author (Darley, 1964) sees appraisal as consisting of a series of steps that may be repeated over time to determine changes in the patient's status. Appraisal is usually used to imply measurement and description of particular behavior, frequently through noting strengths and weaknesses (Peterson & Marquardt, 1981). The term seems to allow for some degree of interpretation in determining what behaviors may be considered normal and disordered, Since appraisal encompasses interpretation, this term would be more inclusive than either testing or examination. Appraisal seems to parallel more completely our first goal of diagnosis, determining the speech and language variation/disorder. That is, appraisal provides not only a description of the variation but also interprets the gathered data to determine the presence of a speech and language disorder.

Evaluation

Evaluation as used by most writers incorporates both descriptive and interpretive functions. Behavior is described and then interpreted through reference to normative data and other patient considerations. Although some writers (Palmer, 1970) suggest that evaluation carries a negative value judgement, for us this term again seems to refer most closely to our first goal of diagnosis, determining the characteristics of the speech and language variation/disorder.

Assessment

Assessment is the term chosen by several authors to imply a description of the nature, severity, and prognosis of the problem as well as a plan of remediation. We see assessment as including our goals of determining the speech and language disorder and proposing patient management. What is lacking, usually through deliberate omission by some authors (Palmer, 1970; Perkins, 1977), is inclusion of probable causal factors. As stated, we feel all three goals should be addressed by speech–language pathologists during their diagnostic activity.

Thus, we see testing, examination, appraisal, evaluation, and assessment as terms used to refer to only parts of the more total professional activity that we choose to term diagnosis. Diagnosis not only represents the most complete meaning of the activity we intend to discuss but also carries the orientation to which we subscribe.

SUMMARY

Chapter 1 has presented the three goals that make up the diagnostician's job functions:

1. Determining the nature and severity of the speech and language disorder;
2. Understanding historical and contemporary causal factors;
3. Proposing appropriate patient management.

In order to perform his job functions the diagnostician must have three primary personal and professional characteristics:

1. An organized fund of knowledge and a frame of reference that are readily applied to the practicalities of diagnosis. This fund of knowledge includes information about:
   a. Normal speech and language development and use;
   b. Disorders of speech and language;
   c. Causal factors that disrupt normal speech and language;
   d. Various management alternatives;
2. A skilled problem-solving ability that stems from scientific methodology;
3. Patient concern as his ultimate professional responsibility.

This chapter also considered the terminology used in our profession to refer to the diagnostic process.

STUDY QUESTIONS

1. Rees (1978) and Darley and Spriestersbach (1978) have addressed the philosophy that guides the clinical process of diagnosis. Compare these authors' positions to the orientation presented in the present chapter.
2. Compile a list of journals which provide information in each of the areas delineated under funds of knowledge needed by the diagnostician. For example: Normal Speech and Language: *The Journal of Child Language;* Variations and Disorders of Speech and Language: *Journal of Speech and Language Disorders;* Causal Factors: *Cleft Palate Journal;* Management Alternatives: *Seminars in Speech, Language and Hearing.*
3. Schultz (1972, Chap. 3) discusses the professional status sometimes accorded the diagnostician versus the therapist. React to Schultz's discussion.
4. Compare the use of the terms diagnosis, assessment, and evaluation by the following authors to the view of diagnosis presented here: Perkins, 1977; Darley and Spriestersbach, 1978; Salvia and Ysseldyke, 1981; Emerick and Hatten, 1979; and Sanders, 1979.
5. In this first chapter we described speech and language behavior in three ways: (1) as speech and language variations, (2) as speech and language disorders, and (3) as speech and language problems. The diagnostician's job is to view his client from these three perspectives. Compare other definitions of terms used to signify disordered speech and language with the three levels of description we discussed. See the contributions of Emerick and Hatten (1979), Leonard (1972), Rees (1978), and Van Riper (1972).
6. Lass, McReynolds, Northern, and Yoder (1982) have edited a three-volume book in which an attempt has been made to bring together information needed by professionals in speech, language, and hearing. In reviewing these books, how completely do they address the funds of knowldege required by the diagnostician as discussed in this chapter?

Chapter 2

The speech and language processing model as an organizational framework for the diagnostician's funds of knowledge

MODELS AS ORGANIZING PRINCIPLES

Unless the data in the diagnostician's field of study is organized into a structured frame of reference, the information cannot be effectively applied to clinical problems. Bits of scattered data cannot be readily and selectively recalled. As a behavioral scientist and problem solver, the diagnostician must go beyond the "chunking," cataloging, and purely descriptive phases of scientific development. The diagnostician must organize and integrate the bits of knowledge into facts, inferences, hypotheses, theories, theoretical constructs, and conceptual frameworks in order to ask the most pertinent questions about speech and language disorders.

Models offer a potentially useful organizing principle for the diagnostician's funds of knowledge. The use of models to portray and organize information and to serve as strategies of inquiry has become prevalent in many disciplines, including communication sciences and disorders (Perkins, 1977).

Numerous models exist exemplifying different perspectives on the communication process, from interactive communication models that represent senders and receivers of information to more specific models of human information processing (Massaro, 1975). There are models that focus on human communication modalities (Porch, 1971); on the anatomic and physiologic basis of speech and language (Whitaker, 1971); on receptive and expressive language processes (Morley, 1972; Porch, 1971); on the interface between anatomy and language processing (Mysak, 1966); and on a specified speech or language process such as speech production (Mysak, 1976), auditory processing (Lemme & Daves, 1982), the neuroprocessing basis of language (Buckingham, 1982), and fluent speech production (Zimmerman, 1980c).

THE SPEECH AND LANGUAGE PROCESSING MODEL

The Speech and Language Processing Model (SLPM) to be presented here represents one way of conceptualizing the many different facets that make up the study of speech and language disorders, placing the individual in a biological perspective. It is considered a human information processing model that can serve as a framework for organizing and retrieving information about normal and disordered speech and language and as a measurement framework for establishing cause–effect relationships. The SLPM was constructed by applying seven considerations for critically evaluating a model's usefulness to the speech–language pathologist. These seven considerations were

1. **For a model to be maximally useful it should focus on speech and language.** While the broader context of communication, particularly human communication, is important, speech and language is the diagnostician's primary area of expertise. Because of this central interest, a model needs to allow for detailed specificity in organizing this most relevant fund of knowledge. If a model does not allow integration of considerable in-depth information related to speech and language, the model may easily become superfluous, and the diagnostician will need to rely on alternative ways of integrating information. In other words, a diagnostician's model needs to organize maximally the relevant knowledge he commands or the model will not aid him.

2. **Since the auditory–oral modalities are the basic modalities of speech and language and the first to develop, these modalities may justifiably serve as the primary modalities explicated in a model.** This is not to say that a diagnostician does not need to maintain awareness of other modalities of input and output. Rather, it simply says that a detailed specification of information needs to be provided foremost for the auditory–oral modalities. Although the auditory–oral modalities will have the most specific application for the diagnostician, those working largely with special populations, such as the hearing impaired or adult aphasics, may also wish to have a general representation of other modalities in addition to the auditory–oral modality.

3. **A diagnostically useful model should carefully describe and delineate observable speech and language behavior.** The observed speech and language behavior needs to be dealt with in considerable specificity, not merely labeled output or speech and language behavior. The diagnostician in viewing the behavior presented to him needs a consistent framework that guides his observations and forces consideration of numerous observable parameters. A diagnostic model must provide for expansion of the observed speech and language characteristics.

4. **A model should allow for specification of the anatomy and physiology underlying speech and language—the hypothesized internal process.** Much of a diagnostician's needed funds of knowledge concern the patient's processing of speech and language; therefore a useful model must be able to expand on this crucial area.

5. **The diagnostic model should assist in developing the interface between the physical basis for speech and language—anatomy and internal processing—and the observable speech and language behaviors.**

6. **The model should help the diagnostician understand causal factors and hypothesize cause–effect relationships.** Speech and language input and the larger environmental context need to be organized in relation to internal processing and observable speech and language parameters. Through representation of these three aspects the diagnostician can examine all potential causal factors and relationships. He can suggest relationships between input factors, internal processing, and observable speech and language. Such a model should aid the diagnostician in seeing, for example, that a patient's observed pitch is related to laryngeal processes but may be related as well to input factors such as the pitch of another person who has a significant interpersonal relationship with the patient.

7. **A diagnostician's model should help him develop ways of measuring speech and language disorders.** A model that contributes to distinguishing between observable versus inferred behavior, factual versus theoretical information, helps the diagnostician in developing measurement strategies and in weighing the validity of the information obtained. For example, in diagnosing a stutterer's speech disorder, the diagnostician may decide to describe and measure the observed speech behavior or inferred processes. Measurement of observed behavior may give him data about the frequency, length, and contexts of repetitions and prolongations. The diagnostician might, however, hypothesize that the stutterer's nonfluencies are related to delayed auditory feedback processes and set out to measure and describe this inferred dimension. Given these two sets of information, one concerning observed behavior and the other inferred processes, the diagnostician must keep in mind the level of abstraction and inference in arriving at each.

Components of the speech and language processing model

Focusing on the above seven considerations the SLPM (Figure 2-1) was constructed specifically for application to the clinical process of diagnosis. The SLPM has three major components.

1. *The speech and language environment component* emphasizes those environmental events, either historical or contemporary, that help explain the individual's current development and use of speech and language.

2. The *speech and language processing component* offers a schema for understanding the underlying anatomy and processing events that occur when the individual uses speech and language. Within the processing component there are three segments representing anatomical and processing boundaries. Within each segment we present measurable behavioral correlates and the physical processes from which they are derived.

3. The *speech and language product component* specifies the observable parameters of the speech and language behavior that result when an individual speaks.

We will now provide some elaboration of the three components of the SLPM. Our focus will be on information that is considered most useful for carrying out the purposes and tasks of the diagnostic process. This information will be vital when studying later chapters dealing directly with the steps of the diagnostic process.

SPEECH AND LANGUAGE ENVIRONMENT COMPONENT

The speaker/first-language learner functions in a multidimensional environment filled with innumerable influences that can affect speech and language. As diagnosticians we want to understand how environmental factors affect speech and language since they have causal and remedial implications. The SLPM assists in this task by viewing the environment in continued interaction with the individual speech and language user. The SLPM considers two major divisions of the speech and language environment component: (1) the *speech and language input* and (2) the *multidimensional environmental context*. This component is now expanded and is represented in Figure 2-2.

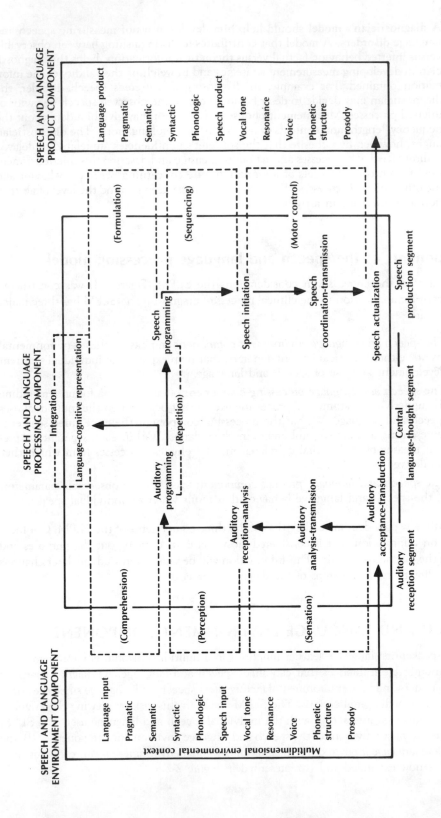

Figure 2-1. Speech and language processing model.

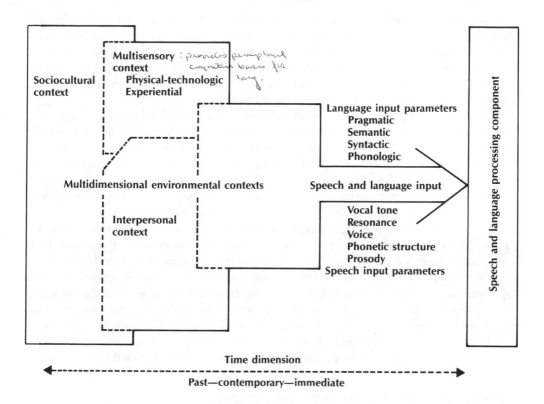

Figure 2-2. Speech and language environment component of the SLPM.

Speech and language input

For our purposes, the primary task of a language user is to learn to speak as others in his environment speak. From his direct sensory experiences and interpersonal communicative interactions the child receives his primary speech and language stimulation (input) for processing. He thereby learns the language practices of those around him. To acquire a complete speech and language system the child must be exposed to all the parameters and levels of speech and language. He must have exposure to the *communicative intentions, sentences, words, sounds, voice qualities, resonance patterns,* and *prosodic features* of those important people in his environment if he is to learn to communicate effectively.

In developing our framework for the environment component we wanted to keep the diagnostician's major concern paramount—speech and language. Therefore we can use the parameters of speech and language as a focal point around which to organize and scan the diverse, potential environmental influences and determinants.

The environment component of the SLPM incorporates the same set of speech and language parameters for input as it does for the speech and language product. Thus, paralleling the product component of the SLPM, speech and language input has been broken down into the *language input* and the *speech input*.

The language input has been subdivided into the *pragmatic, semantic, syntactic,* and *phonologic* levels. Pragmatics concerns how language is used in the environment, the effects various factors have on the use of language, and what functions or purposes language serves. Semantics includes the meaning underlying words and the meaningful relationships between words. Syntactics focuses on the grammar of language, including word order and morphology; while phonology deals with the sounds and rules for ordering sounds in a language. Speech input has been subdivided to include the parameters of *vocal tone, resonance, voice, phonetic structure,* and *prosody.* All of these parameters will be discussed more thoroughly later in the product component.

Using these speech and language parameters, we can then order and interpret the diverse environmental information available to us. Much may be learned about a patient's environment—the maternal grandmother is an alcoholic, the mother is a working woman, the older brother is a delinquent, and so forth. Although helpful in understanding the client as a totality, unless these bits of information can be related to speech and language input, they are not especially helpful to the diagnostician's purpose of attempting to understand causal factors and may, in fact, be extraneous to his central concern.

This approach to considering the environment forces the diagnostician to carefully examine just what it is about a specific environmental factor or event that may have had an effect on speech and language. Often it is difficult to discern the relationship between an identified factor and its effect on speech and language. Frequently it appears that the specified factor is not the most direct influencing factor but rather serves as an umbrella term to cover a variety of experiences that may affect speech and language more directly. Consider, for example, the isolated terms *divorced parents, bilingualism,* and *lower socioeconomic status,* all terms that are frequently used to explain speech and language disorders, and yet in themselves provide insufficient information for causal interpretation.

Multidimensional environmental context

There are multiple environmental factors to consider in relation to speech and language; for example, factors such as family constellation, ethnic membership, and birth order. Perhaps every environmental variable is in some way relevant.

The literature cites numerous factors that at times have a high statistical correlation with certain measures of language; however, we generally do not know how these environmental factors influence the development or use of language. It is not easy to determine what relationship, if any, specified factors have to the onset, development, and use of speech and language. For example, how does a numerical figure reflecting socioeconomic status relate to an adult's restricted use of syntax or a child's limited vocabulary? As McCarthy (1954) indicated some time ago, we need explanatory concepts to assist in our interpretation of statistical correlations.

While the complex contributions of various environmental influences defies clear understanding, the overall context in which language is learned and used includes at least three significant interacting contexts: (1) the *interpersonal context;* (2) the *multisensory context;* and (3) the *sociocultural context.*

First, we know that language originates and is used largely in an *interpersonal context.* In order for a child to develop and use speech and language appropriate to his environment, people in his interpersonal environment must talk to him; he must be exposed to the speech and language of his language community. To understand the interpersonal contribution to speech and language development and use the diagnostician relies on his broad knowledge of human communicative interaction. Wood (1976), Snow and Ferguson (1977), and Waterson and Snow (1978) provide a large body of information about speech and language input in interpersonal contexts.

Second, the speech and language environment has a *multisensory context*. Multisensory influences include *physical–technologic* and *experiential* factors, that is, the environmental stimuli and sensory explorations that form the real world represented by language. For the young child this may mean the sensory information he discovers through his explorations that provide perceptual categories represented by his early words. In addition, multisensory experiences may initiate speech and language within a speaker; for example, an adult may see a cloud or a horse race that prompts him to comment on these sensorily derived events. Thus, the multisensory context may provide the perceptual–cognitive basis for language or may act as a stimulus to instigate speech and language within the speaker.

Third, the interpersonal and multisensory contexts are embedded into a broader *sociocultural context*. However, it is generally the continuous interpersonal environment that transmits sociocultural practices and values. The people in a child's environment provide him with the information that allows him to know the sociocultural practices involved in how, when, and where to use speech and language appropriately. Byrne and Shervanian (1977) and the Naremore chapter in Hixon, Shriberg, and Saxman (1980) provide useful resources for reviewing sociolinguistics.

From this interacting multidimensional environmental context the speaker/first-language learner must abstract the pertinent speech and language data. However, speech and language stimulation is not always in the form of a clear, uncomplicated message. Language, as spoken, is frequently indistinct and fragmented. Rarely are the language rules made explicit; rather, the language learner and speaker must piece together the fragments to deduce the regularities of the system that he is to learn and use. To complicate matters further, the spoken message is only one of a number of competing auditory stimuli. From the noise of the television, street, children playing nearby, the listener must bring to the foreground the speech and language directed toward him. The listener's task, then, is to abstract the relevant speech and language data from disjointed interpersonal, multisensory, and sociocultural contexts that make up his speech and language environment.

In examining the patient's environmental contexts the diagnostician searches for factors that may have contributed to the patient's speech and language disorder. He needs a framework such as depicted here for interpreting environmental determinants as potential causal factors.

Time dimension

In addition to structuring environmental factors that may affect speech and language input, the environment component also incorporates a time dimension. The time dimension is divided into (1) the *historical speech and language environment* and (2) the *immediate speech and language environment*.

This time dimension is seen as a continuum. It encompasses the patient's cumulative past experiences ranging from Day 1, the *distant past,* to the *contemporary environment,* to those events that are *immediate,* that is, currently occurring in the diagnostic setting. Viewing the time dimension on this continuum allows the diagnostician to note changes in environmental circumstances and forces him to consider carefully what effect he and the tasks he uses have on the patient's speech and language behavior. The historical continuum and the immediate diagnostic situation give the diagnostician a *time of occurrence* organization to events within the speech and language environment.

Historical speech and language environment

Our historical time dimension considers all the past interpersonal, sociocultural, and multisensory experiences that have contributed to an individual's speech and language history; it is an accumulation of experiences from the distant past through contemporary events. Yet, the importance of the environment to language acquisition is a point of disagreement among theorists. The position we hold as represented by the SLPM is that the environment provides information—a model from which the child learns language. The environment has a role in providing the data that allows the child to learn the special characteristics of speech and language as used by those around him. And the child's specialized biological self allows him to readily learn the language system available to him.

While we do not have conclusive answers to questions of quality, quantity, source, and timing of speech and language input, for the present we can operate with the assumption that the historical speech and language environment must provide some degree of stimulation pertaining to all parameters of speech and language.

Whenever the diagnostician is considering any past or contemporary environmental influence on speech and language input, he is considering the historical speech and language environment, whether the event occurred 10 years or 2 days earlier. The historical continuum, then, allows examination of these environmental factors within a time-related frame. When a historical factor occurs that may restrict any parameter of speech and language input, this factor becomes causally suspect. The more extreme the limitation or deviation of speech and language input created by the factor, the more probable an effect on speech and language. The diagnostician will have to cull information from his funds of knowledge that supports the environment's historical role in the learning and disrupting of the various parameters of speech and language.

Immediate speech and language environment: the diagnostic setting

The immediate speech and language environment is concerned with the present diagnostic situation. The diagnostician becomes the central figure in the patient's immediate environment. Too often the influences of immediate environmental variables on the patient's speech and language behavior go unexamined by the diagnostician. Therefore the immediate speech and language environment time dimension directs attention to the specific speech and language tasks presented and to the interpersonal characteristics of the diagnostician. This topic will be expanded later when we discuss diagnostic procedures.

SPEECH AND LANGUAGE PROCESSING COMPONENT

The diagnostician must make an attempt to understand what intervenes between the speech and language input and output of his patient. Environmental influences only account for some of the causal factors contributing to disordered speech and language. Disruptions of the physical basis for speech and language account for a large number, perhaps the largest number, of the speech and language disorders seen. Therefore, if the diagnostician is to understand disordered speech and language and its causes he must develop a schema that considers how the physical basis of speech and language relates to speech and language disorders. He must be concerned with the "hidden processes," that is, the internal physical events taking place that are generally not directly observable. This schema must be open-ended, allowing for easy adaptation as knowledge accrues about the physical basis for speech and language.

Many controversies have occurred concerning whether or not an anatomic and physiologic basis can be specified for given speech and language behaviors. Many specifics continue to be disputed, but some commonality can be seen. Unanimity of thought is greater in the peripheral than the central systems. Thus, virtually all theorists viewing speech and language agree that reception of the auditory stimulus within the auditory modality and speech production through movement of the structures of the speech mechanism are indisputable aspects of speech and language processing. What goes on in the brain is much less clear and far from universally agreed on. Its representation may range from the "black box" approach to highly inferential, complex processing concepts.

Even though we must be cautious when attempting to delineate the interface between anatomy, physical processing, and behavior, the available data allow us to make some tentative statements about these relationships. The speech and language processing component of the SLPM (Figure 2-3), abstracted from a large body of information, is *our* statement of these relationships. Its intent is to help the diagnostician do two things:

1. Infer potential physical disruptions from observed behaviors.
2. Predict potential speech and language disorders from knowledge about physical disruptions.

Segments of the speech and language processing component

Our schema is based on the assumption that different internal processing events take place at different anatomic levels within the human being. From this assumption we have divided the speech and language processing component into three segments. These three segments representing anatomic and processing boundaries are (1) the *auditory reception segment,* (2) *central language–thought segment,* and (3) *speech production segment.*

Anatomically, we are concerned with those primary structures by which speech and language are processed. Therefore, in general, the auditory reception segment is made up of the structures of the *auditory modality;* the central language–thought segment is composed primarily of those brain structures frequently called *central language mechanisms;* the speech production segment is made of those structures generally viewed as the *speech modality,* the motor systems responsible for speech production.

Processing events occur within these anatomic boundaries. Our processing schema incorporates two major concepts. First, our schema incorporates what we have termed *physical processes.* From our study of the anatomy and physiology of speech and language we have derived and named a series of physical processes within each segment of the processing component. These physical processes have been hypothesized to account for the events that take place internally when the individual uses speech and language. For the most part they are *not directly observable* to the diagnostician. They are processes that occur on an anatomic–physiologic basis; thus, they are abstracted from many ideas about the physical basis for speech and language. We have attempted to keep the specified processes clinically useful, those that we consider most helpful to the diagnostician in looking at underlying reasons for the speech and language disorders they observe. We are interested in a parsimonious, although theoretical, view of speech and language processing. Therefore, on the SLPM we present a series of *nine primary physical processes.*

Second, our schema incorporates what we have termed *behavioral correlates.* Behavioral correlates are sets of behaviors *observable* to the diagnostician. From the patient's behavioral responses to specified tasks the diagnostician gains information about the patient's ability

SPEECH AND LANGUAGE PROCESSING COMPONENT

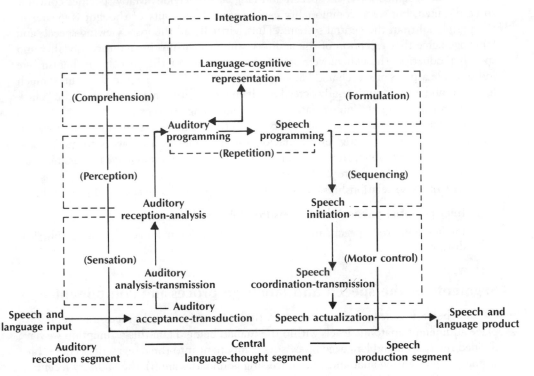

Figure 2-3. Speech and language processing component of the SLPM.

to process speech and language. Thus, the behavioral correlates are viewed on the SLPM as the patient's observable responses to tasks that are intended to measure the internal physical processes. It is the physical processes that give rise to the sets of behaviors measured as behavioral correlates. In our schema, behavioral correlates are considered as behavioral stages or behavioral processes reflective of the internal physical processes within each segment of the processing component. What we are calling behavioral correlates often have been called psychological processes or stages of information processing. Each behavioral correlate presents different information to the diagnostician for observation. On the SLPM we present a series of *eight primary behavioral correlates.*

Table 2-1 demonstrates the relationship of the eight behavioral correlates to the nine physical processes within each segment of the speech and language processing component of the SLPM. The dashed lines represent the anatomic and processing overlap that exists among the segments.

At this time we present in greater detail some of the information from which the speech and language processing component was derived. Our focus is on the behavioral correlates that serve as the basis for observations and measurements made by the diagnostician. However, the reader must keep in mind that our schema views these behavioral correlates as arising from underlying physical processes.

Table 2-1. Schema for the speech and language processing component demonstrating how physical processes for speech and language give rise to a set of behavioral correlates within each segment of component

Segment	Physical processes	Behavioral correlates
Auditory reception segment	Auditory acceptance-transduction Auditory analysis-transmission Auditory reception-analysis Auditory programming	Sensation Perception
Central language-thought segment	Language-cognitive representation Speech programming	Comprehension Integration Formulation Repetition
Speech production segment	Speech initiation Speech coordination-transmission Speech actualization	Sequencing Motor control

Auditory reception segment

The anatomy of the auditory reception segment is made up of the *bilateral structures of the auditory modality,* from the outer ear to Heschl's gyrus, the primary auditory cortex. The auditory reception segment is considered as a *primary recognition system.* The physical processes that take place here are referred to as *prelinguistic processes,* that is, analyses that take place before spoken messages can be understood.

The four physical processes within the auditory reception segment are (1) *auditory acceptance-transduction,* (2) *auditory analysis-transmission,* (3) *auditory reception-analysis,* and (4) *auditory programming.* These processes are involved in receiving, coding, analyzing, transmitting, and programming the auditory stimulus. They code and analyze the incoming physical characteristics of the auditory stimulation, ultimately turning the data into phonetic feature patterns. These processes prepare the speech data for linguistic analysis, which takes place in the central language–thought segment. Table 2-2 summarizes the physical processing activities within the auditory reception segment. For further information regarding auditory processing activities summaries are provided by Lemme and Daves (1982), Goldstein (1982), and Kuhl (1982).

Sensation and *perception* are the two behavioral correlates that result from the prelinguistic physical processes taking place within the auditory reception segment. Measurement of the sets of behaviors that define sensation and perception allow the diagnostician to say something about his patients' ability to process auditory information prior to language comprehension.

Table 2-2. Physical processing activities within the auditory reception segment

Anatomy	Physical processes	Description
Outer ear to hair cells in cochlea	Auditory acceptance-transduction	Accepts and transduces acoustic energy for further neurologic processing
Cochlea, auditory pathways to primary auditory cortex	Auditory analysis-transmission	Prelinguistic neural coding and analysis of frequency, intensity, and durational characteristics of the auditory stimulus
Primary auditory cortex	Auditory reception and analysis	Coded auditory data further analyzed and restructured into complex auditory patterns and compared with previously established patterns
Primary auditory cortex in interaction with Wernicke's area	Auditory programming	Prelinguistic functions include sorting speech from non-speech patterns, changing auditory patterns into phonetic (feature) patterns, storing these phonetic features.

Sensation

On the SLPM, sensation is tied to the physical processes of auditory acceptance-transduction, auditory analysis-transmission, and auditory reception-analysis. Sensation is viewed as a low-level *behavioral response to the presence of sound.*

Sensation does not occur until cortical activation has taken place—auditory reception-analysis. As Luria (1966) says, it occurs in the first stages of arrival at the primary auditory cortex. Sensation, in this view, is a "preliminary" behavioral response to the neural activation that occurs when the intensity, frequency, and durational characteristics of the stimulus are received by the primary auditory cortex. Sensation is associated with the primary selection, sorting out, and registration of the essential components of the auditory stimulus.

Theoretically, at this stage the auditory stimulus is not interpreted by the listener; he cannot give the stimulus meaning relative to other auditory stimuli. The listener can report if he is aware of the presence or absence of sound, but supposedly he cannot identify the sound (Chalfant & Scheffelin, 1969). Sensation is rather an on–off registration process; the sound is or is not heard.

Thus, when the diagnostician measures sensation, he is particularly interested in his patient's ability to hear. He searches for the patient's threshold of hearing. He wants to know if the patient can respond to the presence of a sound without regard for recognition of the characteristics of the sound. If the stimulus is presented at the threshold of hearing, the listener usually only says that he hears (senses) sound. Even if words were presented at the threshold of hearing, the listener probably does not recognize or interpret the phonemic and semantic features of the words presented; he would again only hear sound. Therefore, when diagnosticians are interested in discovering if there are disruptions in the auditory processing system that affect the ability to hear, they usually present nonlinguistic stimuli—pure tones and noise.

Perception

On the SLPM, perception as a behavioral correlate occurs when the prelinguistic auditory programming process has been added to the process of auditory reception-analysis. Auditory perception is modality bound; it occurs as the end result of the activities taking place within the auditory modality. Thus, perception is dependent on the sequencing, grouping, and storing of innumerable auditory patterns.

For most types of auditory stimulation an active listener is able to report more information about its auditory characteristics than just hearing it. In everyday listening, reports of sensation seldom occur alone. Thus, as the next "highest" behavioral correlate after sensation, perception differs from sensation in that the listener can now recognize and sort the auditory information as well as compare and discriminate it in relation to previously stored information. In short, the listener can *derive significance* from the characteristics of the auditory stimulation.

Luria (1966) views perception as a complex, active process that includes the identification of individual signals, integration of like signals into categorical groups, selection of their meaning from a series of alternatives, and discrimination of the components of the signal that are essential to the listener from those components that are considered unessential.

Many tasks go into perception, making a clear delineation of the nature of perception difficult. Operationally, perception has included *measuring a set of behavioral responses to tasks defined as* auditory attention, stimulus recognition, localization, auditory closure, categorization of auditory patterns, discrimination, temporal ordering, temporal judgment, and patterning the auditory stimulation into significant features.

Aram and Nation (1982) explored the literature on speech perception and auditory processing, and enumerated five perceptual operations that appear to be basic to language processing and implicated in language disorders. They described these five operations as (1) *auditory attention,* the ability to select and alert to one stimuli over another; (2) *auditory rate,* accommodating to a rapid temporal pattern of acoustic input; (3) *auditory discrimination,* sorting between speech and nonspeech signals; (4) *auditory memory,* retention of auditory information; and (5) *auditory sequencing,* holding auditory information in order of presentation. Diagnosticians study the perceptual abilities of their patients by selecting specific stimulus tasks that ask for specific response patterns, depending on what aspect of perception they wish to study.

Central language–thought segment

The brain–language–cognitive relationship has undergone extensive study since the excitement generated by Broca's (1861a, 1861b) presentation of the relationship between "articulated language" and the cortical area now known as Broca's area, the third frontal convolution. While the left hemisphere appears to be dominant for most aspects of syntactic processing, the right hemisphere has been found to contribute to other aspects of language—cognitive processing.

On the SLPM the central language–thought segment is considered as a linguistic–cognitive processing system. This segment processes the prelinguistic information from the auditory reception segment by the interaction of three physical processes: (1) *auditory programming,* (2) *language–cognitive representation,* and (3) *speech programming.* These physical processing interactions allow the individual to understand (decode) what he hears, to integrate previously learned cognitive–language information and experiences with new information, to create (encode) messages to be spoken, and to repeat what he hears.

These physical processes could be considered *ideational* (symbolic) in nature; that is, the central language–thought segment may interpret the auditory patterns by *deriving representational meanings.* This process of building up representational forms within the central language–thought segment is developmental; rules are learned over time, children responding differently than adults.

Table 2-3 summarizes the physical processing activities within the central language–thought segment. For further reading about the physical activities of this segment the reader can consult Lemme and Daves (1982), Buckingham (1982), Massaro (1975), Caplan (1980), and Segalowitz (1983).

The physical processes within the central language–thought segment give rise primarily to four measurable behavioral correlates. As measurable sets of behaviors, the correlates of comprehension, formulation, integration, and repetition reveal the individual's ability to represent and process linguistic–cognitive information.

Comprehension

Comprehension is seen to occur on the SLPM as a result of interactions between the physical processes of auditory programming and language–cognitive representation. These processes decode the auditory patterns into linguistic information.

Table 2-3. Physical processing activities within the central language-thought segment

Anatomy	Physical processes	Description
Wernicke's area in interaction with remainder of auditory association cortex	Auditory programming	Linguistic functions include both decoding and encoding, e.g., decoding phonetic features into phonemes and phonologic sequences; decoding some aspects of syntax; encoding the phonologic pattern and certain syntactic units into the message being expressed.
Angular and supramarginal gyri in interaction with auditory, visual, somesthetic association areas bilaterally through various association pathways	Language-cognitive representation	Language decoding, integration, and encoding. Linguistic processing of the message occurs as well as other higher order language-cognitive interpretations of messages. Multi-modality analysis and synthesis of past and present language-cognitive information.
Broca's area in interaction with auditory association areas and primary motor cortex	Speech programming	Process of changing the auditory program of the message into a motor program; i.e., a series of motor speech commands; an auditory-motor transducer; "reads" the phonologic representation of the message and transduces it into a series of motor speech representations incorporating both phonologic and prosodic features.

Language is comprehended because the listener applies linguistic rules to his auditory perceptions. We are taking here a more liberal view of comprehension as a behavioral correlate than the view expressed by Rees and Shulman (1978), thereby reserving more complex ideational comprehension for the behavioral correlate of language integration (Aram & Nation, 1982). This literal view of comprehension implies that the listener has analyzed the phonologic, syntactic, and semantic structure of the message and understands what has been said relative to lexical meaning and syntactic word order.

In order to do this the listener must be able to turn the prelinguistic phonetic features into phonologic, semantic, and syntactic representations for comparison with stored information. The data suggest that different processes are responsible for decoding different components of the message. Processing of linguistic information for comprehension is suggested to "begin" with phonologic comprehension that primarily occurs as a result of the auditory programming process. Syntactic and semantic comprehension follows that results primarily from the language–thought representation process.

Thus, the diagnostician interested in measuring comprehension can develop tasks that isolate the linguistic levels of language comprehension. At the same time he can work toward separating comprehension problems that stem from prelinguistic disruptions versus those that stem from disruption of the linguistic processes.

Integration

Language integration introduces the most complex form of message interpretation. The underlying physical process of language–cognitive representation allows the language user to integrate complex multimodality information from the past and present to derive more pragmatic meanings imbedded in communication, as well as to create and plan a message to be spoken. As stated by Aram and Nation (pp. 118–119, 1982):

> The [behavioral correlate] of integration allows the listener to apprehend the pragmatics of the language to which he is exposed, allowing him to be aware of the intentions involved in communication directed toward him, and aids in interpreting the communicative context. Similarly, it is from integration, or a juxtaposition of language and thought, that a speaker arrives at the intentions for his own communication and the contextual modifications required to make his message appropriate to the time, place, and persons present.

Other than the pragmatic aspects of language the behavioral correlate of integration implies that the listener derives more complex meanings from messages, that is, meanings beyond the linguistic structure of the message. These complex meanings are related to the variety of cognitive–linguistic situational experiences the language user has encountered and apprehended. Wiig and Semel (1976) and Blank, Rose, and Berlin (1978) have presented views on what we consider as complex language integration. These authors all implicate the role that cognitive processes, sensory–perceptual information, and previous learning have on complex message interpretation and use.

Our view of complex meaning was presented in detail as a continuum that becomes increasingly complex along the dimensions of (1) abstraction, from a one-to-one concrete instance of a word to no external reference, (2) the number of comparisons that need to be made to integrate the information, and (3) the number of rearrangements or transformations of information that need to be made to relate incoming language with past information and experience (Aram & Nation, 1982).

Language integration therefore implies an additive synthesis of information from more than one modality. It is a meeting and exchange between auditory, visual, and somesthetic experience that is stored and becomes available for future interpretation and retrieval. Relationships are formed among the various types of information. The human develops the capability of relating words to words and words heard to objects seen; he can label a visual event and visualize an auditory event; he can interpret and discuss his sensory world through language and thought.

In measuring behaviors that reveal a patient's language integration abilities the diagnostician must go beyond the literal meaning of messages. The tasks chosen must go beyond comprehension and formulation of the structure of messages and incorporate pragmatic dimensions and interpretation of the complexity of messages such as presupposition and inference, illocutionary acts, discourse analysis, and other cognitive–language relationships.

Formulation

Formulation is the behavioral correlate that reveals the speaker's linguistic structuring of a message in accordance with the standards of his language community. To formulate a message the speaker must first know his intent and from this intent he can plan the linguistic structure of the message. Formulation, therefore, implies that the speaker implements the linguistic rules by which messages are structured. He selects the appropriate words (lexical retrieval), orders the words into appropriate syntactic patterns, and selects the appropriate phonologic sequences.

As in comprehension, there is information suggesting that different underlying physical processes are responsible for encoding different components of the message during formulation. Thus, processing of linguistic information for semantic and syntactic formulation is a result primarily of the language–cognitive representation process, followed by more syntactic and phonologic formulation from auditory programming. Final phonologic formulation occurs when the speech programming process turns the phonologic program received from auditory programming into a motor speech program. Therefore, the diagnostician interested in measuring the behavioral correlate formulation observes the language product. He can design tasks to isolate the various levels of language and from his observations potentially determine the physical processes that may be disrupted.

Repetition

Repetition implies that a language stimulus presented is reproduced with no assumptions made regarding the meaningfulness or purposefulness of the response. The SLPM suggests that repetition may occur in one of two ways.

First, repetition may proceed through the usual comprehension–integration–formulation sequence that would involve all central language–thought processes. In this case, the language stimulus would be comprehended as well as purposefully reproduced—*meaningful repetition*.

Alternatively, repetition may result via a shortcut. Information can be *shunted* directly from auditory programming to speech programming, thus bypassing language–cognitive representation—*nonmeaningful repetition*. But for repetition to be intact, the auditory programming process must arouse the appropriate sequence of sounds to be sent to the speech programming process for motoric representation. Anatomically, Wernicke's area (auditory programming) possesses conduction links with Broca's area (speech programming) via the arcuate fasciculus. This route permits transmission of auditory–verbal sequences without reference to meaning. An individual shunting information across this route presents behavior observed essentially as a rote response, independent from meaningful comprehension or purposeful formulation.

Speech production segment

The anatomy of the speech production segment is made up of the bilateral structures of the speech modality—from the primary motor cortex to the muscles and structures of the speech mechanism. The speech production segment is considered as a *primary production system*. The processes that take place in this segment are referred to as *postlinguistic processes,* that is, *motor events* that occur after a message has been formulated. These processes turn the message into spoken form.

To produce a formulated message a series of interrelated physical processes occur within the speech production segment. The physical processes of (1) *speech programming,* (2) *speech initiation,* (3) *speech coordination-transmission,* and (4) *speech actualization* are responsible for the motoric production of the formulated message; that is, they allow for speech to occur. Table 2-4 summarizes the physical activities that take place within the speech production segment. For further reading on the physical activities within this segment the reader can consult Abbs and Kennedy (1982), Kahane (1982), and Folkins and Kuehn (1982).

The processing component of the SLPM specifies two behavioral correlates reflective of the physical processes within the speech production segment. The behavioral correlates of *sequencing* and *motor control* assist the diagnostician in determining how well the speaker can carry out the postlinguistic motor activities needed for speech production.

Sequencing

As a result of the physical processes of speech initiation and speech programming where the motor plan has been transduced and instigated the speaker would be able to produce an appropriately sequenced message. A sequential ordering of speech acts would occur, including flow of speech, timing of speech, and ordering of phonetic and syllabic strings. Kent (1976) states that seriation is one of two major control problems in the production of speech. He goes on to say that

> Seriation is a category that deals with the general problem of patterning or sequencing, and probably finds its most obvious expression in the assembly of phonetic or syllabic strings. Also included in this category are certain phenomena that have been labeled as problems of articulatory timing. (p. 79)

Thus, sequencing as a behavioral correlate focuses on ordering the parts of the speech event as opposed to muscular control of the motor event.

Motor control

The final behavioral correlate of the speech production segment is motor control tied to the physical processes of speech initiation, speech coordination-transmission, and speech actualization. This behavioral correlate allows the diagnostician to observe if *on-target, precise movements* of the speech-producing structures have occurred.

Together all the physical processes of the speech production segment are responsible for initiating, transmitting, coordinating, and actualizing the motor activity required for

Table 2-4. Physical processing activities within the speech production segment

Anatomy	Physical processes	Description
Broca's area in interaction with the primary motor cortex	Speech programming	As a postlinguistic process it transduces the motor program of the message into a series of motor commands to be initiated as a sequence of neuromotor impulses.
Primary motor cortex and corticobulbar pathways within central nervous system	Speech initiation	Initiates neuromotor impulses that result in sequential muscular movements for speech production; both segmental and suprasegmental features.
Extrapyramidal, cerebellar, reticular motor systems in interaction with the primary motor cortex and pyramidal system	Speech coordination-transmission	Mediates, transmits, modulates, coordinates, facilitates, and inhibits neural impulses to allow for controlled, smooth, on-target sequential muscular movements.
Structures that make up the speech mechanism including the peripheral nervous system, primarily motor cranial nerves	Speech actualization Breathing for speech Phonation Resonation Articulation Prosodation	The organized, controlled, and coordinated neuromuscular activities of the speech mechanism that result from all previous motor processes, allowing for accurate force, timing, and speed of contractions; range of movement, direction of movement, etc.—all controlled in relationship to other bodily activities taking place while an individual is talking.

producing a spoken response. The speech actualization process is the final physical process for producing the speech event. It involves the actual movements of the speech mechanism. *Breathing for speech, phonation, resonation, articulation,* and *prosodation** are subprocesses of speech actualization.

The diagnostician can observe patterned movements, tension, position, manner of production, and so forth, to arrive at an estimate of muscular activity and control. There are also instrumental measures available for gaining information about motor control during speech production (Folkins & Kuehn, 1982). Cinefluorography, electromyography, and laryngoscopy are among those extrasensory measures that provide rather direct instrumental analyses of the processes within the speech production segment.

The diagnostician also can observe these correlates directly by listening to the parameters of the speech product (see discussion of speech and language product component). For example, he can see if the tongue, lips, and jaws move in the right direction and with appropriate tension for producing any specific sound of the language; or he can listen for excess resonance or inappropriate pitch.

When observing the behavioral correlates of motor control and sequencing, it must be kept in mind that they are reflections of physical processes that are carrying out a preprogrammed message (speech programming). As Kent (1973) has indicated in his development of a preprogramming model for speech movements, the motor program inherently includes timing control. He adds that once the program is triggered (speech initiation in the SLPM) the serial movements of speech are produced in the planned sequence.

SPEECH AND LANGUAGE PRODUCT COMPONENT

When a speaker utters a message, the resulting product is an *acoustic waveform* made up of physical dimensions: frequency, intensity, spectrum, and duration. This end *acoustic product* can be structured for analysis differently depending on the purposes of the observer. For example, a speech scientist may be interested in using various types of instruments to study the frequency or intensity characteristics of the acoustic waveform. A voice teacher may be interested in listening to the pitch, loudness, and quality characteristics of the voice. A psycholinguist may be interested in describing the syntactic structure of the speaker's message. The diagnostician of speech and language disorders may be interested in any or all of the above observations of the acoustic product, along with many others, to help define his patient's speech and language disorder.

What is or is not heard in the patient's speech and language product at any stage during his learning and use of speech and language usually forms the basis for identification of a speech and language disorder and also serves as the basis for a diagnostic referral. The parameters of the speech and language product are typically the diagnostician's initial concern. From what he hears and observes of the patient's speech and language product, the diagnostician then considers the processing basis and environmental factors that may account for the disordered product. Thus, the diagnostician often first uses information

---

*We have developed a somewhat artificial subprocess of speech actualization that we have termed prosodation. It is a unified, integrated process incorporating aspects of the other subprocesses of speech actualization. This process is responsible for the speech product we later view as prosody. We know of no literature that specifically discusses a prosodation process. However, there is beginning to be more study of the underlying physiologic events that result in the product we call prosody.

from the speech and language product to identify, classify, and uncover the causal basis for speech and language disorders.

Acknowledging that many viewpoints exist about speech and language behavior, we have designed the speech and language product component of the SLPM to assist the diagnostician in ordering the many details of the speech and language behavior he may observe when a patient speaks. The details of this component are expanded in Figure 2-4 where the speech and language product component has been divided into two levels: the *speech product* and the *language product.*

The speech product is seen as a direct reflection of the processes that occur in the speech production segment. The five basic parameters of the speech product are *vocal tone* and *resonance,* which in combination provide us with the third parameter, *voice.* The fourth parameter of the speech product is *phonetic structure.* Adding phonetic structure to voice provides the fifth parameter, *prosody.*

The language product is viewed as a direct reflection of the series of processes responsible for message creation and formulation within the central language–thought segment. The language product includes four parameters or levels of language: *phonologic, syntactic, semantic,* and *pragmatic.*

Although the component represents our current thinking, we in no way expect every diagnostician to adopt all aspects of this particular framework. But we do consider the speech and language product component to exemplify a number of strengths.

1. It is comprehensive and terminologically consistent.
2. It is theoretically consistent—It relates speech and language behavior to underlying speech and language processes.
3. It is adaptable to disorder classification systems.
4. It is adaptable to multiple measurement approaches.

With these four considerations in mind, the primary emphasis of this section is a description of the speech and language product to which the diagnostician can direct his measurements. What follows is an explication of the terms used in the speech and language product mponent of the SLPM. Figure 2-4 should be consulted regularly throughout this discussion.

Speech product

Vocal tone

Produced by vocal fold movement, vocal tone relates most directly to the speech actualization subprocess of phonation. While the subprocess of breathing for speech provides the underlying breath stream for phonation, sound is not produced until there is laryngeal participation. Although breathing for speech provides the power source for phonation, phonation contributes most directly to vocal tone.

In analyzing vocal tone the diagnostician describes three primary physical and perceptual parameters: *intensity,* or its perceptual correlate, *loudness; frequency,* perceived as *pitch;* and *spectral complexity,* perceived as *vocal quality.*

To obtain physical measurements of the characteristics of vocal tone requires instrumental analysis. Instruments such as the spectrograph, pitch meter, and sound level meter give information about the intensity, frequency, and spectrum of vocal tone.

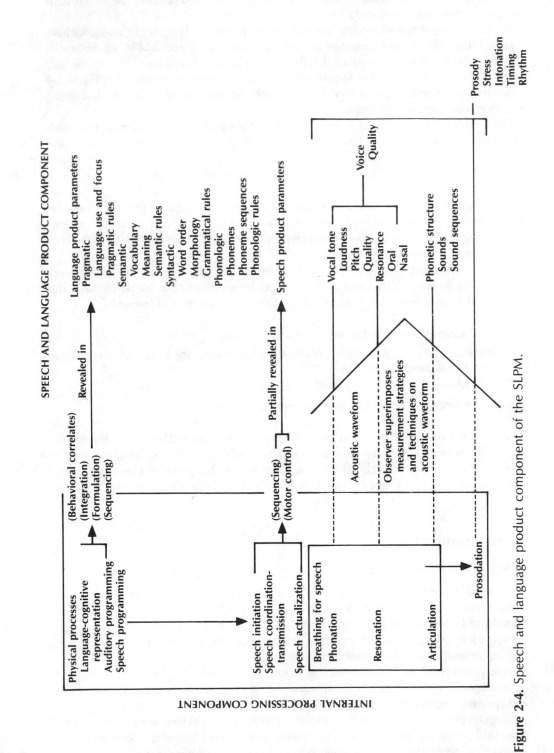

Figure 2-4. Speech and language product component of the SLPM.

Diagnosticians, however, generally measure the *perceptual correlates* of the physical characteristics. *Loudness* is typically judged as appropriate or inappropriate for a given situation. Judgments of too loud, too soft, or fading generally serve as rough indicators of the unacceptability of the loudness dimension of vocal tone.

Pitch, the perceptual correlate of vocal fold vibration, refers to the highness or lowness of vocal tone. Diagnosticians describing this aspect of vocal tone are generally concerned with the total possible pitch range, the optimum range (the range of most easily produced tones), the habitual range, and the modal pitch. Inappropriate pitch fluctuations and breaks in the tone as well as a monotone or stereotyped use of pitch may be noted if present.

Quality disorders introduced at the laryngeal level generally result from hyper- or hypotension of the laryngeal mechanism or aperiodic vibration of the vocal folds. Laryngeal hypertension may produce qualities described by some as harshness and glottal shock. Laryngeal hypotension frequently results in excessive loss of air, producing a breathy quality. Aperiodic vocal fold vibration introduces noise elements creating qualities such as hoarseness.

In addition to describing the loudness, pitch, and quality of vocal tone, diagnosticians also encounter patients who produce no vocal tone. The two most common occurrences of absence of vocal tone are in hysterical aphonia, where the structural mechanism is intact but the patient does not phonate normally, and in laryngectomized patients, where all or part of the laryngeal mechanism has been removed.

Resonance

Before the vocal tone exits from the speaker, it is modified by contributions of the pharyngeal, nasal, and oral cavities and their interactions—the resonation process. The primary functions of these cavities are to increase the loudness of the vocal tone and to add quality modifications, the sounding board and open cavity effects.

The study of resonance as a speech product has been emphasized primarily from an interest in the acoustic characteristics of the three normally nasal sounds of English, the /m/, /n/, and /ŋ/, and a significant concern for the resonance deviations in speakers with inadequate velopharyngeal closure. Resonance as a speech product, other than these two concerns, has primarily been studied as a feature of voice quality.

There are many instrumental measures that have been devised to study nasal air flow, air and sound pressure, and the acoustic spectrum of nasality as a product (Counihan, 1971a, 1971b; Schwartz, 1971). While resonance contributions can be measured objectively through instrumentation, typically, clinical descriptions are qualitative and note too much or too little contribution of a particular resonating cavity. For example, nasal resonance may be described as appropriate, too great (hypernasality or simply nasality) or too little (hyponasality), or of a certain type (cul-de-sac).

Resonance as a product to be measured by the diagnostician resides primarily in his perceptual judgement. This perceptual judgement must be based on a knowledge of the effects of nasal coupling with the oral cavity. As with all attempts to separate a product for a perceptual analysis, the diagnostician must take into account how his perceptions may be accounted for by degrees of interactions. All that is heard as nasal resonance may not be a simple matter of nasal coupling, rather it may also stem from other characteristics of the vocal and nasal tracts. His judgments should consider how much is related to what.

Voice

Often the voice problem presented cannot be referred easily to vocal tone or resonance alone, but rather as an interaction between these two products. Voice as a speech product and a disorder is clearly an ambiguous phenomenon. Our profession has repeatedly attempted to define voice in relationship to underlying production processes. Voice quality has defied description by speech pathologists. Many types of voice quality disorders are described by terms that are seldom agreed on by those listening to the voice.

We indicated earlier that voice quality is a component of vocal tone related to phonation; now we indicate that voice is a product related as well to resonation. We could add that voice is a reflection of articulation and prosodation; again, we feel we would be correct. For example, Boone (1977) discusses the oral cavity as a single or multiple resonator depending on the position of the tongue and other oral structures. Thus, changes in articulatory structures can have an effect on oral resonance, resulting in changes in perceived voice quality during speech. However, we want to reserve our concept of the voice product to the perceptual quality of the sound we perceive as uncontaminated as possible by these other speech production subprocesses. For our purposes here, then, the voice product comprises the product of vocal tone and resonance in varying degrees of combination.

Perhaps our concept of both vocal tone and voice would be best exemplified by the quality of the voice sound produced when a speaker prolongs vowels at various pitch and loudness levels. The perceptions we make of these productions come closest, for us, to the meaning of voice as an interaction of phonation and resonation. The diagnostician is very likely to hear the many variations in voice quality that are produced by normal and deviant users of the product, voice. For example, laryngeal hypertension may cause a harsh vocal tone quality, but this tone, when coupled with insufficient pharyngeal resonation, resulting in damping of lower frequencies and amplification of high overtones, may yield an overall thin, relatively high, and "tinny" voice quality termed by some as strident.

Phonetic structure

Phonetic structure is most directly referable to the subprocess of articulation, the process by which the voiced and voiceless airstream is modified by the articulators to produce the characteristic acoustic spectrum for the speech sounds of our language. The utterances that we segment in phonetic structure are referred to as phones and are classified in a number of ways.

1. *Production (physiologic) systems* are concerned with the place and manner of articulation.
2. *Acoustic systems* describe the physical characteristics associated with each speech sound.
3. *Perceptual systems* have their basis in an understanding of the sound system of a given language; the listener categorizes a sound produced in comparison to his knowledge of standard sounds.

When analyzing phonetic structure, it is important to distinguish between the phonetic product and the phonemic product. The former has its basis in a physiologic–acoustic analysis, the latter in an acoustic–perceptual–linguistic analysis.

When describing the *phonetic product,* the diagnostician is interested in the way speech sounds are actually produced by the speaker, referred to frequently as motor (physiologic) phonetics. Observation of phones tells the diagnostician about the idiosyncratic production of particular sounds by a given speaker. These are phonetically transcribed using diacritics to aid in recording the actual specific productions of phones. Thus, the diagnostician can note phonetic differences of length, nasalization, lip rounding, tongue height, voicing, and so forth. His interest is in a refined description of how a given sound was produced during the articulation process.

Another branch of the study of phonetics, acoustic phonetics, provides the diagnostician with another form of description. He can, through instrumental analysis, study the acoustic properties of speech sounds, properties such as formant structure, fundamental frequency, duration, and intensity.

The *phonemic product,* on the other hand, is more concerned with the diagnostician's perceptual judgment of speech sounds. He wants to know if a sound that is produced meets the standard for that sound in a given language. To do this he listens to the acoustic characteristics of the sound and determines perceptually if it fits a specific sound category. Thus, the phonemic product is measured by the diagnostician's judgments and is dependent on his knowledge of normal speech sounds.

The phonemic product treats specific occurrences of phones as members of idealized sound categories (phonemes). Phonemic transcriptions ignore fine nonmeaningful distinctions between members of the same phoneme category and only record sounds that function as linguistically different.

While the phonetic and phonemic products may in fact be the same segmented behavior (a phone), it is how the behavior is viewed that gives rise to the phonetic/phonemic distinction. When the concern is the specific production of sounds as they are formed in the speech actualization subprocess, the phonetic viewpoint is primary. When the production of sounds as representative of linguistic differences is the concern, the phonemic viewpoint is primary.

Not only does the diagnostician segment out the vowels and consonants from the stream of speech when he views phonetic structure, but he also observes the sequential relationship of sounds. He is not concerned about meaningful sequences here so much as the influence of one sound on another. That is, he is interested in observing the effect of coarticulation—the phonetic context (Daniloff, 1973; Klatt, 1974).

Prosody

Prosody as a speech product is referable to the subprocess we have termed prosodation. It is an integrated process, incorporating aspects from the other four speech actualization subprocesses. Thus, prosody is related to the other speech products: vocal tone, resonance, voice, and phonetic structure. Prosody is a fundamental aspect of speech behavior, but there is little general agreement as to the boundaries of the actual behavior observed. Sometimes it is called "the melody of speech" or vocal variety. It is made up of both segmental and suprasegmental features, although some writers prefer to exclude the segmental aspects of prosody (Freeman, 1982).

As a perceptual correlate to the process we have called prosodation, there is little definitive information. Prosody as an acoustic phenomenon has sometimes been identified as fundamental voice frequency, voice intensity level, and acoustic phonetic duration. Netsell (1973) operationally defines three prosodic features: intonation, stress, and rhythm. To him, intonation is perceptually related to the fundamental frequency of vocal fold vibration. Stress relates to syllable emphasis, and rhythm is the perception of the phonetic events over time.

Most authors include the following in some combination as features of prosody: pitch, loudness, time, rhythm, fluency, stress, pauses, quality, juncture, duration, intonation, rate, and phrasing. Darley (1964) speaks of stress, rhythm, and pitch comprising the prosodic quality of speech. Fisher (1966) mentions rate, stress, phrasing, and intonation as components of prosody. Perkins (1977) in discussing the "speech flow processes" comments that rhythm, established by patterns of stress and rate, is identified in speech as prosody.

Drawing from these and other authors, prosody seems to include at least two major dimensions: one that focuses on *intonation and stress patterns* and a second that has to do with *timing-rhythm*. Timing-rhythm includes two factors: *rate* and *fluency*. Rate concerns the overall speed of message utterance, phrasing characteristics, pause length, syllable length, and hesitancies. Fluency addresses how smoothly phonemes, syllables, words, and phrases are joined together into longer utterances. Repetitions and prolongations of these features create disruptions in fluency, a prosody variation.

As has been stated, these prosody characteristics are a result of the entire set of speech actualization subprocesses, but as behaviors (products) they can be isolated to some extent and viewed as an independent parameter of the speech product. The dimensions that make up prosody can be observed in the same way that phones and phonemes are viewed. The diagnostician can notate how words are stressed, if a pause occurs between two words, if a sentence was said with a downward inflection, if a vowel was prolonged, or if the rate is fast.

Prosody is more typically viewed as extending over an utterance, suprasegmental, rather than specific instances, segmental. The overall stress patterns used, the overall intonation patterns, the overall timing-rhythm patterns, and the rate and fluency are noted rather than viewing a specific instance of stress, intonation, or time. This is primarily because a specific instance provides little information about the nature of the prosody product, nor would a specific instance of a prosody error, even if consistent, do much to the meaning intended by the speaker. Some speakers may even have an overall variation of prosodic features without interfering significantly with communication. We know of any number of people who speak with little change in intonation, stress, and timing; they sound boring, but we can understand their message.

Prosodic features serve to signal meaningful differences between utterances, for example, the rising pitch used when asking a question. They also signal semantic relationships in certain ambiguous sentences; for example, "He is a French teacher." They also serve in extralinguistic ways to express certain emotions and to give each speaker a distinct vocal quality; they do seem to add to the "beauty" of languages. Here the diagnostician would be looking at the use of prosody to convey subtleties of meaning, to express various emotional states, to ask questions versus making statements, or to distinguish between words that are written alike.

Thus, prosody observations can be made strictly as a production phenomenon; or, on the other hand, they can be observed as a function of meaning. Freeman (1982) provides a detailed discussion of prosodic features relative to linguistic processing.

Language product

Phonologic level

Whereas phonetic structure aims primarily to describe the actual production of instances of phones, the phonologic level treats specific phones as representative of phoneme categories, both segmental and suprasegmental phonemes. The concern shifts more to generalized characteristics and rules of the system that signal meaning rather than individual sound description. Segmental features include the sounds or phonemes of the language and their rules of permissible order. Suprasegmental features include juncture (the difference between giant's eyes and giant size), stress (the difference between cónduct and condúct), and intonation (the difference between "Mary is going" said with a rising intonation pattern as a question or falling intonation as a statement).

In describing the phonologic level of language, then, the diagnostician aims to make an inventory of the patient's phonemic system and to identify the rules by which he selects and joins these phonemes together. He studies the phonologic level of language from the same data (phones) as he uses to study phonetic structure.

When studying the patient's phonemic inventory, the diagnostician may choose to describe the patient's own phonemic system or to note how the patient's phonemic usage differs from mature standard English. If he chooses the former, he identifies all sound categories that signal a change in meaning in much the same manner that a linguist identifies phonemes in an exotic language. More commonly, in clinical situations the diagnostician surveys a patient's phonemic inventory in comparison to standard English, keeping in mind the speech and language environment from which the patient learned language.

For some time speech–language pathologists have been analyzing phonology in the same way that articulation/phonetic structure was analyzed, primarily through place and manner descriptions of errors made (Van Riper & Irwin, 1958). As distinctions began to be drawn between phonetic structure and phonology other analysis systems came into play. First there was a major effort to view phonology from distinctive features and phonologic rules perspectives drawn from the work of Chomsky and Halle (1968), Jakobson, Fant, and Halle (1963), Miller and Nicely (1955), and Oller (1973). These systems of distinctive feature and phonologic rule analysis were adapted for clinical use by McReynolds and Engmann (1975) and Compton and Hutton (1978). Second, emphasis began to be placed on children's use of phonologic processes during development. Their sound system was analyzed in terms of sets of phonologic processes present in speech, such as cluster reduction, nasal assimilation, backing, and fronting. Systems of phonologic process analysis were developed by Ingram (1976), Weiner (1979), and Shriberg and Kwiatkowski (1980). A major work on phonology has been presented by Edwards and Shriberg (1983).

Syntactic level

A description of the syntactic level usually includes two major aspects: *word order* and *morphology*. Word order incorporates the development and use of phrase structure rules and transformations. Phrase structure rules pertain to the expansion and description of noun phrases and verb phrases, while transformations change the phrase structures to produce the surface form of the sentence. Formally, transformations are rules that add, delete, substitute, or reorder constituents in a sentence. Morphology is primarily concerned with markers indicating, for example, plurality and possession for nouns, comparison for adjectives and adverbs, tense for verbs, and derivations for words. Some writers also include the development of some free morphemes such as the copula and the auxiliary.

A number of linguists have presented descriptions of the mature, idealized syntactic system, although Chomsky (1957, 1965) has undoubtedly had the greatest impact on our view of syntax. Others have related formal linguistic theory to both adults' and children's actual use of syntax. Notable among those who have addressed syntax are Slobin (1966, 1970),

Brown (1973), C. Chomsky (1969), McNeill (1970), Menyuk (1977), and deVilliers and deVilliers (1978).

Lee (1974), Menyuk (1969), and Miner (1969) developed procedures for viewing syntactic development at various ages. Lee's work (Lee, 1966, 1974; Lee & Canter, 1971) is a comprehensive presentation for analyzing the developmental aspects of syntax. Lee (1974) first presents a compact discussion of grammatical structure with reference to early development. She then presents a classification of developmental sentence types (DST), procedures for collecting spontaneous language, and elaborate procedures for scoring and analysis. The developmental sentence scoring (DSS) analysis gives the diagnostician information as to the developmental order of pronouns, verbs, negatives, conjunctions, yes/no questions, and "wh" questions.

Many others followed these early leads to systematic assessment of syntax. Among those systems of analysis that appear to be most influential are those of Tyack and Gottsleben (1974), Trantham and Pedersen (1976), and Miller (1981). Leonard (1972) was instrumental in addressing the issue of syntactic delay versus deviance in his approach to syntactic analysis.

Semantic level

The semantic level of language is concerned with meaning, with the use of agreed on symbols of a given language that represent things, concepts, attributes, actions, or feelings. The study of semantics usually includes the *lexicon* (vocabulary), *semantic features, semantic fields,* and *semantic relations.* While vocabulary growth is well documented, study of the development of semantic features and semantic relations is still in its infancy.

The primary focus on semantics, particularly at a concrete level, has been the lexicon, the relationship between words and their external representation. Numerous studies, normative data, and tests have been published that aim to describe and measure vocabulary growth and breadth. Probably the most reported data regarding vocabulary growth in children are given by Smith (1926). An adaptation of that data can be found in Dale (1972).

Investigators are also describing semantic features. Just as phonemes are seen to be bundles of distinctive features, so also are lexical items seen to be bundles of semantic features. Attempts are being made to identify a comprehensive inventory of these semantic features, although to date no one system of features has been widely adopted or gained wide clinical application.

When a child first begins to use words, he does not know their full adult meaning. Rather, semantic development is a process of adding more and more semantic features until the child's meaning matches that of the adult. Clark's semantic feature hypothesis (1973) holds that children's first words are overextended categories based on perceptual experience of characteristics such as shape, size, sound, and texture. The child then forms more restricted word categories through a narrowing down process in which he observes and adds additional features to the words he uses. Clark (1973) also notes that children differentiate various areas of experience or "semantic domains" by learning the most superordinate general features before the more restricted and specific features.

How cognitive categories and lexical entries are related is the topic addressed in semantic field and semantic domain research. Rosch (1973) and Nelson (1973, 1978) have provided important stimulus for work in this area.

The semantic roles or semantic relations between words in sentences have also been the subject of considerable theorizing. Bloom (1970), Bowerman (1973), Brown (1973a, 1973b), Schlesinger (1971), and others have presented schemata for viewing the semantic relations expressed in sentences. Drawing from a number of sources, Miller and Yoder (1974) have presented a table that outlines these early semantic relations and shows their developmental progression. Leonard (1976) summarized much of the work in this area.

Even though theoretical frameworks are still under development, the diagnostician should not be content to collect only vocabulary information, but should try to describe the semantic features observed in lexical items and the semantic relations expressed in utterances.

Pragmatic level

Pragmatics concerns the speaker's functional use of language; that is, how and why does the speaker use language; what are his purposes; and what does he accomplish through different utterances? For example, a reticent adult may simply reply to questions, rarely initiating communication, while an aggressive communicator may issue forth many commands. Or perhaps young children may use language for self-stimulation or to direct their motor behavior.

At present there exists no unified framework that has gained general acceptance for viewing the various pragmatic uses of language, although those provided by Dore (1974, 1975), Halliday (1977a, 1977b), Bates (1976), and Prutting (1979, 1982b) have received considerable attention. Prutting and Kirchner (1983) have presented a protocol developed by Prutting (1982a) for assessing pragmatic behavior. This protocol, which draws from the work of Bates (1976), Searle (1969), Austin (1962), Ervin-Tripp and Mitchell-Kernan (1977), among others, is reproduced in Table 2-5.

The pragmatic level of language has a communicative focus and is colored by the individuals multidimensional environment; that is, speakers have numerous interpersonal, sociocultural, and multisensory influences acting on the messages they create. Along with the pragmatic schema presented here, the speech and language environment component of the SLPM (Figure 2-2) helps put a perspective on the analysis of the pragmatic level of language. As well, Prutting (1979) has summarized pragmatic development in children and Miller (1978) has provided a protocol for observing communicative interactions in language disordered children.

SUMMARY

As with all models of speech and language, the SLPM is only a reflection of its authors' viewpoint at the time it was constructed. It, too, has many missing pieces of information about the speech and language process, a process that is incompletely understood. However, as an organizing principle and a measurement framework for the diagnostician, the SLPM is structured to allow for continued modification and interpretation as information about speech and language accrues.

By showing the interface between the speech and language environment, the speech and language processing, and the speech and language product components, we feel the SLPM serves as an important conceptual framework in accomplishing the purposes of diagnosis.

The SLPM provides the diagnostician with

1. A means for viewing the events that have taken place in the speech and language environment that may help explain the patient's current speech and language functioning;

Table 2-5. Pragmatic protocol

Name:_____   Date:_____

Communicative   Communicative
Setting Observed:_____   Partner's Relationship: _____

Communicative Act	Appropriate	Inappropriate	No Opportunity to Observe
UTTERANCE ACT			
A. Verbal/Paralinguistic			
1. Intelligibility			
2. Vocal intensity			
3. Voice quality			
4. Prosody			
5. Fluency			
B. Nonverbal			
1. Physical proximity			
2. Physical contacts			
3. Body posture			
4. Foot/leg movements			
5. Hand/arm movements			
6. Gestures			
7. Facial Expression			
8. Eye gaze			
PROPOSITIONAL ACT			
A. Lexical selection/Use			
1. Specificity/accuracy			
B. Specifying relationships between words			
1. Word order			
2. Given and new information			

Communicative Act	Appropriate	Inappropriate	No Opportunity to Observe
C. Stylistic variations			
1. The varying of Communicative style			
ILLOCUTIONARY ACTS AND PERLOCUTIONARY			
A. Speech acts			
1. Speech act pair analysis			
2. Variety of speech acts			
B. Topic			
1. Selection			
2. Introduction			
3. Maintenance			
4. Change			
C. Turntaking			
1. Initiation			
2. Response			
3. Repair/revision			
4. Pause time			
5. Interruption/overlap			
6. Feedback to speakers			
7. Adjacency			
8. Contingency			
9. Quantity/conciseness			

C.A. Prutting, University of California, Santa Barbara, 1982

*From Prutting, C. A., and Kirchner, D. M. Applied pragmatics. In T. M. Gallagher and C. A. Prutting (Eds.), *Pragmatic assessment and intervention issues in language.* San Diego: College-Hill Press, 1983. Pp. 45–47.

2. A means for viewing any disruptions in the underlying physical basis for speech and language that may explain the observed disorder;

3. A direct organization of speech and language input and output behaviors that can be observed and used to isolate and define the speech and language disorder.

The speech and language product component guides in delineating the speech and language disorder, while the linkage to the environment and processing components aids in understanding potential causal factors and in proposing client management.

STUDY QUESTIONS

1. How has the field of speech-language pathology been organized and structured in the following textbooks: Perkins (1977), Van Riper (1972), Hixon, Shriberg and Saxman (1980), and Shames and Wiig (1982)? Is there a unifying orientation? A similar means of organization?

2. As a project the student might evaluate the SLPM in comparison to several other models of communication to determine how well they meet the seven considerations for construction of a diagnostic model discussed in this chapter (pp. 20-21). Suggested models are those constructed by Mysak (1966, 1976), Porch (1971), and Sanders (1976).

3. Understanding the physical processing basis for language stems from highly inferential information, often based on studies of brain abnormality. Many questions exist regarding the organization and development of cerebral structures for language as they relate to language disorders in children. What positions have been taken by Aram and Nation (1982) and Johnston (1982)?

4. Duchan (1983) has written an insightful article that critiques the use of stage processing models as explanations of language behavior and disorders. From her perspective what issues would you develop in contrast to those proposed in the SLPM?

5. Rees (1973), analyzing literature relating auditory processing to language disorders, developed the argument that "there is no basis for the assumption that the comprehension of heard speech depends on the fundamental ability to analyze the utterance into a string of phonemes—or larger segments—in the order produced." What alternative hypotheses does she offer?

6. Perkins (1977) states, "Whereas glottal vibration rate stands in a direct (though not linear) relation to pitch, and intensity of glottal pulses to loudness, what production process stands in direct relation to perceived quality? None." What dimension does Perkins suggest as basic to the production of the product we call voice quality? How can it be measured instrumentally?

7. Does Moncur and Brackett's (1974) concept of prosody coincide with that used here? Pay particular attention to their discussion of pitch. How does their concept of prosody compare to that of Freeman (1982)?

Chapter 3

The diagnostic process

The diagnostician's job is to help patients with their specific speech and language problems. To do this requires an understanding of the sequence of events that makes up the diagnostic process. In this chapter we present an overview of this process. First, we present the professional activity of diagnosis as reflected in the steps of the method of science. Second, we demonstrate that shifts of diagnostic focus occur depending upon the referral that has been made, the work setting of the diagnostician, and other role modifications. Third, administrative procedures are discussed. The diagnostician does not work in an administrative vacuum. Someone must attend to a range of administrative matters that ensure smooth scheduling, follow-up, and information flow into and out of the work setting. In some circumstances these administrative matters fall to the diagnostician and in others they do not. Diagnosticians must know about and understand the administrative procedures of their work setting. Even when not directly responsible for administration, the diagnostician influences and is influenced by the administrative personnel and practices in his job setting.

DIAGNOSIS: AN APPLICATION OF THE SCIENTIFIC METHOD

Diagnosis of speech and language disorders is a problem-solving skill; therefore the method of science should be applicable to this clinical process. The diagnostician is a clinical scientist; he is attempting to predict and understand the cause–effect relationships of his patient's problem in order to change the future state of the patient. In our view the diagnostician of speech and language disorders does fulfill Brown and Ghiselli's (1955) concepts of a scientist.

> He who rigorously applies the scientific method is a scientist. . .The scientist acts as a probe; his task is to prod nature into displaying her workings. His search, then, must be an active one. He is not a mere passive recorder, registering successions of sensory impressions as events occur before him, but he busies himself in devising all manner of procedures, gadgets, and techniques by means of which he can push into the greater vistas that lie beyond the scope of superficial observation. (Brown & Ghiselli, 1955, p. 10)

Steps of the scientific method

The method of science is often defined and described as the application of a series of steps that are undertaken to complete the method. The exact number of steps varies depending upon the person discussing the method, but the order and intent of the steps remain similar and delineate the constancy of the scientific method. Here we present seven steps. Questions that might be posed by speech-language pathologists using this method are outlined at each step. Our intent here is to have the student think through and reflect on the purposes of diagnosis and the role the diagnostician might perform at each of the seven steps in the process.

Step I	*Definition and delimitation of the problem area: Understanding the subject matter*	What is our problem?
		What are we diagnosing?
		What fund of knowledge do we need as diagnosticians?
		How do we acquire the knowledge we need to do diagnoses?
		How may this knowledge be organized by the diagnostician?
		How much does theory rule our jobs as diagnosticians?
		Since the diagnostician is confronted with so many different speech and language disorders, do you think he needs a broader base of knowledge than the researcher?
		How does the diagnostician use his general fund of knowledge for the purpose of diagnosing an individual patient?
Step II	*Development of hypotheses to be tested*	What are the purposes of diagnosis?
		How can hypotheses be formulated by the diagnostician that fit the concept of the use of the hypothesis in research or in the use of the method of science?
		Are statements of hypotheses appropriate for studying the individual?
		How do we state a clinical hypothesis?
		How do our hypotheses relate to the problem presented by the patient, by the referral source?
		What relationships should be expresssed in a clinical hypothesis?
		Can clinical hypotheses be unbiased?
		A researcher is generally free to study hypotheses of specific interest to him; hypotheses that are as narrowly defined as he feels warranted for predicting events in his field of knowledge. Does the diagnostician have this freedom?
Step III	*Development of procedures for testing the hypotheses: Research design*	What are the clinical tools needed by the diagnostician?
		How are the tools of diagnosis selected for the purposes of diagnosis for the individual patient?

Step III
(Cont)

How does the diagnostician evaluate the appropriateness of his tools?

Can the diagnostician exert control in his testing sessions by selection of his tools?

Do we have tools for diagnosis that meet the requirements for measuring instruments that are so important for research? Do we have to be concerned about precision, reliability, and validity?

Since the diagnostician does not know his patient personally before the time of the diagnosis, how can he consider control over the variables that may be present?

How much time should be allotted for testing procedures?

Is there an order for presenting testing procedures in diagnosis? Are we concerned about the effect one procedure may have on another?

Step IV   *Collection of the data*

What are the clinical procedures of diagnosis?

Can the diagnostician control all the variables during the testing session?

How does he account for variables that he cannot control?

What happens if the diagnostician is not able to use the procedures he initially selected? Does this invalidate the diagnosis?

Young children present significant testing problems? What can a diagnostician do during the testing session to assure that the data that is obtained is accurately recorded?

Can the diagnostician be as systematic in collecting the data needed for diagnosis as the researcher who has control over his experiment? Can the word systematic be interpreted in such a way as to apply to the diagnostic process?

How can the diagnostician observe and record verbal information objectively?

Step V   *Analysis of the data*

How is the information obtained for analysis?

How does the diagnostician score the information?

How do we analyze the information obtained in the diagnostic process?

Do we have measures that are descriptive and predictive?

Can the results obtained in diagnosis be quantified?

Step VI   *Interpretation of the data: Support or reject the hypothesis*

How does the diagnostician interpret the results obtained in the diagnosis?

How can we know if our results are close to the true behaviors we set out to study?

When interpreting the findings of the diagnosis, do we rely only on the specific test findings?

How is the information organized in relationship to the hypothesis?

How is the information synthesized and summarized?

Step VII   *Generalizing from the data: Conclusions*

How does the diagnostician interpret and communicate the findings of the diagnosis?

What applications to other patients can be made from the interpretations made on the patient seen? Can this or should this be done?

In what forms is the information from the diagnosis communicated?

Does diagnosis stop at this point?

How does the diagnostician determine appropriate management plans?

Appropriateness for diagnosis

These seven steps of the scientific method can guide the diagnostic process and at the same time allow the diagnostician to exercise his individual professional decision-making abilities. In our view the method can be applied to the individual patient who can be studied as if he constituted a "mini research project."

Using the method of science requires the diagnostician to be rigorous in his approach to diagnosis, following a logical, orderly process of decision making. The method forces us to be systematic and organized. It helps us plan diagnoses more efficiently and economically.

Through the appropriate application of the method of science, diagnosis should be more precise and more controlled, evidencing less bias and error, thereby allowing for more appropriate interpretations and predictions of behavior. The diagnostician can learn to sharpen his skills of observation and reasoning abilities. Greater sophistication and confidence should come as the method is applied, although, at first, deliberate thought is needed until it becomes the diagnostician's habitual way of thinking through the diagnostic problems he sees. From using the method he will be able to develop greater insights into the accuracy of his decisions. The more questions he asks about the conclusions he makes, the greater will his powers of observation become. His failures should be less frequent, since the method allows for correction of error. The constant use of the method of science in his diagnostic practice will prevent him from having unwarranted biases; therefore inappropriate recommendations for treatment and referral will be prevented.

Using the method of science also has the advantage of helping the diagnostician realize what he knows and what he needs to learn. Information in our profession is continually changing and growing. Realizing that he may never know all he needs to know for the solution of his daily professional problems, the diagnostician applies his present knowledge with the intention of testing and increasing this knowledge. He engages in a continual search for information that allows him to better carry out his professional responsibilities. Thus, in addition to providing a logical guide to diagnosis, using the method of science enables the diagnostician to augment his knowledge.

The adaptation and application of the method of science should provide the diagnostician with an approach useful for all diagnostic problems he confronts. Rather than individual diagnostic approaches for voice problems or articulation problems, he has a method that is applicable to all disorders. It provides a set of unifying principles, thereby addressing Rees' (1978, p. 20) conclusion "that the profession lacks a set of unified principles underlying current approaches to diagnosis." The method of science should prevent the reliance on the "problem-type" diagnosis, which amounts to little more than a testing approach for a disorder rather than a diagnosis. As Darley states

> The clinician devoted to the methodology of science will come at each new patient afresh, bringing his most lively curiosity and careful critical analysis to bear upon the problem. He will not shackle himself to a previously developed conviction of what he will find nor be overly influenced by the connotations of whatever labels come already affixed. (Darley, 1964, p. 10)

Therefore the method of science is not just simply *appropriate* for the *diagnostician*; it is *highly significant* for his development as a professional problem solver. The use of the method and its adaptation to such systems as problem-oriented records (Kent & Chabon, 1980) becomes a major way of helping us to be accountable for what we do. Kamhi (in press) presents this viewpoint in reference to problem solving in child language disorders.

THE DIAGNOSTIC MODEL

Figure 3-1 presents our model for adapting the steps of the method of science to the diagnostic process. Our diagnostic model presents a series of steps that the diagnostician must systematically consider as he solves the clincial problems presented in each diagnosis. The seven steps of the diagnostic model are (1) constituent analysis: definition and delimitation of the clinical problem; (2) clinical hypotheses: derivation of cause–effect relationships; (3) clinical design: development of the measurement plan; (4) clinical testing: collection of the data; (5) clinical data analysis; (6) clinical interpretation, and (7) conclusions: patient management.

These seven steps outline and organize the primary functions the diagnostician performs during a diagnosis. The steps are discrete in that at each step the diagnostician has certain specifiable tasks to perform. The steps, however, are also interactive and cyclic. What occurs at one step influences all others. This interaction is depicted in the model by a converging diamond-shaped figure, showing the cumulative convergence of all steps into conclusions, the tentative solution to the clinical problem.

In addition to outlining the major steps in diagnosis and showing their interaction, the model also illustrates that we can separate the diagnostic process into two major halves, one concerned with causal factors and the other with effects. Thus, if the diagnostician's primary concern for a certain patient is about causal factors, he can proceed to follow the steps on the lefthand side under *cause*, somewhat independent of the *effects* on the righthand side. In other situations, for example, when the diagnostician knows the cause of the speech and language disorder as in an adult with aphasia resulting from a cerebrovascular accident (CVA), he may want to concentrate his efforts on the effect steps.

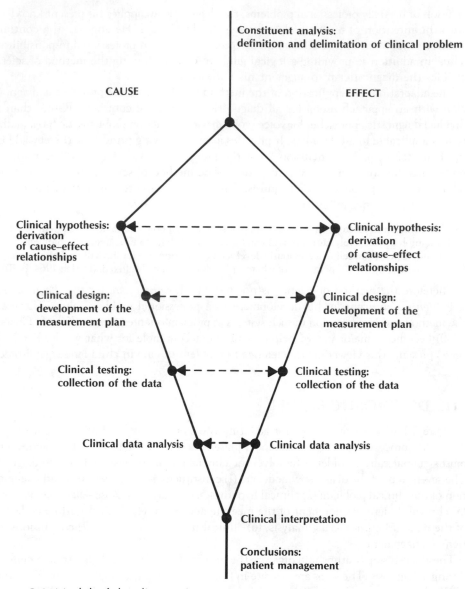

Figure 3-1. Model of the diagnostic process: a scientific framework.

By allowing concentration on both cause and effect, or either one, the model shows how the diagnostic adaptation of the scientific method can be directed to the diagnostic needs of the specific patient.

Constituent analysis: definition and delimitation of the clinical problem

The first step of the diagnostic process, the constituent analysis, can be considered somewhat analogous to the literature review that precedes a research project. It is from studying the information available about a particular subject matter that a researcher develops questions he wishes to address. Similarly, in diagnosis it is from studying what is known about a patient that the diagnostician develops his initial clinical questions.

The definition and delimitation process, the constituent analysis, is a thorough, systematic analysis of each bit of information *(constituent)* that has been made available about the patient. The diagnostician's ability to perform this analysis is dependent on two primary sources of information:

1. The patient information he has available to him from any source prior to actual patient contact;

2. His organized funds of knowledge about normal and disordered speech and language.

At this first step of the diagnostic process, the diagnostician reviews the patient information made available from a number of sources: the referral source, case history forms, and medical records among others.

The diagnostician then categorizes and examines each of the constituents in light of his funds of knowledge to determine if they are significant and relevant for asking appropriate clinical questions. It is on the basis of his constituent analysis that the diagnostician determines what his specific job will be with each patient he sees.

The constituent analysis, then, integrates two important ingredients: what the diagnostician knows about the patient and what the diagnostician knows about normal and disordered speech and language. This step readies the diagnostician for the remainder of the diagnostic process.

Analyze the following constituents. What are the relevant and important constituents? Robert is a 4-year-old child who was referred by his pediatrician. Robert, as far as his mother is concerned, does not have the speech disorder the pediatrician hears. The pediatrician in his referral letter has stated, "This boy's speech is so difficult to understand that I believe something is significantly wrong with his speech development. The mother is against this referral but will follow through with the evaluation. We need to get this boy some help." What mental process will you go through to analyze the constituents?

Clinical hypotheses: derivation of cause–effect relationships

At the second step of the diagnostic process the diagnostician formulates working clinical hypotheses expressing cause–effect relationships. Derived from the constituent analysis, hypotheses are statements of *most likely* cause–effect relationships. Hypotheses can be stated with varying degrees of specificity and assurance, depending on the significance and validity of the constituents used for analysis. For example, from a neurologist's referral stating that James Burcham suffered a severe CVA affecting the left cerebral hemisphere, the diagnostician probably would be more assured that this causal factor contributed to the language disorder than a mother's report that "my neighbor thinks Byron's tongue is lazy."

Although in diagnosis we are generally concerned with both causes and effects, we have noted (Figure 3-1) that the diagnostic process can diverge into a cause (left side) or an effect (right side) emphasis. This divergence develops an important diagnostic perspective; that is, the diagnostician can pursue cause and effect either separately or simultaneously. If he wishes to view the problem in terms of the behaviors that are disordered, the model allows him to emphasize behavioral (effect) disorders independent from concerns regarding causal factors.

Because of the incomplete state of knowledge regarding causal factors of speech and language disorders, diagnosticians must be cautious about making cause–effect hypotheses. We therefore want to present the independence of cause and/or effect while at the same time emphasizing their interdependence. The dotted lines and arrows on the model are our way of showing the interrelationships of cause and effect throughout the diagnostic process. The convergence of these two aspects throughout the remainder of the steps indicates that we are striving to bring together information about causal factors and observed speech and language disorders while at the same time continuing to demonstrate both their dependence and independence.

Cause–effect hypotheses, then, are the diagnostician's best statements or questions about the causal factors and presented speech and language disorders of the patients he sees. While these hypotheses are initially formulated on the information available prior to patient contact, they may be reformulated or revised as further information is made available throughout the complete diagnostic process. The hypothesis is the diagnostician's tentative solution of the patient's problem.

What hypothesis would you derive for Robert? What support would you use to convince another professional that you have developed the most likely hypothesis? Does this hypothesis seem meaningful: "Robert has a severe voice disorder related to vocal abuse?" Why or why not?

Clinical design: development of the measurement plan

In the third step of the diagnostic process the diagnostician plans the diagnostic session in order to test his clinical hypothesis. He designs the diagnosis. He wants to gain information about the patient's hypothesized speech and language disorder and its causes. The diagnostician in this phase selects and develops needed tools to fit his design, and he plans his testing strategy to optimize data collection.

In designing the diagnosis for a particular patient, an overriding concern is the plan for systematically observing and measuring the patient's behavior. In his planning for systematic measurement, the diagnostician draws on the countless tools and procedures available. The interview is a major source of information. The diagnostician must decide what he wants to learn in the interview and how he is going to learn it. Besides the interview, the diagnostician may plan for unstructured situations in which to observe spontaneous behavior, develop his own testing protocols for eliciting desired behavior, or choose from the array of commercial or experimental tools available. There are various ways professionals view the purposes of clinical design. Assessment to some implies the use of standardized tools, which allow for normative comparisons to be made. Others, Muma (1978, 1981) being a major proponent, would say that clinical assessment is a process of discovering and describing how an individual functions in natural contexts. Clinical design must consider these alternatives to systematically observing a patient with a speech and language disorder.

Whatever the specific tools selected, the diagnostician evaluates their usefulness to him for gathering information about the cause–effect relationships he has hypothesized. He must evaluate the importance of each tool he wants to use in relationship to all other tools and procedures considered. How important will the information gained from each tool be for understanding the clinical problem?

Also, in designing the diagnosis, the diagnostician must plan his testing strategy to optimize his data collection. For example, in the interview, how might he best frame his questions to gain the most complete and valid information? In testing, in what order will he present his procedures to best capitalize on his patient's abilities and personal characteristics: Which would be best to start with and end with? How does he plan to record his observations? Just as well-executed research studies come from well-designed research plans, so also do successful diagnoses follow carefully conceived diagnostic plans.

With Robert what tools would you consider because he is 4 years old? Why would age be a consideration for selecting and developing clinical tools? What tools would you consider for the mother? If she is resistant to this referral, does that make a difference?

Clinical testing: collection of the data

The fourth step of the diagnostic process starts the face-to-face contact with the patient and his family. It is here that the diagnostician gains his interview information and administers the tools he has selected to test his clinical hypothesis. He collects his data.

A major concern in data collection is control over the stimuli, responses, and reinforcements. As well, the diagnostician is concerned with the appropriateness of the tools. Will he have to adapt the format of the tool to fit the patient? Will he have to adapt the order in which he presents each of the procedures he has selected? He must also determine if all the procedures selected are needed.

The diagnostician has to understand that many adaptations of the tools and procedures are made during the actual assessment of the patient. Even though he has carefully selected the procedures he wants to use and has a good understanding of the potential clinical problem, he still has to adjust to the specific and actual behaviors of the patient. No diagnostician's anticipatory design ever comes completely true. This flexibility is of major importance, especially when testing young children who do not always behave in a way that facilitates the diagnostician's plan.

Besides his presentation of the tools selected, the diagnostician must be concerned with factors that are a major part of any interview and testing situation. He must be able to relate to each patient, keeping in mind the various background experiences and needs that both he and his patients bring to the diagnostic situation.

The collection of data step also includes recording of the data as it occurs. The diagnostician must capture the data in a form that he can analyze and reflect on at a later time. In effect, he needs some means of making permanent his evidence. Some test procedures provide scoring forms that assist in this process; others do not.

Let us suppose that Robert was very uncooperative. From the moment you introduced yourself to him and his mother he developed clinging behavior, seemed resistant, and would not speak; and when you attempted to take him and his mother to your testing room, he began to scream and throw himself on the floor. What does this do to your selection of clinical tools? How would you manage a situation like this? What tool would you need most at this time?

Clinical data analysis

In the fifth step of the diagnostic process the diagnostician objectifies and analyzes the data he has collected. He scores, categorizes, and orders all the information obtained in the interview and testing sessions.

Scoring of the data is done, basically, to determine how well and how poorly the patient performed in reference to some standard criteria. This standard criteria may be normative data as specified by the test instrument used. Or the standard may be in terms of intragroup comparisons, that is, comparing the patient being seen with other patients with similar problems. In many instances, particularly when "scoring" spontaneous behavior, the standard derives from the diagnostician's background information on normal use of speech and language and his information about the characteristic speech and language behavior in disorders that have been profiled in the literature.

After objectifying the obtained data, the diagnostician then needs to categorize the data in relation to the cause–effect hypothesis. He must order the data that provides information about speech and language behaviors. At this time the diagnostician must consider the validity, reliability, and completeness of the data obtained.

This step in the diagnostic process is meant to be an objective scoring and ordering of data, not an interpretive step. It should be viewed as a prelude to the next step, interpretation of the data. Incidentally, as a discrete step in the diagnostic process, analysis of the data is one of the more arbitrary steps. The same is true in research studies. Seldom is analysis of the data truly separated from either data collection or, more important, from data interpretation. However, we feel the objectivity implied in this analysis step is important enough to make it explicitly separate, especially for the student learning the diagnostic process. We must learn to look at the results of our data collection apart from the interpretation we may then give them.

Information concerning Robert was collected using the screening portion of the Templin–Darley Tests of Articulation (Templin & Darley, 1969), the Northwestern Syntax Screening Test (Lee, 1969), the Peabody Picture Vocabulary Test (Dunn & Dunn, 1981), an audiometric screening test (Northern & Downs, 1978; *Asha* Committee of Audiometric Evaluation, 1975), and the Goldman–Fristoe–Woodcock Test of Auditory Discrimination (Goldman et al., 1970). First, looking backward from the tools used, what would you think the clinical hypothesis for Robert might have been? Next, how would you analyze the information from these tests? How do you go about analyzing data from tests such as these?

Clinical interpretation

After he has analyzed the data, the diagnostician proceeds to an interpretation of the clinical data, the sixth step on the diagnostic model. In this step the diagnostician uses all the information now available, from all sources, to determine its meaning and significance. He wants to know if the data confirms or denies his original hypotheses or if it suggests other interpretations. This interpretation is vital as it sets the course for future management of the patient.

The diagnostician must determine the significance of the results. Here he takes all the data available to him and determines what it means in relationship to his cause–effect hypothesis, to the general purposes of diagnosis, to the referral request, and to the statement of the problem as seen by the patient.

After logically interpreting his data, the diagnostician has to arrive at some conclusion to his thoughts, however tentative they may be. Thus, he is called on to state succinctly what the disorder may be and to implicate probable causal factors; he must formulate, state, and support the diagnosis.

This step of the diagnostic process is not merely a summary of the data. Rather, it is the diagnostician's ability to put the pieces together, an attempt to understand the whole. The diagnostician must use his reasoning abilities to present the most logical interpretation of the available data. Note that we have said the information available; however, missing information may be as important to interpretation as the information that has been obtained.

The diagnostician in the interpretation phase is exercising his highest degree of professionalism. He must be aware of all the variables that have entered into the diagnostic process for each patient, keeping his interpretations within these boundaries, while at the same time using his knowledge and problem-solving skills to arrive at his best answers to the clinical problems presented.

In our analysis of Robert's responses to the testing tools presented in the last step, we discovered that he fell below the mean or average on all of the tests. How might you interpret the meaning of this data? Interpretations, remember, are in terms of your working hypothesis and should take into consideration cause–effect relationships.

Conclusions: patient management

At the seventh and final step on the diagnostic model, conclusions are drawn by the diagnostician that revolve primarily around management considerations. He must decide what is to be done and how it is to be done.

The interpretation of the clinical data from the previous step allowed the diagnostician to identify the nature of the speech and language disorder and its probable causal factors. Now he must decide if the disorder constitutes a problem that needs attention and, if so, what can be done about it. He must formulate a management proposal. The diagnostician must know what management alternatives are appropriate for the disorder and its contributing causal factors. He also must consider the best alternatives considering age, family concerns, other factors, and probable prognosis. He must not arrive at merely an ideal plan but must have practical knowledge of the options available to him in his community within the cost and time restrictions of the client. All phases of the diagnostic process enter into making these decisions, including how the patient may be able to follow through with any management decisions made.

After arriving at a management proposal, the diagnostician must communicate the findings of his diagnosis and his recommended management plan to the patient. The diagnostician must know how to interpret the diagnostic findings to those concerned so that they understand what has been said and what implications the findings have for them. The diagnostician must be able to engage in a two-way consideration of his recommended management proposal. He must determine if his plan is realistic and will be supported by the patient or if alternative plans need to be implemented. At this phase the diagnostician must demonstrate competence in interpersonal communication, the ability to transmit his findings and plan of action and to listen to the questions, concerns, and viewpoints of the patient and his family. As well as communicating with the patient and his family, the diagnostician must be able to communicate his findings and plans to other professionals involved. This includes reporting the findings to the original referral source and making the diagnostic findings available to others concerned with the proposed management of the patient.

The diagnostician also must follow up on the diagnostic decisions that have been made. He must monitor the recommendations that have been developed in the management proposal to ensure implementation. This may include referrals, scheduling for therapy, or whatever steps need to be taken.

Step seven, then, focuses on an action plan for the patient. Here, at last, the diagnostic process has "payoff" for the patient and family. They are helped in developing an understanding of the disorder and its probable causes and join with the diagnostician in determining what can be done about it.

From your interpretation of Robert's problem, you decide that treatment is necessary as well as further testing by an otolaryngologist. Knowing the mother's initial resistance, how might you interpret your findings and recommendations for her, helping her gain the perspective she needs to get something done for the child? As we indicated at the beginning of this example on Robert, the mother was against the pediatrician's referral.

These seven steps of the clinical adaptation of the method of science illustrate the functions of the diagnostician throughout the diagnostic process. All diagnoses require the use of these steps in various degrees of specificity. We have listed each step of the process as a discrete stage in diagnosis. We do this, not because this reflects how diagnoses are "really" performed, but because we feel these steps are necessary components for all diagnoses and can be isolated to some degree for teaching purposes. While the tasks embodied in the seven steps generally occur in all diagnoses, they may not always happen exactly as listed; steps may recur more than once within a single diagnosis. What is important here, however, is to show how an application of the scientific method can guide our diagnostic process as well as guide the teaching of that process.

In conclusion, by following the seven steps of the diagnostic process, the diagnostician should have a comprehensive understanding of diagnosis as it applies to the individual patient, regardless of the type of speech and language disorder presented. As a clinical scientist, the diagnostician should arrive at reasonable solutions to the clinical problems and at the same time know the weaknesses inherent in each diagnosis he performs. Following this method we would expect the diagnostician to

1. Demonstrate his reasoning abilities for deriving an appropriate clinical hypothesis;
2. Be familiar with the literature and current thinking on the clinical problem he has hypothesized;
3. Be able to present supporting evidence for the logic of his clinical hypothesis, including any contradictory evidence;
4. Give careful thought to the best way the patient should be approached in terms of testing procedures;
5. Be aware of the inherent difficulties in his approach to the clinical problem and make educated and judicious decisions about his testing procedures;
6. Give thought to the potential results when he selects his tools and procedures;
7. Develop suitable methods of description and analysis;
8. Know how well the results of his approach and analyses will apply to the solution of the speech and language disorder;
9. Be able to cope with future difficulties and carry out his proposed plans in an acceptable manner.

SHIFTS OF DIAGNOSTIC FOCUS

The diagnostician's job functions can vary depending on his work setting and the intent of the referral. These two factors frequently require the diagnostician to alter the stated purposes of diagnosis to fit the special circumstances of each referral and each work setting. Regardless of the circumstances, however, the diagnostic model as illustrated in Figure 3-1 allows for adaptations of the diagnostic process. Rather than promote different "types of diagnoses" such as the *survey, screening, appraisal, etiologic,* and *differential* diagnoses as some authors do (Mysak, 1976), we feel these "types of diagnoses" and other modifications simply represent a *shift of focus* toward one of the three general goals of diagnosis. We do not believe that a change in the general orientation to diagnosis is needed but rather a differential concentration, adapting the diagnostic design to meet the specific purposes established by the setting or referral request.

Setting modifications

Various amounts of time are allotted to the diagnostic process in different settings. Time, therefore, becomes an important practical consideration in using the steps of the method. In one setting the entire process may be restricted to an hour's duration; in others, several hours or repeated sessions may be permitted. In many school settings and some inpatient facilities, the diagnostic process may extend over many short time periods. With restricted time limits, the diagnostician may emphasize one step of the process more than another. For example he may be called on to "screen" a large preschool population. In this setting he probably would focus more on the speech and language behavior than on causal factors; his hypotheses and diagnostic design would be developed for the group served rather than individuals, and most of his allotted time with each individual would be devoted to data collection.

The type of patient seen in each setting also determines how the steps are used. If, for example, the entire patient population is adult aphasics, the steps would be adjusted to account for their specific needs. The diagnostician would probably specify to a greater extent the speech and language testing procedures for data collection, because the cause–effect relationships would be clearer. A diagnostician in a setting where only trainable mentally retarded children are seen may be primarily concerned with the speech and language behavior of the children rather than causation. (This depends on the security of the diagnosis of mental retardation.) His job may be to specify the amount and type of speech and language behavior the children use with the purpose of providing baselines of behavior for designing language and speech therapy. The diagnostician working in a setting with deaf and severely hard-of-hearing children may be mostly concerned with the development of speech and language behaviors. Or his purpose in this setting may be to determine each child's ability to process auditory information with emphasis on the amount of amplification that may be needed. In settings such as these the diagnostician may be involved primarily with determining how a patient may best learn speech and language rather than in establishing cause–effect relationships.

In other settings physicians and speech pathologists have joined forces to arrive at more exacting descriptions of the speech and language disorder, causal factors, and patient management. Darley (1973) has discussed the interdependent partnership between speech pathologists and neurologists in diagnosis and treatment of neurologic disorders. Thus, demands of a particular setting will require a shift of diagnostic focus among the three stated goals of diagnosis.

Referral modifications

In addition to the modifications dictated by the various work settings, the purpose of the referral may require the diagnostician to modify the diagnostic process. Diagnosticians are not always asked to provide an intensive cause–effect workup of an individual patient. Some referrals are for the purpose of screening large groups of individuals; others may ask for a consultation regarding a likely cause for an already specified speech and language disorder; others may ask for a definitive analysis of the speech and language behavior; still others may ask for the diagnostician's expertise with a specific testing tool. For example, Mr. McOsker, an adult aphasic, is referred by a neurologist with the request that prognostic recommendations be given for language recovery. In this instance the primary speech and language disorder (aphasia) and causal factor (brain damage) are known. What is being requested is a determination of probable future language status of the patient. While the diagnostician has to further describe the nature and severity of the language disorder, as well as look for other possible contributing causal considerations, as a consultant to the neurologist his major question to address, his diagnostic focus, would be patient management. These represent only some of the referral requests that require the diagnostician to modify his use of the steps of the diagnostic process.

Even in screening procedures, although generally not thought of as a diagnostic function, all aspects of the diagnostic model are being used. The intent of speech and language screening is to discover who has a significant variation and who does not. During his screenings the diagnostician may employ tools for both cause and effect. A screening articulation test may provide information about both phonetic structure and speech mechanism function. A routine speech mechanism examination certainly is used to discover any causal relationship between errors in sound production and deviations of the speech-producing mechanism. The audiometric screening test functions both to detect hearing problems in and of themselves or as potential causes for any speech and language disorder that may be discovered. From the information obtained during screening procedures the diagnostician may recommend a more complete diagnostic workup. At times enough information is obtained during the screening to warrant recommendations for immediate therapeutic intervention. Thus, in many instances "screening" procedures encompass the entire set of steps in the diagnostic process.

If the referral source has asked for a detailed specification of the speech and language behaviors, the diagnostician may emphasize the effect side of the diagnostic model. He selects tools to give him detailed information to report back to the referral source. Or the referral source may be more interested in the information the diagnostician may be able to supply about suspected causal factors. The referral source may give detailed information about the speech and language characteristics but wants the diagnostician's opinion about the relationship these characteristics may have to various underlying causal factors. Thus, the diagnostician would study the speech and language characteristics, emphasizing the causal side of the diagnostic model. His clinical question might be, "What are the potential causes for the specified set of speech and language symptoms?" Again, he would devise testing procedures to uncover the relationship between the effects and the potential causes.

Referrals such as these examples require the diagnostician at times to focus on a certain aspect of the total diagnostic process. Even though the diagnostician's job varies depending on referral requests, he still maintains a perspective on all the steps of the diagnostic process. In his verification of another professional's hypothesis he looks at the data that tell him whether the initial referral statement is consistent with his own analysis of the data. If not, he can set up alternative hypotheses for testing or for suggestion to the referral source. Thus, while a diagnostician keeps in mind the three general goals of diagnosis, referral requests may focus his attention on one primary goal of his diagnostic job.

Other role modifications

Our profession also incorporates persons other than professional diagnosticians who may assume limited roles in the overall diagnosis of speech and language disorders. Students are trained to conduct all diagnostic functions; however, early in their training their main focus may be to test for and describe speech and language behaviors or to administer certain tests that pertain to causal factors. While the student later in training tries out his interpretive and decision-making skills, the final responsibility for the diagnosis lies with the supervising professional.

In addition to the roles played by students, we often see nurses conducting hearing screening programs or administering other specific tests at the request of physicians. Frequently, schools utilize parent volunteers to help administer routine tests. Paraprofessionals also perform designated tasks within speech and hearing agencies. In general these personnel are involved in administering a specific test for a specific reason. Their focus is generally on screening a large population or gaining specific, circumscribed information. Test interpretations are generally not part of their role. Rather, judgments and decisions are largely left to the speech pathologist, audiologist, or physician under whose direction they function. While these persons may be able to perform partial functions in the diagnosis, it is only the professional diagnostician who assumes full responsibility; who combines his knowledge and experience, his problem-solving skill, and his patient concern for fulfilling all the diagnostic activities.

Adaptation of diagnostic process to setting and referral requirements

Following the diagnostic model gives the diagnostician the flexibility for fulfilling all his job functions regardless of his setting and the intent of the referrals he receives. The examples in Table 3-1 present a series of potential job functions a diagnostician may have relative to both his work setting and the intent of the referral. The examples illustrate how the diagnostician would focus on different aspects of the diagnostic model, maintaining his overall view of the purposes of diagnosis, to offer tentative solutions to clinical problems.

These are only several among many of the referrals for diagnosis that come to the diagnostician in different work settings. The constancy of the diagnostic model as an adaptation of the scientific method assists the diagnostician in handling the variability that occurs.

ADMINISTRATION AND THE DIAGNOSTICIAN

The scope of the diagnostic process goes beyond the specifics of what the professional does to prepare for and perform a diagnosis with a given patient. In conjunction with the professional diagnostic services offered a patient comes "paperwork." Paperwork is euphemistically used to mean the administrative procedures necessary to process a patient

Table 3-1. Diagnostic shifts of focus based on the referral and work setting.

REFERRAL: *From a public school speech pathologist to a speech and hearing center.*	REFERRAL: *From a mother to a community speech and hearing center.*	REFERRAL: *From the kindergarten teacher to the public school speech pathologist.*
"Devin has a severe articulation problem. I have not been able to determine the extent of his articulatory pattern to plan treatment."	"My son Devin has a speech problem. We want to know if it is significant."	"Devin cannot make the s, sh, ch, z, and j sounds. Should he have therapy now?"

In this referral the diagnostician would most likely initially emphasize the effect side of the diagnostic model. An effect hypothesis has been stated: "articulation problem." The diagnostician has been asked to assist in clarifying the articulatory pattern to assist in treatment. He would consider the products of phonetic structure and phonology for emphasis. However, since no causal factors are stated, the diagnostician would probably design his diagnosis within a causal framework. In a referral like this the chances that the pattern of articulation is related to something other than development are likely. Still his emphasis, as requested, will be the analysis of the articulatory pattern.

He would design his diagnosis to discover as much as possible about the characteristics of Devin's sound system. He would select tools to gain details about the sounds he can produce, which sounds are in error, how the sounds are in error, where they are in error, etc. Because of the causal aspect, he would probably do this with a careful view of Devin's speech production abilities.

He would analyze and interpret his data in terms of the referral and provide the referral source with information that might assist with treatment planning.

If he discovered other information about the child's speech and language system, he would convey this to the referral source, particularly if other important causal factors have been uncovered.

This is a wide-open re-referral with any number of possibilities. The diagnostician would have to consider both the cause and effect aspects of diagnosis. He would have to do a constituent analysis at the time the client came for his appointment and set up tentative hypotheses for testing.

All the steps of the diagnostic model would be used. However, the diagnostician might have to consider the use of tools that sample a wide range of behaviors since so little is known. He would surely want to obtain a good spontaneous speech sample early in the testing to see if he could isolate the basic area of variation. The mother has indicated there is a problem, but she is unsure if it is significant. Therefore the diagnostician must consider as well that the child's speech may be normal for his age.

The diagnostician would select tools and order them in such a way that each tool adds more information and allows the diagnostician to disregard certain cause–effect relationships.

Throughout he is attempting to discover if there is a disorder and what may be causally related in order to analyze and interpret this information to the mother in light of her referral question. "Is the problem significant?"

In instances like these the diagnostician may have to be quite tentative. Much information may be missing. He may have completed the diagnostic session with only a more secure hypothesis that needs further exploration.

Let's presume in this setting the speech pathologist usually does not see kindergarten children except on special referral. His first reaction may be that the child is developing these sounds late. But teachers often know the difference; so, is something else going on? The diagnostician in this instance may want to emphasize the causal side of the diagnostic model. There may be something about the child's speech mechanism that prevents him from producing these sounds correctly.

The diagnostician may elect, first, to sit in the classroom and listen to the child to verify his sound errors. From what he hears he may go no further. He may hear a typical sound substitution pattern that he will reevaluate at the end of the school year. However, he may hear production errors that suggest a closer look. He then may have the child come to his therapy room at another session and select tools which emphasize speech production abilities. His emphasis would be on the why — why these sound errors exist.

He would select procedures that test the articulation process as used in the production of the sound classes in error — affricate and fricative production.

He may select tools to analyze tongue function and dentition. He would most likely be interested in a kinesiologic analysis, how the articulators function in production of these sounds.

From his analysis and interpretation the diagnostician should be able to answer the referral question. "Is therapy needed now?" Or he may have discovered an underlying cause that needs other types of attention.

for diagnostic services. Procedures used are developed primarily as a means for the patient to gain diagnostic services and as record-keeping mechanisms.

When a patient or professional seeks service from an agency, his first contact is usually administrative. If the administrative face of the agency is ambiguous, cumbersome, or "sloppy," the public may develop a faulty impression of the professional activities of the agency, which will be reflected in their use of the agency. Clear, concise processing procedures focusing on the individual requesting service and not on the needs of the agency are essential. Both must be served, but the primary focus should be on the patient. If the patient is required to go through extensive, and to him irrelevant, procedures to obtain an appointment for diagnosis, he may arrive on his appointment day with resentments toward the agency or may not show up at all. These situations must be circumvented. This is not to say that certain paperwork procedures cannot be instituted and used as long as the patient understands how these procedures facilitate the professional service he receives. What people seeking professional services want is someone who perceives their needs and responds to them as directly as possible. Thus, explanations about the required administrative procedures may be needed to alleviate the frustration some patients feel.

The administrative procedures designed for record keeping gather information pertaining to who the patient is, where he lives, his problem, how he came to the diagnostic setting, what his current status is, and whose responsibility it is for follow-up. These records have numerous intra-agency purposes, designed often for statistical reasons and to "keep track" of the patients seen. Records are often necessary for use by other community and governmental agencies. Record keeping has become an absolute necessity in a setting offering diagnostic services to the public, whether in a community agency, a hospital, a school system, or private practice.

Administrative components

The three major administrative components of diagnosis include *intake procedures* (the procedures that are followed for processing information about a patient prior to his appointment), the *diagnostic session* (what occurs from the time the patient arrives for his appointment until the diagnostic "day" is over), and *follow-up* (involvement with the patient following the diagnostic session)

We offer a flowchart (Figure 3-2) that represents the service performed within each component. We will briefly discuss each of the components and then provide an outline for the reader's consideration. Our intent is to give the student an understanding of the importance of administration to the diagnostic process and the different functions he may have to perform in his work setting.

Our development of the three administrative components may fit some settings better than others. However, we feel the flowchart and outlines can be adapted to the specific needs of any work setting. We have also included in Appendix I a set of forms that can be reviewed in conjunction with the flowchart. Each form represents a different administrative function and is designed to assist the agency in carrying out these functions. The forms are not intended to be used as they are by any specific agency; rather they are representative of forms designed to facilitate patient service.

From the outset it is important to keep in mind that many or all of the details within each administrative component may be handled by the diagnostician rather than by supportive administrative personnel. Some settings use administrative personnel, whereas other settings, for example, private practice, may require the professional to handle all aspects

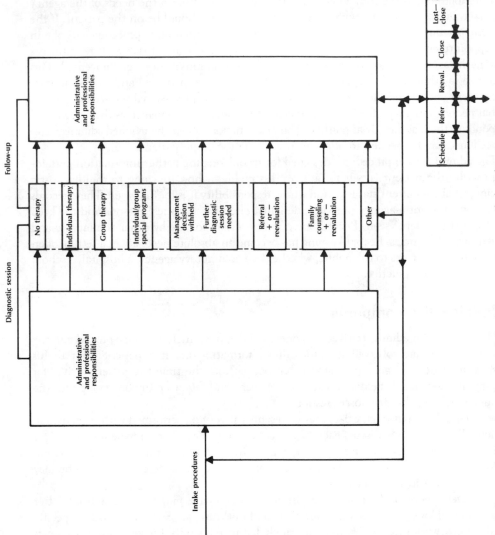

Figure 3-2. Flowchart of the professional and administrative components of the diagnostic process.

of the processing of patients for diagnosis. Our use of the words "professional" and "administrative" in this discussion refers primarily to functions rather than people. For example, the individual who takes incoming referral calls may be either a diagnostician or a scheduling secretary.

Intake procedures

Intake procedures and policies include the patient-processing activities from the time of the initial referring contact until the time the patient is scheduled for an appointment. Within this administrative component a system is instituted for taking information about the patient, the referral source, the problem, and patient concerns.

It is of great importance that the patient knows what is going to happen at this initial stage. Information which allows the patient to feel secure that the agency understands his needs and will follow up as efficiently as possible should be provided. This is relatively easy if an appointment for diagnosis is given at the time of initial contact. Then the patient knows when he is to come and when something will be done. However, if appointments are not given until later, the patient must know when and how the appointment is to come. The use of a follow-up acknowledgment letter (Appendix I) is a useful device in providing such information. The letter can state the conditions of the scheduling process and other information that may be useful. A brochure or letter that describes the agency, its services, and its costs also can be useful for providing a basic understanding of the services offered by the speech and hearing agency.

Another aspect of intake procedures is the intra-agency processing needed to keep track of the patient until he is scheduled for his diagnostic appointment. There is no excuse for losing a patient in the "administrative mill." If paperwork is necessary for providing services to human beings, then the process should be as efficient and economical as possible; patients should not be "mislaid" and costs should not skyrocket because of extensive administrative processes and personnel.

The information that is made available to the diagnostician prior to actual patient contact is a part of intake procedures. How much information is needed prior to patient contact and what administrative procedures are established for receiving, accepting, and processing referrals vary from setting to setting and are more or less dependent on the professional philosophy of the setting. For example, the diagnostician working in a hospital setting may receive the referral (consult request) in the form of a telephone call from the duty nurse who is transmitting the physician's orders for a speech evaluation. In this instance the diagnostician has available to him the patient's medical chart. Whatever is in that chart in terms of general, developmental, and medical history as well as the patient's current medical status is data the diagnostician can use prior to contact with the patient. He will know a great deal about the patient, including whether he is healthy enough to respond to a speech and language evaluation. The diagnostician can also contact the physician for further information and discuss the patient with the nursing staff. Thus, considerable information is available.

Another example is the public school setting where the diagnostician receives a referral from the classroom teacher stating that a child seems to have a speech problem that is interfering with his classroom performance. In this setting the diagnostician may have available the school records on the child, which may be extensive or minimal, depending on the philosophy of the school. At the least the child's records will usually include his academic performance, teacher reactions to him, and perhaps an academic profile indicating how well he does in what subjects. In some instances intelligence test results are available, some health records, and family information that may have been filed by the school nurse or psychologist. The diagnostician may have a good bit of information to use unless it is the policy of the school system not to make pupil records available to the diagnostician, a practice in some systems as well as in some agencies.

A question that sometimes arises about intake procedures is with whom the patient should have his first contact. Should it be a professional or can other administrative personnel function in this manner? It is of prime importance that the first person a patient makes contact with is someone who demonstrates knowledge of the agency and its procedures. If the initial contact person is not a speech pathologist, he should know what questions he can answer and when the assistance of a professional is needed. This initial contact person begins the patient's contract with the agency and should handle this situation sensibly and sensitively. Whoever assumes this role must project warmth, sincerity, and knowledge, especially since this first, crucial contact is usually by telephone. These administrative concerns are of particular importance in large agencies serving many individuals with speech and language problems.

The following outline presents the major considerations within the intake procedures component of the administration flowchart (Figure 3-2).

Administrative

Staff responsibilities and roles
    Professional
    Administrative

Initial referral contact
    Procedures for processing
    Referral data forms
    Processing flow
    Follow-up
        Letters and forms

Information gathering
    Types of information
        Histories
        Other professional services performed
    Procedures for processing
        Requests for information
    Follow-up
        Forms and letters

Appointment scheduling
    Criteria for scheduling
        Patient needs
        Professional staff availability
        Individual
        Teams
        Space and time allocations (see diagnostic session)
    Scheduling procedure
        Patient contact
        Procedures for processing
            Forms and letters
            Follow-up

Professional

Steps 1, 2, and 3 of the diagnostic process

Diagnostic session

The second administrative component (Figure 3-2) begins at the time the patient arrives for his appointment with the diagnostician. There are both administrative and professional aspects within this component.

Someone within the diagnostic setting needs to attend to the practical details of where, when, and with what material the diagnostic sessions will be performed. In a smoothly administered setting these decisions are made well in advance of the diagnostic day so that time and space problems are circumvented and needed diagnostic materials are available. When the patient arrives at the agency, it should be made clear to him where he is to go. Even if he has been given a room number when he was scheduled for his appointment, there should be clearly visible information as to the location of the diagnostic setting within the building. There should be someone to greet the patient when he arrives—in large settings this may be the function of a receptionist; in other instances the professional staff member is present. Just as important as the beginning of the diagnostic session is its ending. The patient may need directions for leaving the setting. In some agencies the patient must go to a business office for fee arrangements, but even in a one-person private practice the patient will want to know fee payment procedures. This information should be given to the patient; he should not have to ask.

The primary activity of the diagnostic session is to conduct the diagnosis. These professional services are achieved through the seven steps of the diagnostic process. Therefore the professional service aspect of the diagnostic session will not be expanded on here.

The following outline presents the major aspects of the diagnostic session component of the administrative flowchart (Figure 3-2).

Administrative

Staff responsibilities and roles
    Professional
    Administrative

Space allocation
    Room availability
    Observation facilities
    Specially equipped rooms
        Audiologic
        Videotape
        Others
    Waiting rooms
    Playrooms

Time allocation
    Unit of time for a diagnostic session
    Block of staggered scheduling

Materials and equipment
    Specially equipped rooms

Availability of diagnostic tools
Acquisition of needed materials
Location of materials
Procedures for use of materials

Initial patient contact
Waiting room location

Business procedures
Fees
Method of payment

Professional

Steps 4, 5, 6, and 7 of the diagnostic process; reconsideration of Steps 1, 2, and 3 as needed

Follow-up

The third component of the administrative flowchart is concerned with those administrative and professional services provided for patients after they have completed the initial diagnostic session. Once the patient has been diagnosed and management proposals have been offered, the primary concern of the diagnostician and the agency is the follow-up needed to see that whatever continued services the patient needs are obtained. These services may include scheduling for therapy, referrals to outside agencies, or parental conferences and assistance. Again, we provide an outline of the major aspects of the follow-up component, and Appendix I provides some forms that are useful for these purposes.

Administrative

Staff responsibilities and roles
Professional
Administrative

Referral processing procedures
Letters and forms
Follow-up

Therapy scheduling
Patient assignment
Needs of patient—diagnosis
Staff availability
Space and time allocations
Scheduling procedures
Forms and letters—scheduling form
Follow-up
Record keeping
Reports
Procedures for maintaining records
Active
Inactive
Accessibility

Professional

Step 7 of the diagnostic process

Setting and administration

The specifics of intake procedures, diagnostic session, and follow-up may differ considerably in a nursing home, a public school, or a community hearing and speech agency. For example, a particular agency may have a multidisciplinary diagnostic clinic staffed by speech pathologists, audiologists, psychologists, and social service workers. The procedures for administration reflect how all personnel interact with one another to perform all the services that might be needed. On the day of the diagnosis there would be a need to establish the leader of the diagnostic team, which might vary from patient to patient depending on the nature of the clinical hypothesis. Or the agency might use several sessions for each diagnosis, particularly for children. The flowchart could reflect this two-session policy for diagnostic procedures. A second block could be added to indicate the follow-up that was to occur in the second session. This type of organization would be more reflective of a team approach or a staffing approach to the diagnosis of patients. A staffing approach to diagnosis is frequently instituted in agencies where the primary patient is the young child who may be severely involved emotionally, mentally, psychologically, or physically.

The flowchart (Figure 3-2), the outlines, and the appendix of forms (Appendix I) can be adapted for use in any diagnostic setting.

SUMMARY

This chapter has served as an overview of the diagnostic process. We developed the view that the method of science can be applied directly to the diagnostic process, demonstrating how the diagnostician can apply the method to the specific instance of the individual patient; the patient becomes his N of 1. The method of science gives the diagnostician a systematic, orderly approach to diagnosis. His problem-solving and decision-making abilities are enhanced through use of the seven steps illustrated.

Two other topics were addressed. First, we considered how the diagnostic process is often modified based on work setting and purpose of the referral. These modifications were considered as shifts of diagnostic focus rather than different types of diagnoses. Second, we presented information about administration and the diagnostician. Some emphasis was placed on utilization of procedures that facilitated the diagnostic process while at the same time providing the agency with needed information for agency record keeping.

STUDY QUESTIONS

1. Compare the steps of the method of science as applied to the diagnostic process to several texts that discuss the method of science in research. Are the same types of questions asked by researchers as those asked by diagnosticians as presented in this chapter?
2. Emerick and Hatten (1979) present a diagnostic paradigm (Figure 1-2, page 21). Compare our Figure 3-1 of the diagnostic process to their paradigm. What are the similarities and differences in the way the diagnostic process is illustrated? Also, compare our Figure 3-1 to McLean and Snyder-McLean's (1978) transactional model for assessment of children with severe language deficits.
3. How do the evaluation process concepts Schultz (1973) has derived from information theory parallel those we have derived from the scientific framework? Are the two compatible?
4. Kent and Chabon (1980) discuss the use of the problem-oriented record in a university speech and hearing clinic. How might this system be adapted to the diagnostic process?
5. Read Moll's (1975) presidential address to the American Speech and Hearing Association. Do you agree or disagree with the common goal he sets forth for the professions of speech pathology and audiology?

6. Weed (1970) has pointed out how careful and systematic record keeping that has its first concern in patient care is important in the medical profession. How might the procedures he has developed be adapted for speech and hearing services?
7. Palmer (1970) discusses important information about referrals as they affect the specific purposes of psychological testing. Are his ideas compatible with those expressed here?
8. Mysak (1976) presents nine diagnostic approaches or combinations of approaches. How might each of these approaches be interpreted in terms of our concept of shifts of diagnostic focus?
9. As we stated in the administration section, patients should not be lost because of lack of concern over administrative structure. What was done at the speech and hearing clinic of the Mount Sinai Medical Center to decrease their no-show rate (Bar, 1975)?
10. Can a secretary be trained to handle the complexities of taking referral information? How much can administrative personnel other than the diagnostician say to a mother who has immediate questions about her child's problem?

Chapter 4

Constituent analysis: definition and delimitation of the clinical problem

The constituent analysis is the diagnostician's first step in the quest for solutions to clinical problems. This analysis becomes the blueprint for planning the remainder of the diagnostic process. From it, all the other steps emanate: derivation of the clinical hypothesis, the selection of tools and procedures, the collection, the analysis, the interpretation of the data, and the conclusions. Inquiry starts with the definition and delimitation of a problem, not a method for solving a problem. As Brown and Ghiselli (1955) put it:

> So much is known about methodology that the solution of many new problems seldom demands a radical change in method. Even research findings of 'world shaking' proportions have arisen from only slight alterations in already well-established and familiar methods. (p. 133)

If the diagnostician makes errors in the constituent analysis, he will likely make errors in the remaining steps of diagnosis, unless corrective procedures can be applied during the ongoing process. The constituent analysis is as objective and systematic as possible, thereby minimizing diagnostician error.

THE DIAGNOSTICIAN'S TASKS

We are using the term "constituent analysis" to refer to those tasks the diagnostician performs from the information obtained *prior to the patient's appointment.* In this sense the constituent analysis is analogous with what others call the case study (Dickson & Jann, 1974). No single source provides the diagnostician with all the types of patient information he may need. The information gathered from the different sources must be inventoried; each bit of information must be categorized and evaluated against all other bits of information. Gaining information from multiple sources increases the reliability and validity of the information. What information usually is available, at the very least, is a referral statement. At other times extensive information is available, including history forms filled out by the patient or his family and other medical, psychological, and educational information. This information is used to discover past and present events, facts, attitudes, situations, and conditions that relate to the speech and language disorder. The information is used to determine the way other people or the patient himself views the problem.

Whatever the amount of information, the diagnostician considers the constituents in reference to his funds of knowledge about normal and disordered speech and language. For example, if Mrs. Cronise requests a speech and language diagnosis for her 3-year-old daughter Celeste who "does not talk yet," the diagnostician evaluates this statement in reference to normal language development: What language patterns do most 3-year-old children use? Thus, at the heart of the constituent analysis is the juxtaposition of specific patient information against the diagnostician's constantly growing and changing funds of knowledge about speech and language.

The diagnostician performs two constituent analysis tasks. He (1) categorizes the available constituents, and (2) determines the significance of the constituents. It should be made clear that these two tasks are not distinct and separable. More realistically they occur simultaneously. However, to facilitate learning to do the analysis and demonstrate its relevance to the overall planning of the diagnosis, we are treating these tasks as if they were distinct.

CATEGORIZES THE AVAILABLE CONSTITUENTS

A constituent is any piece or pieces of information drawn from the patient information base. These constituents come in many forms: reliable, personal, theoretical, situational, inferential, factual, abstract, meaningful, nonmeaningful, explanatory, valid, and unreliable.

The diagnostician must ascertain what each constituent reveals to him and how valid and reliable it is. For example, a constituent may be factual and reliable (Pamela is 3 years old), theoretical and explanatory (Fred does not talk because he does not want to), abstract (Judy has a speech disorder), personal and situational (Todd talks like his father), and non-meaningful and unreliable (Jill's speech problem started at birth). Of course, no constituent is only in one form; the same constituent could be abstract, reliable, personal, and situational. All constituents require examination and validation; the diagnostician must evaluate all the constituents that come to him.

As well, the diagnostician should remember that any single constituent might be evaluated in more than one way; a causal constituent can also be used as an effect constituent. For example, 4-year-old Noel who is only speaking in one-word utterances is obviously having trouble with language (an effect constituent). This extremely slow language development might also be signaling a causal constituent—mental retardation, hearing loss, and so forth.

The diagnostician's first task in the constituent analysis, categorizing the constituents, can be thought of as taking an inventory of the available patient data. As in all inventories, the diagnostician must develop a format for taking his inventory. This inventory should reflect the purposes of diagnosis—to differentiate the patient's clinical problem from all other speech and language disorders. Therefore his inventory should be listed within categories relevant to this job.

To facilitate categorizing the constituents we have designed a constituent analysis form (Form 4-1). This form has been devised to categorize information around (1) the job of the diagnostician and (2) the SLPM which emphasizes cause–effect relationships. It includes categories that assist the diagnostician in keeping in mind a number of important considerations for defining and delimiting the patient's clinical problem. They are

1. Identification data,
2. General purposes of diagnosis,
3. Specific purpose of each diagnosis,
4. Characteristics of the speech and language disorder,
5. Causal factors to be considered,
6. Management considerations,

Form 4-1. Constituent analysis format*

Patient Identification

Purpose of Diagnosis

General: Diagnostician's job

Referral: Note purposes asked by referral source

Statement of Problem

Note how the problem has been stated by different people concerned with the patient

Further Information Needed

Interview: Consider questions you may want to ask to gather more information

---

SLPM: Cause–Effect Categorization

Environment Component	*Processing Component*	*Product Component*
Categorize speech and language input, total environmental context, and causal factor information.	Categorize anatomy, physical processes, behavioral correlates, and causal factors for all segments.	Categorize characteristics of speech and language products affected at all levels
Make use of causal factor scanning mechanism	Make use of causal factor scanning mechanism	

Management Considerations

Note information that leads you to think about possible management needs

Behavioral Considerations

Note information that may help you manage the patient's behavior during the diagnostic session

Other Information

Note information that may be useful but is not categorized elsewhere

---

*This format basically presents categories under which constituents can be inventoried.

7. Sources and types of further information that may be needed,
8. Information that may assist in controlling behavioral problems that might occur during the diagnostic session,
9. Incidental information that might prove relevant but cannot be categorized elsewhere on the form.

Using Form 4-1 in parallel with the SLPM allows the diagnostician to view each patient as if he were a *mini SLPM*. The categories on the form are derived directly from the components of the model, thereby facilitating integration of the information for derivation of cause–effect relationships. With this in mind we will discuss in greater detail the use of the SLPM as a schema for categorizing cause–effect constituents.

SLPM schema for categorizing cause–effect constituents

We know that many causal factors both internal and external to the individual can affect his ability to learn and use speech and language appropriately. However, classification and categorization of speech and language disorders and their causal bases historically has been quite fragmented. Different and inconsistent bases of classification have developed over the years (Nation & Aram, 1977).

As has been pointed out, the constituent analysis step of the diagnostic process has a forward reference to the remaining steps of the process. A major task in the constituent analysis is the categorization of cause–effect factors, needed for the derivation of the cause–effect relationships expressed in the clinical hypothesis. The diagnostician must have a schema by which he can categorize these cause–effect factors that allows as well for the development of consistent, useful nomenclature and classification systems.

This section is devoted to the presentation of a schema for categorizing cause–effect constituents based on the Speech and Language Processing Model presented in Chapter 2. It develops and expands the use of the SLPM as a consistent organizing schema for naming, categorizing, and classifying speech and language disorders, and for searching out and classifying causal factors. We consider the diagnostic classification system presented in this section to be of major importance to the diagnostician for developing an understanding of the complex cause–effect relationships that exist—information that is vital to both diagnosis and management of speech and language disorders. This system should be applicable to various speech and language disorders and has been adapted by Shriberg and Kwiatkowski (1982) in their development of a classification system for phonological disorders.

Categorization of effect constituents

From the SLPM, internally consistent categorization systems can be devised. The model provides for three levels of classification. They are the product level, the behavioral correlate level, and the processing level. We will briefly develop the use of each level of classification for categorizing effect constituents, those that reveal information about the characteristics, the symptoms of the patient's speech and language disorder.

Product level

In a behavioral science the first and foremost basis for a classification system should stem from the most observable set of behaviors. Since speech and language behavior is the diagnostician's major interest, the product level of categorization reflects this primacy. The product level specifies the observable parameters of disordered speech and language that are heard when a patient speaks. As described in Chapter 2, the product level has two divisions: the speech product and the language product. Within each of these divisions the SLPM provides the diagnostician with sets of speech and language parameters that can be used to categorize product (effect) constituents. Here we would categorize such specific constituents as "he talks funny," "he can't say his (r) sounds," "he only uses one word," and so on.

Categorize the following patient's behavior on the product level. When Mrs. Weiss was asked to define words, she defined *have* as "to have and to hold." When asked to try again she said, "What all of us have we should appreciate (long pause) the best." For the word *bridge* she responded, "Access over the river—little more than access because you (not completed)." When asked to describe a picture of a boy flying a kite she said, "He's holding the——that's attached to the flying object—the kite; yes, he's holding the ribbon."

Behavioral correlate level

The SLPM provides a second effect level, the behavioral correlate level, for categorizing speech and language constituents. Based on sets of observable behavior that are operationally defined by tasks, this level tells the diagnostician about a patient's auditory reception, central language and thought, and speech production abilities. Chapter 2 provides a discussion of behavioral correlates as externalized behaviors, hypothesized as reflective of physical processes.

With the addition of the behavioral correlate level, greater insights can be gained into speech and language disorders. For example, through the behavioral correlate level the diagnostician can categorize the language behaviors reported within comprehension, integration, and formulation categories, or he can specify speech behaviors as sequencing or motor control difficulties. Depending upon how behaviors were reported he could categorize the comprehension disorder as related primarily to the pragmatic, semantic, or phonologic aspects of message comprehension.

As has been stated, the behavioral correlates are hypothesized as externalized behaviors to physical processes. This gives the diagnostician another dimension to categorization of behavior. The disruptions of the behavioral correlates provide him with information about potentially disrupted physical processes as a basis for the disorders he observes. Thus, the diagnostician can categorize behavioral correlates as contemporary causal factors for the speech and language disorder. For example, disruptions of sensation or perception can be cited as the basis for the current comprehension disorder.

Therefore, having the behavioral correlate level along with the product level gives diagnosticians a better grasp of cause–effect relationships. In essence, the behavioral correlate level can help diagnosticians explain the products they categorize or it can help them infer disrupted physical processes.

Categorize the following patient's performance on the behavioral correlate level. When asked to point to pictures of a dog, a cat, and a chair, 7-year-old Diane pointed incorrectly to all of them. When asked her name, she responded, "No-no." When asked if she wanted a cookie, she shook her head in a positive manner but did not reach out for the cookie held before her. When the examiner was behind her and called out her name in a whisper, she turned to face the examiner. Two bells were placed before her of the same size. One bell rang; the second did not. The examiner "rang" the two bells and replaced them before Diane. She responded by picking up the bell that rang, holding it to her ear, and shaking it.

Physical processing level

In addition to the speech and language product and the behavioral correlates, an effect categorization system based on physical processing can be devised. When using this system, we must keep in mind its highly theoretical, inferential, basically nonobservable basis as discussed in Chapter 2. This level does not tell diagnosticians what the disordered speech and language behavior is. It does not describe speech and language disorders. Rather, its primary usefulness resides in ordering underlying disrupted processes and therefore contributing to discovering cause-effect relationships.

If the diagnostician can infer disrupted processes from the disordered product, or if he can predict disordered products from knowledge about disrupted processes, he can develop more sophisticated hypotheses about cause-effect relationships. It is the diagnostician's knowledge of the relationships among the physical processes, the behavioral correlates, and the speech and language products that allows for this sophistication.

Categorize the following information on the physical processing level. Four-year-old Paxton was seen by the diagnostician to determine why he was using only one-word responses. At 4 months of age he sustained a severe blow to the left side of the head resulting in a skull fracture; he was hospitalized for 1 month under careful observation following procedures for removal of a hematoma that had spread over a large portion of the temporal lobe. His subsequent physical development was almost within normal limits; however, speech and language were as stated: when he responded, it was with single words, not always intelligible. He did not always follow directions appropriately, but he did point to some pictures that were named at the 3-year level.

These three effect categorization levels have distinct advantages for the constituent analysis. First, because they stem directly from the SLPM, they have a built-in consistency that is logical, understandable, and practical. Each of the levels is internally consistent; the terminology at each level was specified and defined in the construction of the SLPM. Thus, the use of this nomenclature and these categorization systems reveals how the diagnostician arrives at the diagnostic labels he uses. Also, the levels allow the diagnostician to represent the difference between what was observed and what was inferred from the reported constituents.

Second, the diagnostician does not need a special set of nomenclature to specify the disorders he encounters. The SLPM nomenclature can be used simply by applying the noun "disorder" or the adjective "disordered." For example, the product, voice, can be discussed as a voice disorder or disordered voice; the behavioral correlate, formulation, can be discussed as a formulation disorder or disordered formulation; and the physical process, speech programming, can be discussed as a speech programming disorder or disordered speech programming.

Third, these levels allow diagnosticians to incorporate other nomenclature without undue difficulty. It requires knowing how a specific term used to specify a disorder came about, but in most instances its relationship to the SLPM categories is apparent. True, certain labels for disorders will probably remain for many years to come; for example, stuttering has a strong historical reference and implies to many people a specific type of speech behavior. This term can retain its clinical usefulness, but at the same time it can be incorporated into the SLPM as a disorder of prosody. It may be doubtful whether the term "prosody" will ever be favored over the tradition-bound term "stuttering;" but we also must remember that in the past stuttering was called "psellismus" (Rieber & Brubaker, 1966).

Fourth, each of these levels provides the diagnostician with different information about the speech and language disorder he is investigating. How he uses each level for categorization of effect constituents depends on his diagnostic emphasis and the data made available to him. Thus, these levels help the diagnostician to determine the relationship among behaviors, processes, and causal factors.

Categorization of causal constituents

As well as a fragmented view of classification, our historical heritage has left us with a limited view of causation. The focus has often been on a static view of etiology rather than a dynamic view of complex cause–effect interactions. Diagnosticians must have knowledge of the potential causes of speech and language disorders as a first step in hypothesizing cause–effect relationships and as a final step in the diagnostic process, whereby the disorder is specified as a cause–effect relationship.

A consistent schema must be developed for diagnostic use, emphasizing how the causal factors were responsible for the speech and language disorder, not a search for a causal factor in and of itself. In this view the diagnostician searches his patient's history for causal constituents that may have influenced the learning and use of speech and language over time. The schema presented here assists the diagnostician in categorizing causal constituents by juxtaposing the factors in relationship to the components of the SLPM.

Basis for classification

It becomes quickly obvious that the number of interacting factors that could affect speech and language learning and use is innumerable. In fact, it may be accurate to say that any indentifiable factor, extrinsic or intrinsic to the human, has the potential of becoming causally related to the speech and language disorder. As well, a factor that may be causally related to a disorder in one individual may have no relationship to a similar disorder seen in another. Many patients are seen with "a causal factor" in their history, but that factor has no bearing on their speech and language disorder. No assumptions can be made that a given set of causal factors can account for or encompass the range of speech and language disorders seen. It is likely that the study of causal factors may defy any single organizational attempt at cataloging, nor will any organizational attempt satisfy all segments of the profession (Sameroff, 1975).

However, some guidelines for organizing a schema for causal factors are essential. The schema should

1. Stress discovering cause–effect relationships, not just causal factors,
2. Delimit the number of causal categories needed for a causal search mechanism,
3. Demonstrate how a specific causal factor exerts its primary effect,

4. Facilitate the diagnostician's purposes,
5. Accommodate the current and future literature about causal factors,
6. Be open-ended to allow for development of future perspectives regarding causation.

Essentially, then, diagnosticians need a means of reviewing the vast range of potential causal factors and demonstrating how any specific factor exerts its influence on speech and language. The emphasis must be on a consistent schema that facilitates the diagnostician's search for causation, allowing for appropriate interpretation of cause–effect relationships (Blalock, 1971). The diagnostician needs to know how the causal factors have interacted with the human being and/or his environment to create the behavioral disorder seen. The diagnostician must stress the effect of the causal factor, not the causal factor in and of itself.

To this end, we will first present a *scanning mechanism* based on the SLPM for searching out and categorizing causal factors.

Scanning mechanism for causal factors

The scanning mechanism emphasizes causal factors that primarily affect the speech and language environment component and causal factors that primarily affect the speech and language processing component. Table 4-1 presents the scanning categories developed within each of these components; it is a mechanism for searching out and categorizing causal factors.

In deriving the scanning mechanisms we attempted to "factor analyze" causal factors cited in the literature, looking for the commonalities among factors that could be grouped and meaningfully related to the speech and language environment and processing components. From this "factor analysis" we developed major scanning categories for causal factors; although not mutually exclusive, redundancy among the categories was kept to a minimum. These are superordinate categories that can be subdivided into increasingly more specific factors. Using this scanning mechanism the diagnostician can search for factors that have already affected his patient's speech and language environment, physical processing system, and the interactions among the causal factors.

The following discussion is designed to demonstrate the use of the scanning mechanism, not as an exhaustive discussion of causal factors. Our intent is to provide an organizational schema for later use in analysis and interpretation of cause–effect relationships.

• **Factors primarily affecting the speech and language environment.** To begin this discussion a word of caution is important. Little is known about how speech and language environment factors act as "causes" of speech and language disorders. What is known comes mostly from analyses of environmental variables that have been correlated with the speech and language product of children at various ages and stages of development. Therefore we suggest when the diagnostician considers causal factors primarily affecting the speech and language environment component that he emphasizes their correlational aspect rather than their causal aspect. (Kenny, 1979).

Speech and language environment factors are considered as extrinsic to the individual and are viewed in the SLPM primarily in terms of their effect on the quality and quantity of speech and language input (Figure 2-2). To some degree an individual may create part of his own speech and language input through external feedback; for example, when an infant's babbling acts as a stimulus to continued babbling or when a child engages in a

Table 4-1. Scanning mechanism for categorizing causal factors based on SLPM

Environment	Processing
1. Factors primarily affecting the speech and language environment component	II. Factors primarily affecting the internal speech and language processing component

A. Interpersonal context factors
  1. Parents and parenting
  2. Sibling relations
  3. Other significant relationships
B. Sociocultural context factors
  1. Income, economic status
  2. Education-occupation of parents and client
  3. Racial, ethnic practices
C. Multisensory context factors
  1. Physical-technologic factors
    a. Physical environment
    b. Technologic possessions and use
  2. Experiential factors
    a. Significant abrupt changes
    b. Sensorimotor stimulation and exploration
	A. Given biological makeup
	B. Structural defects and growths
	C. Nutrition
	D. Diseases, infections, and allergies
	E. Physical traumas and accidents
	F. Drugs and irradiation
	G. Psychological-emotional mechanisms

dialogue with himself, being both listener and speaker. For the most part, however, the speech and language environment is largely established by others, imposed on an individual by someone or something in his environment.

Table 4-1 presents the major categories in the scanning mechanism for environmental causal factors. These categories are necessarily interdependent; for example, sociocultural influences are primarily executed through interpersonal relationships. Similarly, experiential factors are largely provided by the interpersonal and physical–technologic influences. As well, physical–technologic factors are often concomitants of sociocultural factors. The reader should review the material presented in Chapter 2 that discussed the speech and language environment component of the SLPM.

Interpersonal factors. Interpersonal factors are probably the most important influences on speech and language input. Here the concern is directed toward the *parents and parenting*—their psychological and physical characteristics, attitudes, behaviors, and child-rearing practices. Consideration of *sibling relations* is also included in interpersonal factors, including such influences as numerical birth order, multiple births, and sex of siblings. Finally, the diagnostician considers *other significant interpersonal relationships* that the individual has, such as with a spouse, a caretaker other than the parent, teachers, and extended family members. Gallagher (1983) has addressed some of these factors in her discussion of language in relation to the communicative partner.

Sociocultural factors. The sociocultural factors may function through individual interpersonal relationships, notably the family, or as the result of more general ethnic and cultural influences. Such immediate factors as the *income* and *economic status* and the *educational–occupational status* of an individual and his family may contribute to the amount and kind of speech and language used in the environment. Similarly, *racial and ethnic practices* in terms of verbal behavior, and value attached to speech and language differ.

Physical–technologic factors. Probably the most "concrete" set of factors affecting the multisensory context of the speech and language environment are those relating to the physical–technologic environment. How an individual is influenced by the *physical environment* may aid and abet appropriate speech and language development. The physical characteristics of the immediate environment may include such factors as available space, cleanliness, and diversity. *Technologic possessions* and *use* relate to industrial and mechanical means of expanding and altering the immediate environment such as televisions, radios, and cars. While these technologic possessions may change the immediate environment, the changes are not necessarily in the direction of providing appropriate speech and language experiences.

Experiential factors. The final category, experiential factors, includes *significant abrupt changes* (hospitalization, death, divorce, etc.) and *sensorimotor stimulation* and *exploration*. While these experiences occur as well within the interpersonal context, the importance of these experiences for speech and language development and use is highlighted in our scanning mechanism by considering them within the multisensory context.

- *Factors primarily affecting speech and language processing.* Many causal factors can disrupt the biological basis for speech and language (Darby, 1981). These factors, directly or indirectly, affect the physical processing system for language. For example, damage to the left cerebral cortex can have a direct effect on the patient's ability to comprehend, integrate, and formulate language. However, the effects of something like kidney disease may be more indirect. The illness may be so physiologically debilitating that many biological systems of the body are affected, including the speech and language processing system.

When the diagnostician categorizes causal factors affecting physical processing, he will have to know if and how the factor affected one or more of the three segments of the processing component. Was it a direct effect, or did the causal factor affect another bodily system, which then exerted an effect on speech and language processing? Therefore, the diagnostician must have specific knowledge about the physical basis for speech and language, as well as more general knowledge about human biological systems. The reader should review Chapter 2 which discusses the speech and language processing component of the SLPM and Darby's book (1981), *Speech Evaluation in Medicine.*

Table 4-1 presents the scanning mechanism for categorizing causal factors affecting the physical basis for speech and language. As with environmental factors, the categories are interdependent. For example, a child born with a cleft lip and palate has a structural defect as a part of his given biological makeup. Although a specific causal factor may be placed into more than one category in the scanning mechanism, we believe that by the use of these categories the diagnostician will not overlook significant causal factors affecting physical processing.

Given biological makeup. An individual is born with, and continues to have, a basic biological makeup. This biological makeup consists of a number of bodily systems that constitute the individual's anatomy and physiology. There are many ways these bodily systems can be organized; for example, they can be divided into motor, skeletal, neurologic, or vascular systems, depending on the professional specialty viewing the individual. The speech and language processing component of the SLPM is our organizational view of the bodily system of most importance to us. Of course, this system incorporates many of the same structures that make up other bodily systems, for example, the neurologic system. Therefore, when viewing given biological makeup as a potential causal factor for speech and language disorders, the diagnostician may have to consider the effects of disruptions in any bodily system on the speech and language processing system.

Within this category the diagnostician is concerned with all the normal and abnormal structural and functional (physiologic) conditions of the patient that may affect the ability to process speech and language. An individual's given biological makeup is viewed as that anatomy and physiology present at the time of birth. The basis of this category is the belief that all individuals have an inherited (innate) set of anatomic and physiologic characteristics—some good, some unfortunate—that are his given biological makeup. This category includes those conditions that occurred during gestation and conditions that occurred because of the birth process. Thus, this category has potential overlap with all other categories of our scanning mechanism, particularly the categories of structural defects and growths, and physical traumas and accidents. This overlap of categories, for example, categorizing cleft lip and palate as both a given biological makeup factor and as a structural defect factor, maintains focus both on the condition and the time of occurrence.

The given biological makeup factor helps the diagnostician maintain an important perspective on biological conditions he sees; a perspective that says all these conditions are not necessarily "abnormal." For example, mental retardation is generally interpreted as "abnormal." Remember, however, that mental retardation is a definition based primarily on an IQ score. Given that mental abilities are presumably variations from a mean and range of mental abilities, we should expect in our general population a certain number of individuals who biologically fall below the range of the defined "normal IQ." These individuals then would have a given biological makeup that becomes defined as mental retardation—usually for educational purposes because these children cannot respond to the same methods of teaching as "normal" or "bright" children. However, are they "abnormal"? It may be more appropriate to consider them as having the potential to learn within their given biological makeup. If they are acquiring speech and language within their ability levels, then certain children defined as mentally retarded do not constitute children with speech and language disorders; mental retardation in these instances would not be an abnormal biological causal factor.

There are other instances where variations in structure and function are viewed in the same way, for example, dentition, physical development, tongue size and shape, palatal dimensions, and diadochokinesis of the oral structures; all of these and many others can be examined in light of the causal factor, given biological makeup. This view helps diagnosticians determine if the condition has a relationship to the speech and language disorder, if the patient has adapted to or can compensate for the variation, or whether other types of management may be required.

Structural defects and growths. The individual may incur a structural defect or growth. He may be born with a congenital malformation such as a cleft palate or congenital atresia or he may acquire structural alterations later in life, as occurs with a laryngectomy, vocal nodules, or removal of brain tissue. Depending on which segment of the processing system is affected, the diagnostician will expect different processing disruptions with resultant disorders of the behavioral correlates and the speech and language products.

Nutrition. During the course of development the biological individual will be influenced by the quantity and quality of the food intake both pre- and postnatally.

Diseases, infections, and allergies. The biological individual may be invaded by virus, bacteria, and allergies that interfere with development and ongoing functioning. These diseases could be contracted via the mother during pregnancy or during the course of the individual's life.

Physical traumas and accidents. The individual may experience physical traumas or accidents that disrupt functioning. These traumas or accidents may be created by external agents as in birth injuries and skull fractures or occur as abrupt internal disruptions as in a cerebrovascular accident.

Drugs and irradiation. The individual may ingest drugs or be exposed to excessive radiation, which may have an adverse effect on biological structure and functioning.

Psychological–emotional mechanisms. Finally, the individual's intrinsic psychological and emotional mechanisms also influence his processing of speech and language. Included within the psychological–emotional mechanism category of causal factors are intrinsic processes that are often thought of as more behavioral than biological. Psychological mechanisms such as attention, motivation, and memory affect the individual's ability to process speech and language. Similarly, emotional factors such as emotional lability and self-concept influence how an individual will receive and create language. We are placing psychological–emotional mechanisms into factors primarily affecting physical processing since we view these mechanisms as a part of the individual's makeup, even though these mechanisms may be disrupted by factors extrinsic to him, that is, environmental causal factors.

PATIENT INFORMATION BASE: NATURE AND SOURCES

In order to categorize the constituents we need to study the nature and sources of information that make up the patient information base and that provide the constituents for analysis. For each patient this represents new information to the diagnostician and the amount of information gathered can vary greatly. In teaching the diagnostic process we proceed throughout this book from the position that the diagnostician has several sources of information available to him, usually (1) a referral statement, (2) a completed case history questionnaire, and at times (3) letters and reports from other concerned professionals. We feel that a student who masters the diagnostic process using comprehensive material will be far better prepared to perform diagnoses in settings where only minimal information is obtained.

Referrals

Referrals come in many forms. In some settings a person may simply call and request an appointment for a diagnosis and may be asked to give little information other than the prospective patient's name, age, address, and telephone number. Other settings may require that the referral for services come only from a physician or other recognized professional. Such "official" referrals range from a brief note on a prescription pad, "I recommend evaluation of Aiko for a speech problem," to detailed descriptions of the presenting problem. In some settings the referral may be quite informal, as when the classroom teacher stops the speech–language pathologist in the hall and asks him to "look at Philip; his voice has been hoarse for a month." Other settings may require elaborate intake procedures before services can be obtained (see discussion of intake procedures Chapter 3).

Whatever the policy for receiving referrals, there is certain basic information the diagnostician should have for categorization on Form 4-1. This information would include

(1) the source of the referral, (2) patient identification, (3) statement of the problem, (4) characteristics of the problem as seen by the referral source, and (5) diagnostic expectations of the referral source.

The diagnostician must have a clear understanding of the origin of the referral; he must verify whether he is receiving a direct or an indirect referral. There is a difference between asking for diagnostic services at someone's suggestion versus being referred directly. For example, a mother who calls for services on the suggestion of the pediatrician may be the direct referral source. The pediatrician's suggestion may have been only to alleviate the mother's undue concern about the child. If, however, the diagnostician receives a letter, report, or call from the pediatrician concerning services for the child, the pediatrician becomes the direct referral source and most probably will become directly involved with the overall management of the child. How the referrals come requires the diagnostician to follow up in different ways.

The referral source should provide basic information about the patient. Identification data is crucial. Without the name, age, address, and telephone number, a referral is difficult to follow up. It is amazing how many referrals do come without this basic identifying information.

The referral source should provide the reason for making the referral. Sometimes the referral source will provide detailed causal information and minimal descriptions of the speech and language behavior. For example, a physician referring a child with a medical diagnosis of cerebral palsy may give detailed information about physical growth and development, the type of cerebral palsy, the etiology of the condition, and then say only that the child does not talk. Form this the diagnostician may not know the specific intent of the physician's referral. Yet the physician may be interested specifically in the capabilities of the child to develop speech or if muscle function is sufficient to produce speech. Not knowing the phyician's specific intent, the diagnostician, in turn, may not provide the physician with the information wanted.

How would you state your diagnostic purpose on the basis of the following two different referrals? Is it clear what the referral source is asking for in each case?

1. Dr. David Link referred Mr. Howard Hardie, a 58-year-old white male, who has been medically diagnosed as having multiple sclerosis. Dr. Link has asked if Mr. Hardie can be taught to compensate for his deteriorating speech-producing abilities.

2. Dr. Joe Deli referred Mrs. Ann Rome, a 32-year-old white female, for a voice evaluation. In his letter of referral Dr. Deli stated that Mrs. Rome has been hoarse for about 2 months.

At times the referral source does not have a specific intent for his referral but, instead, is asking for a diagnosis and recommendations at the discretion of the speech and language diagnostician. Implicit in such a referral is the referral source's interest in knowing if a problem exists and what to do about it. In these instances the diagnostician proceeds to provide services in line with the overall purposes of diagnosis.

The diagnostician must also be aware that at times referrals will come that are not entirely appropriate. He then must decide how to handle the referral. Sometimes the inappropriate referral is not discovered until the case history questionnaire is returned by the family; at other times it is recognized when the referral letter arrives. For example, in speech and language settings it is not uncommon to receive a referral to help someone with their public speaking skills. At other times the referral may be from someone who thinks the speech–language pathologist can diagnose mental retardation or emotional disturbance. When it is discovered that the primary problem is not a speech and language disorder but an educational, emotional, psychological, medical, or other problem, the diagnostician must know what to do with these referrals. Often there is a speech and language disorder associated with the individual's more prevasive problem that has led to referral to the speech–language pathologist. In some of these instances the diagnostician may follow through with the diagnostic process in order to effect a more appropriate referral, to assist the patient in obtaining more appropriate services. At other times he will have to discuss his concerns with the referral source and assist in redirecting the referral. The referral source should, if possible, provide his impressions of the patient's speech and language disorder and causal factors related to it as well as any other information about factors that, to him, are important to the patient's problem.

Consider this referral from a physician: Alex Robin has had a speech disturbance since birth. He has had no serious disease in the past. He does have congenital esotropia and secondary diplopia in the right eye. What are your reactions to this referral? What do you think the significance of the information about the right eye might have? How would you interpret a speech disturbance that has been present since birth?

The following referral was received from a clinical psychologist. Categorize the constituents in terms of the type of information provided. How are subject matter and time presented? What would you do from this point? What is not included in the referral letter that you might like to know before proceeding?

On February 19, 1980, Lee Newton was seen at the psychological clinic in regard to his slow development. Lee obtained an intelligence score of 67 and a mental age of 3 years, 3 months on the *Stanford–Binet Intelligence Scale*. Lee has a vocabulary age of approximately 2½ years. His best subtests were memory (for hidden objects) and identification of objects. No other tests were passed at the 4-year level.

On March 19, 1980, Dr. Anthony administered an EEG to Lee who was 4 years, 10 months of age. I have seen the record, and it shows a low degree of abnormality with irregular diffuse delta activity. Another EEG has been administered recently, but I have not yet seen the results.

I would appreciate a report of your evaluation of Lee. If I can be of further help to you, please do not hesitate to contact me.

History questionnaire

A history questionnaire in this context refers to a questionnaire completed by the patient, his family, or agency personnel prior to the initial meeting with the diagnostician. The use of case history forms is particularly common in settings that do not have immediate access to patient information. Thus, we find history questionnaires particularly common in university speech and hearing centers, community agencies, and private practice. Hospitals, other inpatient settings, and multidisciplinary agencies often make less use of questionnaires in advance, as much of the requested information becomes available in the medical or intra-agency records.

The use of questionnaires to gather historical information for case studies has been standard practice in our profession (Johnson et al., 1963; Milisen, 1957; Emerick & Hatten, 1979), although professionals may differ in the value they place on such tools. Some prefer to gain historical information only in a face-to-face interaction with the patient, feeling that they can then better judge the importance and accuracy of the information they obtain. Other limitations have been pointed out in gaining information via questionnaires: not allowing the patient to state what may be most important to him, wording questions in such a way that the informant does not understand or know how to respond, and the difficulty of adapting a form suitable to patients of all ages with varying problems. A further problem with the history questionnaire is the patient's lack of understanding of why certain information is requested. Often a parent has no idea why a form asks for birth information and may simply choose not to answer such questions. Finally, one of the chief criticisms of questionnaires is the questionable accuracy of the information obtained.

We believe that many of the criticisms can be overcome by carefully designed questionnaires. Questions can be framed and vocabulary selected in a straightforward manner that can be understood by most people without offending their sense of privacy. To circumvent the need for lengthy responses and to increase the reliability of responses, questions can be framed that require checking an appropriate blank, yes or no responses, or minimal written responses. Leaving space at the end of the questionnaire for open-ended responding allows the respondents to discuss any aspects of their problem not covered by the questionnaire. Cover letters can also accompany the questionnaire to explain its purposes and to alleviate a patient's concern about not understanding all aspects of the questionnaire. If the questionnaire is presented as being helpful to the diagnostician in doing a more thorough job, it will be acceptable to most people asked to respond.

A major difficulty encountered in questionnaire construction is in making them appropriate for agencies serving large numbers of patients of all ages and with all types of speech and language disorders. It would be quite impossible to develop anything suitable for all the patients except the most general of questions. For example, how could a form be constructed that would be appropriate for a 3-year-old child with a suspected language disorder and a 23-year-old person suspected of a prosody disorder? Thus, in some settings more than one case history form must be constructed to use with the different patients to be seen.

Some setttings choose to send out questionnaires that have been devised for specific "problem types." For example, if it is known that the child referred has a repaired cleft palate, a history form designed for that potential causal factor may be used rather than a general history form. There are instances where this is appropriate, but it requires immediate verification of the special "problem type" before the questionnaire can be sent. Johnson et al. (1963) and Darley and Spriestersbach (1978) suggest supplementary case history information for a number of problem types including cerebral palsy, cleft palate, dysphasia, and postlaryngectomy.

Notice how these supplementary histories tend to be organized around etiologic (causal) factors. They assume a certain cause–effect relationship exists. If such etiologic information is known at the time of referral and is considered valid and reliable, there may be justification for sending specific history questionnaires related to these causal factors. In most instances, however, a general history form, perhaps one constructed for children and one for adults, would serve the setting most efficiently. Even this division may cause some difficulty; most children's case history forms do not seem appropriate for the adolescent, nor does the adolescent fit into many of the adult histories. The adolescent and the geriatric client are often "in limbo" when it comes to the construction of case history questionnaires.

Our view about the use of questionnaires is that they provide a primary source of information for the constituent analysis. They should be designed to motivate the informant and to provide sufficient information about the patient: Who he is and where he fits in the world? What is his world like? What has he got going for him? Against him? What has already been determined about the problem and its causes? What has the family been told? How do they and others perceive the problem? What importance do they give it? What do they want from the diagnostician?

In the context of the total diagnostic process, questionnaires have several distinct advantages. In general, they increase the overall efficiency of diagnosis. They provide many constituents for categorization in advance. They allow the diagnostician to identify areas of missing information and particular problem areas around which he can focus his subsequent interview. The questionnaire serves as a springboard for the interview, helping to establish rapport since the patient feels the diagnostician already knows something about the problem. We also find that completing a questionnaire at home often gives informants time to think about the questions asked and allows them to consult sources such as the baby book or pediatrician's record for specific information.

All in all, we maintain that the advantages of questionnaires outweigh the disadvantages. If it is used in conjunction with the interview, the reliability and validity of the information can be cross-checked. For example, Gallagher (1983) has developed a tool she calls the "Pre-assessment Questionnaire" designed specifically to obtain information about the child's communicative behavior.

A children's case history questionnaire

We now discuss in some detail an example of a children's case history questionnaire to demonstrate how and what information can be obtained from this source. This history form has been completed on a patient named *Katherine Compardo,* who serves throughout this book as an example patient for demonstrating the various diagnostic tasks at each of the steps of the diagnostic process.

This history form is a general questionnaire useful through the early teenage years, but perhaps most useful for preschool children and children up to 10 years of age. Its construction allows for gathering detailed information about the many types of children's speech and language disorders stemming from many different causal factors. Each item on the form has been found useful for doing the constituent analysis.

The children's case history form asks for several major categories of information and, where possible, develops questions chronologically. The categories of information are (1) identification, (2) statement of the problem, (3) speech, language, and hearing history, (4) general development, (5) medical history, (6) behavior, (7) educational history, and (8) home and family information. For each category we discuss the subject matter and its ordering, suggesting ways it might be useful to the diagnostician for doing his constituent analysis. For the reader's convenience we reproduce each of the sections of the case history form as it is discussed. For a complete history form see Appendix I.

Identification section

Identification information (Form 4-2), including the referral source, is presented first on the children's case history. It gives the diagnostician immediate information about the informant, the child, his parents, and medical supervision. He will know if the informant is the mother, father, another family member, or perhaps the physician, social worker, or other agency personnel.

FORM 4-2

Identification section of the children's speech, language, and hearing history

Date _June 1, 1983_

Person completing this form _Lois Compardo_ Relationship to child _Mother_

I. IDENTIFICATION

Name _Katherine Compardo_ Birth date _March 2, 1981_ Sex _F_ Age _27_

Address _One St. Mary's Court_ Phone: _644-5454_

Mother's name _Lois_ Address _Same_ Age _38_

Father's name _Frank_ Address _Same_ Age _42_

Referred by _Dr. Wasser_ Address _McGee Medical Building_

Family doctor _None_ Address _____

Child's pediatrician _Dr. Wasser_ Address _McGee Medical Building_

From these items the diagnostician can begin to categorize the environmental background of the child. This section, used in conjunction with the home and family section of the history, provides insight into causal factors that may have affected or be affecting the speech and language environment. Such information as parental addresses and ages tells us about the family structure: is the family unit intact; are both parents living together; is there a wide age discrepancy between the parents; are these young or old parents? If the person completing the form is the father rather than the mother, is this important? Perhaps it is a social worker or a physician. What do these constituents tell the diagnostician about the family? The address begins to provide information helpful for socioeconomic considerations. Of course, the diagnostician will have to know his own community before an address registers any information about style of living for the family. In categorizing this information, we are trying to evaluate the sociocultural, the multisensory, and the interpersonal context that make up the speech and language environment of the child being seen—what effects causal factors have on the past and current speech and language input received by the child.

The identification section does not give direct information about speech and language products. But, it does provide indirect information. For example, if the child is a 4-year-old girl, the diagnostician would immediately have an expectation reference point. He knows what speech and language normal 4-year-old children should have acquired. So knowing only the age and sex of the child being referred, the diagnostician could categorize this information in the speech and language product categories to serve as an inference about expected speech and language development.

FORM 4-3
Statement of the problem section of the children's speech,
language, and hearing history

II. STATEMENT OF THE PROBLEM

Describe as completely as possible the speech, language, and hearing problem.
Only speaks a few words. Can say ma but won't call me unless I'm there. Points to

Daddy and says it. Understands everything she is told. She won't say anything

else.

When was the problem first noticed? _____*Quiet as an infant*_____

How has the problem changed since you first noticed it? _____*She just isn't*

talking.

What has been done about it? Has this helped? *Nothing*

What do you think caused the problem? _____*No idea*

Are there any family members or relatives who have or had speech, language, or
hearing problems? _____*My nephew didn't start talking till he was 29 months.*

If there is both a pediatrician and a family doctor, or neither, it gives data about the general health care provided for the child. The information about the referral source, as seen by the informant, gives the diagnostician information for doing a reliability check on the source of referral.

Statement of the problem section

In the statement of the problem section (Form 4-3) the family is asked to present their perceptions of the speech and language problem and its causes. Presenting this section early on the history form allows the family to present their basic concerns about the child prior to having to respond to questions that may not seem as relevant, for example, birth history.

The informant is asked to describe the problem somewhat chronologically—at the present time, when first noticed, how it has changed, and what caused it. This time dimension, which creates some redundancy, may help to validate the perceptions of the family.

If this section is filled out completely by the informant and if the diagnostician considers it reliable and valid, he begins to form possible cause–effect constituents. Depending on the responses made to these open-ended questions, the diagnostician should also gain significant insight into the informant's ability to describe the child's speech and language behavior. Any type of problem stemming from any type of cause may be presented here. The diagnostician may also discover that the informant is only presenting another's impressions of the child's problem; quite often a parent will report information gained from the child's pediatrician or his teacher. Thus, the diagnostician may obtain information here about the speech and language product, the speech and language environment, and speech and language processes as well as causal factors that affect speech and language processing.

If the parent reported, "My son cannot be understood when he talks," the diagnostician would suspect something different than if the parent reported, "My son doesn't understand what is said to him." If the informant has indicated the child does not comprehend what is said to him and also states that it is because of a hearing loss, the diagnostician can begin to establish certain potential cause–effect relationships through categorization of this information within the structure of the SLPM. In this instance the hearing loss information fits within the auditory reception segment; whereas the comprehension problem would be categorized within the central language and thought segment.

Speech, language, and hearing section

The speech, language, and hearing history (Form 4-4) follows immediately after the statement of the problem section. This allows the informants to continue providing information that they can easily see is directly relevant to the problem with which they are concerned. This section then continues to build motivation for completing the remainder of the history form. The speech, language, and hearing history section is developed with a time dimension in mind—from past development to current use of speech and language. Adding this section to the statement of the problem, the diagnostician begins to get more details about the speech and language disorder and when it occurred. As well, he develops more insight and confidence into possible cause–effect constituents.

From the additional information provided in this section the diagnostician can better categorize the product that may be disordered. There are specific items about voice, prosody, phonetic structure, and all the parameters of language. Knowing the history of speech and language development not only gives information about the characteristics of the speech and language product, but, depending on the analysis of the information provided, it can give clues as to possible causal factors and underlying speech and language processes.

The information about hearing provides essential data both about hearing loss as a problem and as a probable cause of a speech and language disorder. The diagnostician also might categorize within the speech and language environment such items as, "How well can he be understood by his parents, by his brothers and sisters, by his playmates, and by relatives and strangers?" If the child cannot be understood by those around him, it may tell us something about his overall communicative interaction with people in his environment. The question "Does he imitate speech but not use it?" is intended to help discover if a child may be repeating but not comprehending, integrating or formulating speech and language. Other questions are also designed to provide information about speech and language processes.

FORM 4-4.

Speech, language, and hearing section of the children's speech, language, and hearing history

III. SPEECH, LANGUAGE, AND HEARING HISTORY

How much did your child babble and coo during the first 6 months? *not much*

When did he speak his first words? *2 yrs.* What were the child's first few words?
Here—Daddy—Hi

How many words did the child have at 1½ years? *none* When did he begin to use two-word

sentences? *none*

Does he use speech? Frequently _____ Occasionally __✓__ Never _____

Does he use many gestures? (Give examples if possible.) *gestures—knocks on me for my*
attention, then pulls me

Which does the child prefer to use? Complete sentences _____ *Phrases* _____

One or two words __✓__ *Sounds* _____ *Gestures* _____

Does he make sounds incorrectly? *yes* If so, which ones? *most of them*

Does he hesitate, "get stuck," repeat, or stutter on sounds or words? _____

If so, describe. _____

How does his voice sound? Normal____ Too high____ Too low____ Hoarse____ Nasal____

How well can he be understood? By his parents *everything* By his brothers and sisters

and playmates *everything* By relatives and strangers *everything*

Did your child ever acquire speech and then slow down or stop talking? *no*

Does he imitate speech but not use it? *no*

How well does he understand what is said to him? *understands everything*

Does your child hear adequately? *yes* Does his hearing appear to be constant or does it

vary? _____ Is his hearing poorer when he has a cold? *I don't think so.*

Has your child ever worn a hearing aid? *no* Which ear? _____ How long? _____

Hours per day? _____ Does it seem to help him? _____

NOTE: If the child has a hearing aid, please bring it and the earmold along with you when you come in for your appointment.

General development section

A two-part section on general development (Form 4-5) follows the speech, language, and hearing history. The first part is concerned with the pregnancy, birth, and first few weeks of the child's life—the prenatal, perinatal, and immediate postnatal history. The second part continues the general physical development of the child, including more specific information relevant to the auditory reception and speech production aspects of speech and language. Again, this information is ordered or asked for within a time-dimension framework. For the informants it is still apparent that these items are relevant to their primary concern, their child's speech and language problem.

The general development section is, for the most part, causally oriented. These items assist the diagnostician in categorizing causal factors that may have primarily affected the speech and language processing component. From the funds of knowledge the diagnostician knows that a child who had a difficult birth or is having physical development problems also may have associated speech and language disorders. Therefore these items can particularly assist in uncovering potential structural and neurologic deficits that may be causally related to the speech and language disorders. From this section the diagnostician should discover such potential factors as the presence of a cleft lip and palate, cerebral palsy, other neurologic problems, and mental retardation.

The chart presented in Part B of Form 4-5 is more specific to the auditory reception segment and the speech production segment of the speech and language processing component of the SLPM. Items here are designed to "look at" and categorize certain behaviors that often reflect underlying hearing and speech mechanism disruptions. For example, the items "Talked through nose" and "Food came out nose" obviously relate in some way to palatal function; where the items "Difficulty using tongue" and "Difficulty moving mouth" relate to lip, jaw, and tongue activity.

Medical history section

The next category of information presented on the case history form is medical history (Form 4-6). The concern of this section is additional specific data on the health status of the child, including information about the general medical care received. The items are asked in such a way that the informant supplies the time dimension. Information about the ages and severity of certain medical events that took place over time is requested.

The medical history section continues to add more information concerning possible causal factors. The list of diseases and illnesses incorporates those that may be directly or indirectly related to speech and language disorders. A series of, or even single, illnesses, diseases, operations, and hospitalizations can account for certain speech and language disorders. Knowing when these events occurred and for how long gives the diagnostician a time perspective on interacting situations in the life of the child that may be causally related to the speech and language disorder.

This section, again, assists in determining the validity and reliability of other data previously presented. If, for example, the child had tonsillitis, a tonsillectomy, and ear infections in the medical history, we then refer back to the general development section to see if he was a mouth breather or if he was indifferent to sound for a period of time. Thus, certain aspects of the data reported can be verified and cross-checked.

FORM 4-5
General development section of the children's
speech, language, and hearing history

IV. GENERAL DEVELOPMENT
A. Pregnancy and birth history

Total number of pregnancies _____5_____ How many miscarriages, stillbirths? _____None_____

Explain. _____

Which pregnancy was this child? __Last__ Length of pregnancy? __9 mo.__ Was it difficult? __No__

What illnesses, diseases, and accidents occurred during pregnancy? __None_____

Was there a blood incompatibility between the mother and father? __No_____

Age of mother at child's birth _____36_____ Age of father at child's birth _____40_____

What was the length of labor? __5 hrs.__ Were there any unusual problems at birth (breech birth,

caesarean birth, others)? If so, describe. _____No_____

_____

What drugs were used? __None__ High or low forceps? __No__ Weight of child at birth _____

Were there any bruises, scars, or abnormalities of the child's head? __No_____

Any other abnormalities? _____No_____

_____

Did infant require oxygen? _____No_____ Was child "blue" or jaundiced at birth? _____No_____

Was a blood transfusion required at birth? _____No_____

Were there any problems immediately following birth or during the first 2 weeks of the infant's life (health,

swallowing, sucking, feeding, sleeping, others)? If so, describe. _____
None

_____

At what age did infant regain birth weight? _____

B. Developmental

At what age did the following occur? Held head erect while lying on stomach _____2 or 3 wk._____

Rolled over alone _____ Sat alone unsupported __3 mo.__ Crawled __10 mo.__ Stood alone __15 mo.__

Walked unaided __15 mo.__ Fed self with spoon __1½ yr.__ Had first tooth _____ Bladder trained

_____ Bowel trained _____ Completely toilet trained: Waking _____ Sleeping _____

Dressed and undressed himself_____ What hand does he prefer? __Both__ Has handedness ever been

changed? _____ If so, at what age? _____ How would you describe your child's current

physical development? _____*She seems much slower than my other children.*_____

FORM 4-5—cont'd			

Check these as they apply to your child.

	Yes	*No*	*Explain: give ages if possible.*
Cried less than normal amount		✓	
Laughed less than normal amount		✓	
Yelled and screeched to attract attention or express annoyance	✓		*all along*
Head banging and foot stamping			
Extremely sensitive to vibration			
Very alert to gesture, facial expression, or movement	✓		*since she was a baby*
Shuffled feet while walking			
Generally indifferent to sound		✓	
Did not respond when spoken to		✓	
Responded to noises (car horns, telephones) but not to speech		✓	
Difficulty using tongue	✓		*when she talks*
Difficulty swallowing		✓	
Talked through nose		✓	
Mouth breather		✓	
Tongue-tied		✓	
Difficulty chewing		✓	
Drooled a lot		✓	
Food came out nose		✓	
Constant throat clearing		✓	
Difficulty breathing		✓	
Large tongue		✓	
Difficulty moving mouth	✓		*when she talks*

FORM 4-6
Medical history of the children's
speech, language, and hearing history

V. MEDICAL HISTORY

Is your child now under the care of a doctor? __Yes__ Why? __general check-ups__

Is he taking medication? __No__ Type? _____ Why? _____

At what ages did any of the following illnesses, problems, or operations occur? Please indicate how serious they were.

	Age	Mild	Mod.	Severe		Age	Mild	Mod.	Severe
Adenoidectomy					Earaches				
Allergies					Ear infections				
Asthma					Encephalitis				
Blood disease					Headaches				
Cataracts					Head injuries				
Chickenpox	1½	✓			Heart problems				
Chronic colds					High fevers				
Convulsions					Influenza				
Cross-eyed					Mastoidectomy				
Croup					Measles				
Dental problems					Meningitis				
Diphtheria					Mumps				
Muscle disorder					Rheumatic fever				
Nerve disorder					Scarlet fever				
Orthodontia					Tonsillectomy				
Pneumonia					Tonsillitis				
Polio					Whooping cough				

Has the child ever fallen or had a severe blow to the head? __no__ If so, did he lose consciousness? ____ Did it cause a concussion? ____ Did it cause: Nausea ____ Vomiting ____ Drowsiness ____ Describe any other serious illnesses, injuries, operations, or physical problems not mentioned above. _____

_____

What illnesses have been accompanied by an extremely long, high fever? ____

Temperature _____ How long did the fever last? _____

Which of the above required hospitalization? __none__ _____

Where was the child hospitalized? _____ For how long? _____

Who was the attending physician? _____

Behavior section

The behavior section of the case history form (Form 4-7) is a chart asking the informant to respond to a series of items that describe the essential aspects of the child's behavior, both from an intrapersonal and an interpersonal viewpoint. The time-dimension framework is built in by asking the informant to specify the ages at which any of the items (behavioral signs) may have been significant.

From the responses to these items the diagnostician gets information about the social, emotional, psychological, and behavioral aspects of the child's life. These behaviors may signal an associated problem often seen in children with speech and language disorders. Sometimes these problems are causally related to the speech and language disorder; at other times they are only coincidental with the speech and language disorder, both existing side by side. Still at other times both the behavioral disorder and the speech and language disorder stem from the same underlying causal factor. At any rate, by the time the diagnostician sees the child the two are interacting in the total intra- and interpersonal life of the child. Associated behaviors, as well, give indications of various underlying causal factors for speech and language disorders. They may provide a direct link to psychological–emotional mechanisms as well as to certain mental and neurologic conditions. For example, mental retardation and brain injury tend to produce certain types of behavioral responses, as do hearing loss and deafness.

The behavioral information provides added ingredients for the diagnostician's interpretation of the child's speech and language environment. For example, if he discovers that the child is happy, laughs easily, gets along with other children and adults, and makes friends easily in spite of a reported severe speech and language disorder, it tells the diagnostician something about the child's overall communicative interaction, his overall intra- and interpersonal relationships.

Educational section

The educational history (Form 4-8) provides information about educational experiences that add to the child's environmental background. Knowing if he is in school, how he is doing, and how he feels about school tells us more about him as an individual within an environmental context. As in all the sections, these items give information to the diagnostician about cause–effect relationships as well as potential management concerns.

Of significance from this section is information obtained about mental abilities, learning abilities, and overall intellectual abilities of the child that may have a bearing on the speech and language disorder. For example, knowing that a child is in a special class for the retarded, the diagnostician develops expectations about the speech and language products that may be disordered. His fund of knowledge about mental retardation as a causal factor for speech and language disorders allows him to infer potential problems he may encounter. Tying the information obtained in this section with previous sections, the diagnostician might also learn the basis for the child's mental retardation; for example, it may have resulted from brain injury sustained at birth or in utero rather than being familial.

Again, certain items can be used for a reliability–validity check. For example, the information provided about adjustment to school can be related to previous information about the behavior of the child. This section, like others, also provides the diagnostician with sources from which to obtain further information.

FORM 4-7
Behavioral section of the children's
speech, language, and hearing history

VI. BEHAVIOR

Check these as they apply to your child.

	Yes	No	*Explain: give ages if possible.*
Eating problems		✔	
Sleeping problems		✔	
Toilet training problems		✔	
Difficulty concentrating	✔		*she runs around a lot*
Needed a lot of discipline		✔	
Underactive		✔	
Excitable			
Laughs easily			
Cried a lot		✔	
Difficult to manage		✔	
Overactive	✔		*runs around a lot*
Sensitive			
Personality problem		✔	*she just won't talk*
Gets along with children	✔		
Gets along with adults	✔		
Emotional			
Stays with an activity			
Makes friends easily	✔		
Happy			
Irritable			
Prefers to play alone		✔	*plays alone and with other children*

How do you discipline your child? _____

What are the child's favorite play activities?   *picture books—bike—outdoors*

FORM 4-8
Educational section of the children's
speech, language, and hearing history

VII. EDUCATIONAL HISTORY

Did the child attend day care or nursery school? _No_ Where? _____ Ages _____

Kindergarten? _____ Where? _____ Ages _____

School now attending _____ Address _____

Grade he is now in _____ Grades skipped _____ Grades failed _____

What are his average grades? _____ Best subjects _____ Poorest _____

Is the child frequently absent from school? _____ If so, why? _____

How does child feel about school and about his teacher? _____

_____

What is your impression of your child's learning abilities? _____

_____

_____

Has anyone ever thought he was a slow child? _____

_____

Describe any speech, language, hearing, psychological, and special education services that have been performed including where this was done. How often was your child seen in this service? _____

_____

_____

Home and family section

The home and family section (Form 4-9) adds to the information provided in the identification section, giving more insight into the family life style. This section continues to provide information about cause–effect constituents. The emphasis here is on environmental factors that, in some way, may have affected the child's learning of speech and language—causal factors that affect the input stimulation received by the child. The occupation of the parents, the home and neighborhood, levels of education, source of income, and the address of the family can provide the basis for estimating socioeconomic status using the

FORM 4-9
Home and family section of the children's
speech, language, and hearing history

VIII. HOME AND FAMILY INFORMATION

Father's occupation *Senior Lieutenant* Last grade completed in school ___12___

Mother's occupation ___*Housewife*___ Last grade completed in school ___12___

Brothers and sisters:

	Name	Age	Sex	Grade in school	Speech, hearing, or medical problem
1.	Jennifer	6	F	1	
2.	Nancy	5	F		
3.	Diane	18	F	12	
4.	Frank	20	M	College	
5.					
6.					
7.					
8.					

Are there any other languages spoken in the home? ___*No*___ If so; by whom and how often?
_____

Home and neighborhood (check all that apply): Residential ___✓___ Business area _____
House ✓ Rural ___ Above average ___ Housing development ___ Excellent condition ___
Apartment area ____ Average ✓ Crowded ____ Suburban ✓ Number of rooms? _6_
Members of household other than family? ___*None*_____

Primary source of income (check the appropriate blanks): Salary ___✓___ Hourly wages _____
Commission _____ Welfare _____ Profits and fees _____ Savings and investments _____
Other _____

Please add any additional information you feel will help us in understanding your child and his problem:
I am calling you because my doctor suggested it. When baby was infant, I questioned her hearing because she

was so quiet. Now I am sure she can hear. I have just convinced myself there was nothing wrong; now I have

to start thinking otherwise.

Warner et al. (1960) scale (see Johnson et al., 1963). Knowing the number, ages, and health status of the siblings and other members of the home as well as other languages spoken adds information about family living conditions. Interpersonal interactions and sociocultural information can be interpreted from these items. If there are other normal siblings, the parent's statement of the problem gains validity since they do have points of comparison, that is, the other children who have developed normal speech and language. Knowing as much as possible about the life style of the family assists in planning the interpersonal approach to the diagnosis; diagnosticians must adapt their personal approaches, depending on the background of the families that seek their services. If financial considerations are important, the information provided in this section can be useful for determining the family's ability to pay for the services requested.

Letters and reports from other professionals

A final major source of information for the diagnostician is from other professionals who have had contact with the patient. This source of information is usually the primary one in inpatient settings and other multidiscipline agencies. Often these reports are maintained in an intra-agency file, for example, a medical chart accessible to any professional in that setting. At other times letters or written reports are sent directly to the diagnostician. This information may accompany the professional referral, or the request for such information may be initiated by the diagnostician.

The responses the diagnostician receives from his requests understandably reflect the specialty of the professional or agency contacted. For example, if information is requested from a neurologist, he will provide data about the medical status of the patient, emphasizing the neurologic disease or condition. He may also present some information about speech and language behavior and, perhaps, indications of management and prognosis. If information is requested from hospital records, a duplicate copy of the medical charts of the patient during his hospitalization may be received, sometimes including the day-to-day nursing chart.

When the diagnostician is requesting information from other professional sources, he can specify, to some extent, the information that he feels has a specific bearing on the patient's speech and language disorder. A form letter can be constructed to serve this purpose; however, at times a personalized letter of request will be needed. This procedure varies with the diagnostician and the work setting (see request for information form in Appendix I).

Verbal reports and consults may also be obtained. Often when the diagnostician has an ongoing relationship with another professional who has seen the patient, information is exchanged over the telephone. These phone contacts are initiated by either professional. In multidiscipline settings information is often transmitted verbally. For example, the diagnostician in a school setting may informally talk with the classroom teacher about the problem of a particular child.

Categorize the constituents from this brief report from Dr. Dixon, a pediatric neurologist who referred 5-year-old Trevor for a speech and language diagnosis. His findings included poor gross motor development, head circumference greater than the 98th percentile, a family history on the father's side of megaloencephaly, and motor problems. The result of the computerized tomography (CT) scan revealed normal dilatation of the ventricles with no shift of the midline structures. No areas of increased uptake were observed. EEG results revealed generalized slowing for age with no paroxysmal discharges present.

DETERMINES THE SIGNIFICANCE OF THE CONSTITUENTS

Once the diagnostician has categorized the constituents according to the format provided, he is ready for the second task, determining the significance of the available constituents. The diagnostician wants to find out if he has relevant and secure constituents (theoretically and factually) for defining and delimiting his clinical problem.

Reliability and validity of the information base

Since the information used in the constituent analysis comes from various sources, its validity and reliability must be established. The diagnostician must take into account the biases, memory, and the accuracy of the reporter. All the information available must be viewed as just what it is—the perceptions of one or more people about another person, reported to a third person. This information contains all the flaws that exist in human perception—biases, inaccuracies, loss of details, judgments, and overextensions. Since the diagnostician only has some of the important information, he must evaluate it carefully. He knows that the data is second hand, filtered through other people, parents, and professionals.

Information reported by parents may be about events that occurred some years before. The diagnostician can presume that the parents made the observations at the time they occurred, but how well can they recall the events that took place? At times this depends on the significance of the event in the parents' and patient's life. For example, parents usually remember fairly accurately when their child took his first step, an event that is awaited by parents. But all developmental events are not reported with such accuracy. Do the parents recall when the child said his first word, spoke in two-word sentences, and other details of their child's growth and development? Parents may also present certain biases when they report information about their child. Do they want us to believe that the child is more able than he is and, in some instances, less able than he is?

Professionals from whom information is obtained are not immune to perceptual inaccuracies. They too make errors in observing, measuring, and reporting information. The reports that are written are sometimes a recollection from sketchy notes of a visit that took place some time before. As much as we would like to, we do not always write reports immediately following contact with the patient. Professionals, too, have biases and make errors of judgment. For example, a physician may have a bias for viewing all language-delayed children as aphasic.

If the diagnostician is to develop an accurate interpretation of the information available, he must recognize all these possible sources of distortion. The sources of error must be checked out by the diagnostician when examining and determining the significance of the constituents, since the resulting hypotheses can only be as sound as the data from which they arise.

Constituent "Bruce's father died when he was 3 months old and that is why he doesn't talk."

That Bruce's father died is factual; however, as a cause for Bruce's not talking, it is not theoretically secure. We would be hard pressed to discover either from our clinical experience or from the literature such a direct cause–effect relationship. We have to approach this constituent from a more indirect route; for example, did the death of the father create other problems, which in turn more directly affected Bruce's speech and language development?

The diagnostician must develop the relations that exist among the constituents. This lets him see how the parts relate to the whole. He must develop a unitary picture that encompasses all the relationships among the pieces of information. He must extract as much meaning as possible from each bit of information relative to every other bit of information if he is to gain a clear perspective of his patients' clinical problem.

Constituent[2] "Gretchen did not walk until she was 20 months old."
Constituent[3] "Gretchen did not say her first word until she was 24 months old."
Constituent[4] "Gretchen is now 6 years old."
Constituent[5] "Gretchen only has 50 words that we understand."
These constituents could be analyzed as a group. Each offers important information, but as parts of a whole, the diagnostician can draw a better determination of their significance. A child who does not walk until this age is quite late in motor development. What are the potential reasons for such late development? How can this information be related to the data about speech and language development that were also quite late (the normal age of the first word is more like 10 to 12 months, and at 6 years of age normal children have a relatively complete, sophisticated use of language)? Since these constituents are factual and some describe the speech and language characteristics, how can they be used by the diagnostician to infer certain causal factors? What literature might he want to explore to secure his inferences?

When determining the significance and relevance of the constituents, the diagnostician proceeds to designate the strength each constituent has for explaining the clinical problem. Within a given category he may "rule in" and "rule out" certain constituents. Those constituents that appear to bear no explanatory relationship to the problem are disregarded (ruled out), while those that appear to demonstrate a relationship are retained (ruled in) for further investigation. The constituents retained are those that offer a more secure explanation of the speech and language disorder.

Constituent[6] Mother: "Dorothy isn't talking well because her two older sisters talked for her."
Constituent[7] Teacher: "Dorothy doesn't talk much because she is shy and doesn't want to talk."
Constituent[8] School psychologist: "Dorothy's speech is difficult to understand because she talks softly."
Constituent[9] Dorothy: "I don't talk much because I'm afraid I will stutter."
How many of these statements of the problem as constituents are factual and theoretically secure? Each source of information provides different reasons for what they all agree on—something seems to be wrong with Dorothy's speech. How would the diagnostician go about ruling in and out these various constituents? Can any literature support be found for the causal factors stated? For example, what role do older siblings play in the development and use of speech by a younger sibling? Would a series of interacting factors rather than a direct cause–effect relationship be more likely?

The diagnostician must constantly return to the professional literature if he is to keep abreast of information that helps explain the significance of the constituents he is examining.

It is in this task, the determining of significance of the constituents, that the diagnostician continues to expand his professional knowledge and, in turn, his expertise as a diagnostician. This constant expansion of clinical expertise keeps the diagnostic error rate down; it helps prevent misdiagnosis from occurring, jumping to unwarranted conclusions about cause–effect relationships.

Constituent[10] "My boy Robin stutters because his father does."
This is an inferential constituent, an explanation provided presumably by the mother. This constituent also has potential factual data; that is, "my boy stutters." This could be an accurate behavioral observation based on the mother's ability to observe and know what stuttering is in children. To give significance to this constituent, the diagnostician could explore his professional literature to answer such questions as, What is stuttering in children? What is the occurrence of stuttering in children? At what age is it seen? Also of importance is the direct cause–effect relationship stated by the mother. Is it probably that a child learns to stutter because his father does? How would Robin's stuttering behavior be similar to, or different from, his father's? Can stuttering be learned? Or is something else learned; that is, does the child learn from his father that speech is difficult? What do the theories say about stuttering as a learned behavior? Further, what is known about the genetic basis for stuttering? All of this information must be considered regarding this constituent to determine how secure it may be for clinical purposes.

Errors in diagnosis can occur. The only way to circumvent these errors and potential misdiagnosis is to develop our funds of knowledge to the greatest extent possible, knowing what we know and what we do not know, making it our professional responsibility to learn what we need to know. For example, if a diagnostician is confronted with a child who, unknown to him, is hearing impaired, and the diagnostician has little information about the relationship between hearing loss and speech and language, he may miss hearing loss as a causal factor. But he may go on and make a diagnosis since that is his job. Thus he may come up with a misdiagnosis. For him, the child might be mentally retarded, emotionally disturbed, or brain injured—whatever seems to best tie the patient's behavior to the diagnostician's fund of knowledge.

This task of the constituent analysis step of the diagnostic process helps circumvent these diagnostic errors. It requires the diagnostician to constantly review the constituents presented about his patient and to seek out information from the literature that helps him determine the significance of the constituents (e.g., Shriberg & Smith, 1983). The exacting use of this step should prevent the occurrence of too many errors.

Constituent[11] "Mrs. Metz has aphasia."
This constituent would most likely come from a physician who has made a medical diagnosis of aphasia. It is a constituent that is both factual and inferential but highly theoretically secure. A cause-effect relationship is stated in the constituent. Aphasia is a language disorder due to brain injury. But the diagnostician should not be completely secure. In our experience we have received referrals like this only to discover that the patient was not aphasic but rather dysarthric. There are many considerations that go into an analysis of this constituent. What is aphasia? What causes the aphasia? For this patient, we would want to consider how the aphasia is manifested; does it need to be differentiated from other speech and language disorders resulting from neurologic damage? Undue assumptions about a referral constituent can lead to misdiagnosis.

Once the diagnostician has categorized all the constituents, it becomes most efficient for him to determine their significance and examine their relevancy according to the categories on the constituent analysis form (Form 4-1). He can choose to examine the significance of individual constituents within a category, look at groups of constituents within a category, or examine the entire category simultaneously.

CONSTITUENT ANALYSIS WITH LIMITED PATIENT INFORMATION BASE

Because the constituent analysis as a part of the scientific framework must be adaptable to varying amounts of information, we also want to briefly discuss how the diagnostician might proceed to think through a constituent analysis with only a referral statement as the source of information. In instances where little information is available on which to do a constituent analysis, the diagnostician must rely completely on his funds of knowledge and clinical experience.

For example, consider the following referral statement from a mother about her 4-year-old boy, "Devin has a speech problem." Depending on how this referral is viewed, there is either a single constituent (Devin has a speech problem) or five constituents (name, age, sex, speech problem, and referral from the mother). How can this be categorized and examined for significance? The referral statement says speech rather than language. But do referral sources make a differentiation between these two as the professional diagnostician might do? How do parents make referral statements?

In our experience, parents, using their own terminology, often do state different problems in different ways. For example, in terms of speech versus language problems we have received statements that do lead in one direction or another such as: "He doesn't understand what I say to him." "He doesn't talk good." "He doesn't make his sounds right." "I can't understand him when he talks." "He can't say anything like he should." "He doesn't move his tongue when he talks." An interesting statement of the problem was presented by one mother about her daughter. She stated, "Sandy uses nasal sounds and puts an *e* on the end of words." Puts an *e* on the ends of words was difficult to interpret at the time. However, after the diagnosis the accuracy of the mother's description was noted. The child was extremely unintelligible, producing strings of vowel sounds with glottal stops to signal syllabic production. Many of the vowels were produced nasally, increased in duration, and the final vowel of the string was a prolonged /i/. A transcription of several words looked something like this: /æ̃: ʔ ĩ:/ for rabbit and /ũ: ʔ ĩ:/ for music.

Devin's referral constituent requires the diagnostician to review the types of speech and language disorders that occur in children and how often they occur. From this he could list in order the most probable areas of disorder. The incidence data available might lead him to first expect a disorder in phonology, in our framework a language disorder on the phonologic level, and in more general terminology an articulation disorder. However, since so little is known, alternative potentials must be considered. Devin might have a language disorder on more than the phonologic level. The incidence data might point to a different language disorder. Thus, from his fund of knowledge the diagnostician can determine the significance of this referral constituent and develop from it a series of hypotheses from most to least likely. How likely is it that Devin stutters or has a voice disorder? In our experience it is not too likely, since parents tune into stuttering and voice, and seldom express it simply as a speech problem; rather they come right to the point of their concern, "Devin stutters."

Even if limited information is available prior to diagnosis, the diagnostician can develop an approach to the constituent analysis that would be more efficient than if he just waited until the person came. Another way of viewing the constituent analysis when no other information comes would be to order the analysis to tap all the probabilities that may exist. From knowledge about speech and language as reflected in the SLPM a constituent analysis could be set up that leads to a global hypothesis; all behaviors and processes may be affected, which would require systematic sampling of the various speech and language behaviors and processes.

What might you consider the general problem to be in the following referrals? What are the constituents? (1) From the second-grade teacher, "Sue isn't doing well in my class because of her speech problem. Will you see her for me?" (2) From the pediatrician, "Mrs. Starr will be calling you about her daughter Brenda who isn't talking. Please see her as soon as you can." (3) From the neurologist, "Mr. Grogan has a strange speech pattern, but we haven't found any neurologic basis for it. Does he need speech therapy?"

In these referrals a number of clinical questions can be developed and examined for relevancy. For example, from Mr. Grogan's referral we can assume that we are going to be seeing an adult (why?) who for some reason went to a neurologist. The speech pattern has been described as strange. Does this mean the neurologist has never heard speech like this? Surely if Mr. Grogan was stuttering, the neurologist would have recognized that pattern of speech behavior, but perhaps not; it may be a very atypical pattern of nonfluency. If the speech pattern were neurologically based would the neurologist not have recognized it? Not necessarily, since speech sometimes deteriorates in neurologic disease before the disease can be diagnosed by neurologic testing. Could Mr. Grogan have sustained a minor cerebrovascular accident (CVA) that went undetected except for this speech pattern, which the neurologist did not recognize as related to a possible CVA? These are only some of the questions that can arise from the diagnostician's fund of knowledge about this specific referral. What are others you may want to examine in this referral as well as in the other examples?

SUMMARY

The constituent analysis, the first step of the diagnostic process, consists of two major tasks performed by the diagnostician.

1. He categorizes the bits of information he obtains about his patient.
2. He determines the significance of these constituents for defining and delimiting his clinical problem.

The diagnostician's overall goal in this step is to develop a baseline of relevant information about the patient he is to see. To do this he uses two primary sources of information—his professional knowledge and the specific patient information base he has gathered. Available to him for gathering information are referral sources, case history questionnaires, and letters and reports from other professionals.

For doing the constituent analysis we have provided a method, based on the SLPM, for categorizing cause and effect constituents and examining them for significance. We also suggested the use of a scanning mechanism for viewing causal factors emphasizing

1. Factors primarily affecting the speech and language environment, and
2. Factors primarily affecting the speech and language processing system.

When he has completed the constituent analysis, the diagnostician knows what relevant information he has available about his patient's speech and language disorder—its characteristics and its potential causes. From this he is now ready to derive his clinical hypothesis, his clinical perspective on the most likely cause–effect relationship. He has begun to meet the goals of diagnosis—to determine the nature of the speech and language disorder, to understand its causes, and to propose appropriate client management.

KATHERINE COMPARDO

Categorization of constituents

Katherine Compardo, whose case history form has been presented in this chapter, will be used throughout the remainder of the book as our primary example for illustrating the diagnostician's tasks at each step of the diagnostic process.

Katherine Compardo was referred to a community speech and hearing agency by her mother at the suggestion of Katherine's pediatrician. The information obtained was the telephone data on the request for service form (Appendix I) and a children's case history questionnaire (See this chapter) that was sent out, completed by the mother, and returned to the agency. No further information was received or requested prior to the diagnosis.

From this information we have selected certain constituents to demonstrate the diagnostician's task of categorization. Table 4-2 presents these constituents. The second column on the table indicates the categories where we placed the constituents (see Form 4-1). This table is to be used by the student to justify the categorization decisions we have made and to complete the categorization of the other constituents presented in Katherine's history.

Determining the significance of the constituents

Table 4-3 presents a selection of constituents accompanied by a discussion of their significance. We present them in different ways to demonstrate this task. Some will be individual constituents and others grouped within categories. *The way we have chosen to group certain constituents within categories is in no way meant to be standard practice.* Constituents can be grouped in any number of ways by using the SLPM orientation. Grouping can be based on single behavioral correlates, a series of physical processes, combinations of physical processes and behavioral correlates, specific causal factors affecting one of the components of the SLPM, and so forth. The diagnostician is assisted in his delimitation of the clinical problem by viewing the constituents within a variety of categories; however, no categorization will answer all the clinical questions.

PATIENT PROJECTS

Following are a series of patients representing various speech and language disorders stemming from different causal bases. Along with Katherine Compardo, these patients can be used by students for implementing the steps and tasks of the diagnostic process presented in this book. The patient information base for each of them is located in Appendix II.

William Gafford

Reverend William Gafford, 46 years old, called the clinic on October 17, 1983, immediately following his ear, nose, and throat examination. Information was obtained from Reverend Gafford and recorded on the request for service form. His physicians, Dr. Gershon and Dr. Lefkoff, made the recommendation. Because of his chief complaint of hoarseness that was affecting his occupation as a pastor, he was given an immediate appointment 2 days later. A call was placed to Dr. Gershon and Dr. Lefkoff who provided verbal information that was then included in a referral letter that arrived on the day of the diagnosis. No history questionnaire was sent out.

Because of the limited amount of information available on Reverend Gafford, the student will have to explore the literature carefully and develop many of his own constituents for exploring potential cause–effect relationships. The following could serve as primary resources (Aronson, 1980; Boone, 1977; Cooper & Cooper, 1977; Hirano, 1981; Moore, 1971a, 1971b).

Isadore Alexander

Sixty-eight-year-old Isadore Alexander was referred by Dr. Jarius Lambert, Chief of Otolaryngology, University Hospitals, to the hospital's speech–language pathologist. When checking Dr. Lambert's consult notes, the

(Text continued on page 114.)

Table 4-2. Categorization of selected constituents from the information available about Katherine Compardo.*

Selected Constituents	Categorization From Form 4-1
Four older siblings with no speech, hearing, or medical problems	Speech and language input
Gets along with other children and adults	Speech and language input Behavioral considerations Speech and language product (?)—what role does her speech and language play in getting along with others?
Family lives in a residential, average, suburban neighborhood in a six-room house	Speech and language input—environment
Pediatrician listed as referral source	Further information needed Other Information—if pediatrician referred, there is reinforcement for the presence of some type of speech and language disorder
Understands everything she is told	Behavioral correlates—comprehension and integration Further information—interview Behavioral considerations
Only speaks a few words	Speech and language product Behavioral correlates—integration and formulation
Makes most sounds incorrectly	Speech and language product—phonetic structure and phonology Physical processing—speech programming and remainder of speech production segment
When baby was infant, I questioned her hearing because she was so quiet; now I am sure she can hear; I have just convinced myself there was nothing wrong; now I have to start thinking otherwise	Physical processing—auditory reception segment Further information—interview Purpose of diagnosis Statement of problem

*The student should justify these selected examples and then complete the categorization of Katherine Compardo's constituents.

Table 4-3. Determination of significance of selected constituents from patient information about Katherine Compardo*

Constituents and Categories	Significance
Only speaks a few words	Katherine is now 27 months of age. The following sources indicate that a child this age should have a vocabulary of 300 to 400 words and be speaking in two- or three-word phrases, using nouns, prepositions, verbs, adjectives, and pronouns (Anderson et al., 1963; Dale, 1972; Hopper and Naremore, 1973; Lee, 1966; Lenneberg, 1967; Stark, 1981). With this constituent we can at least say that Katherine is far behind the normal in use of words. There is much more that could be discussed regarding the significance and relevance of this single constituent as it relates to the SLPM. Of relevance is what the constituent says about Katherine's language formulation and, by inference, the physical process of language–thought representation. Berry (1969), Eisenson (1972), Irwin and Marge (1972), Morley (1972), and Wyke (1978), consider that such a delay may signal the disorder labeled childhood aphasia.
Makes most of her sounds incorrectly	Children Katherine's age usually have a fairly well-developed repertoire of speech sound usage (Menyuk, 1971; Sander, 1972; Templin, 1957a; Winitz, 1969; Ingram, 1976). This constituent also adds to our information about late acquisition of the speech and language system. Again, Katherine appears to be far behind what would be expected. This constituent should be considered for its relevance to the speech production segment of the SLPM, beginning with the physical process of speech programming as well as to the speech and language product component. Eisenson (1972), McCarthy and McCarthy (1973), Morley (1972), Perkins (1977), Yoss and Darley (1974), and Aram and Nation (1982), discuss the late acquisition and difficulty with speech sounds as a characteristic of the disorder labeled apraxia of speech in children.
Sensation, perception, comprehension Some of the constituents that help determine if Katherine hears and comprehends speech and language using behavioral correlates as a basis for grouping Hears adequately now but mother concerned about hearing as an infant; quiet as an infant No lack of response when spoken to; responds to noises and voice Responds to telephone and car horn Not indifferent to sound Yelled and screamed to attract attention Alert to gesture, facial expression, movement Did not babble and coo much during the first 6 months Did not imitate sounds during the first and second years Had no words at 1½ years of age	From these constituents we can determine some things about Katherine's ability to hear, perceive, and comprehend. A variable history is presented, the mother at one time seeing signs that made her believe Katherine was not hearing as an infant. However, the constituents indicate that she hears appropriately at this time. (See constituents about her responses to sound and ability to comprehend.) We might be able to conclude from this that Katherine's hearing mechanism is intact—the physical processes of auditory acceptance-transduction, auditory analysis-transmission, and perhaps auditory reception-analysis. Thus the behavioral correlates of sensation and certain aspects of perception may be relatively intact. There may be a question about the behavioral correlate of perception as it relates to the

*These examples in no way reflect all the constituents available on Katherine Compardo nor their examination for significance and relevance. Many more clinical questions need to be asked. The student should continue the examination of the constituents available until they feel they are ready to derive and support a clinical hypothesis.

Continued.

Table 4-3. Determination of significance of selected constituents from patient information about Katherine Compardo*—cont'd

Constituents and Categories	Significance
Sensation, perception, comprehension—cont'd	
Spoke her first word at 2 years of age Understands everything she is told Currently prefers to use one or two words Makes most of her sounds incorrectly Uses speech occasionally; prefers to use gestures	physical process of auditory programming. Katherine's difficulties with developing language and producing speech sounds may signal problems in auditory processing. The literature on the relationship of speech and language acquisition to auditory perception is equivocal, depending on the studies read (Rees, 1973; Aram & Nation, 1982). What do our constituents offer us in regard to auditory perception? The report that Katherine, although responsive to sound, did not babble and coo, was a quiet infant, did not imitate sounds, was late in language acquisition, and makes many sounds incorrectly, indicates that the behavioral correlates of perception of the language stimulus may be a problem. Lack of speech and language development may occur because of auditory processing deficits even when there is no hearing loss. Eisenson (1972), McReynolds (1966), Morley (1972), Myklebust (1954), Yoss and Darley (1974), Hubbell, (1981), and Aram & Nation (1982), all point to auditory processing problems in children labeled as aphasic children who have a significant delay in speech and language acquisition. However, the constituent that Katherine understands everything she is told looms in front of us. Does she really comprehend everything? What is she asked to comprehend? So the question regarding auditory processing, the relationship between the behavioral correlates of perception and comprehension, should remain open.
Language–cognitive representation—speech programming	
Constituents that help us determine if Katherine can create, formulate, and sequence speech and language using physical processes as a basis for grouping.	Many of the constituents listed within this category are the same as used for demonstration in the previous category. How might these constituents be used to examine the relevancy and significance for language formulation and sequencing?
Quiet as an infant Did not babble and coo much during the first 6 months Did not imitate sounds during the first and second years Had no words at 1½ years of age Spoke her first word at 2 years of age; first words were "here," "daddy," and "hi" Currently prefers to use one or two words—only speaks a few words Uses speech occasionally; prefers to use gestures Just isn't talking Makes most of her sounds incorrectly Difficulty using her tongue and moving her mouth when she talks	
Mother reports Katherine understood by parents etc., response is "everything" to all the items	We would question the validity of this response by the mother. It seems as if she interpreted the question to mean How well does Katherine understand these people? See mother's responses elsewhere that Katherine "understands everything."

continued.

Table 4-3. Determination of significance of selected constituents from patient information about Katherine Compardo—cont'd

Constituents and Categories	Significance
Causal factors affecting speech and language processing system See Table 4-1 for the rationale for grouping the constituents under this category, for this grouping we will not include any constituents about the speech and language product, physical processes, behavioral correlates, or speech and language environment that might be relevant to causal factors for Katherine's speech and language disorder; our interest in this categorization is the relationship between certain causal factors and bodily systems that can have an effect on the speech and language processing system.	First, as mentioned, there are many other constituents that may tell as much if not more about disruptions of the physical processing system than those categorized here. We are simply providing another example of how constituents can be examined for relevancy to a patient. Each patient requires different forms of categorization for delimitation.
Length of pregnancy, 9 months No accidents or illnesses during pregnancy No blood incompatibility Five pregnancies; no history of miscarriages or stillbirths No problems with delivery; no drugs or instruments used Mother 36 years of age at time of birth Length of labor, 5 hours No unusual problems at birth No oxygen required for infant No immediate postnatal problems Held head erect (2 to 3 weeks); sat alone (3 months); crawled (10 months); walked unaided (15 months); fed self with a spoon (1½ years) Seems much slower (physically) than my other children Prefers both hands Difficulty using her tongue and mouth when she talks Mild case of chickenpox No serious medical history No severe blows to the head Quiet as an infant No eating, sleeping, toilet training problems Not difficult to manage Yelled and screeched to attract attention (all along) Alert to gesture, facial expression, and movement since she was a baby Difficulty concentrating—runs around a lot Overactive—runs around a lot Makes friends easily; plays both alone and with other children; gets along with other children and adults Mother's nephew did not start talking until he was 29 months old	Each of the constituents listed here can be fitted into the categories given in Table 4-1, factors primarily affecting the speech and language processing system. Each of them can be reviewed in relationship to the professional literature. For example, Katherine did not walk until she was 15 months of age. From Church and Stone (1973), Frankenburg and Dodds (1967), and Mussen et al. (1969), we get a range for onset of walking from 12 to 18 months. Therefore walking as an isolated constituent may give little information and must be examined in relationship to other physical development. What do these same sources give as an age for crawling? Review the constituents presented here in light of the information about physical development, birth history, and general behavior of children classified as aphasic and apraxic. (See Chase, 1972; Eisenson, 1972; Johnson and Myklebust, 1967; McCarthy and McCarthy, 1973; Morley, 1972, Yoss and Darley, 1974,Horwitz, 1984). What would these constituents offer regarding mental retardation? (See Lillywhite and Bradley, 1969.)

diagnostician discovered that Mr. Alexander had been referred to Dr. Lambert by another otolaryngologist, Dr. William Fowles. Mr. Alexander had also seen Dr. Lee Uransky, a neurologist. Before seeing Mr. Alexander, the diagnostician felt it was necessary to obtain further information from Dr. Fowles and Dr. Uransky. No history questionnaire was sent. Some resources the student might find useful are Aronson (1971), Aronson et al. (1964, 1966), Berry (1983), Darley et al. (1969a, 1969b, 1975a, 1975b), and Johns (1978).

Derek Park

Derek Park, age 5 years, 3 months, has just been enrolled in kindergarten at Iles Elementary School. Ms. Eckelmann has asked Mr. Posch the speech–language pathologist to see Derek. Mr. Posch is at Iles twice a week only in the mornings. Because of his case load, he seldom is able to take kindergarten children except on special referrals. On his initial consult with Ms. Eckelmann, he learned that Derek was difficult to understand and that he had a repaired cleft lip and palate. He called Mrs. Park and informed her that he was to see Derek and obtained the name of his plastic surgeon. Mrs. Park also told him that Derek had been seen by the St. John's Hospital cleft palate team. Before seeing Derek, Mr. Posch obtained letters of information from both these sources. The following resources can be useful to explore for doing Derek Park's constituent analysis (Bzoch, 1979; Edwards & Watson, 1980; Peterson-Falzone, 1982; Wells, 1971).

James E. Matkin

James E. Matkin has been referred to the Eastern Speech and Hearing Clinic as a part of the vocational services offered by the Bureau of Vocational Rehabilitation. Currently, Mr. Matkin is unemployed. According to the referral, Mr. Matkin is a stutterer and he confirms this in the history form. The following resources can be consulted (Conture, 1982; Bloodstein, 1981; Gregory, 1979; Van Riper, 1971).

Marie Abadie

Marie Abadie was admitted to the rehabilitation unit of Kankakee General Hospital 3 weeks following the onset of her condition. She was brought over from 6 West, the neurology ward. In Appendix II her discharge summary report as dictated by Dr. Denise Aronson is reproduced. Also included in Appendix II are the results of tests given by Dr. Sandra Mayfield, speech–language pathologist, who has used selected items from various tests of aphasia following a processing schema. Analyze the results of the testing. What significance do her findings have to a classification of processing deficits in aphasia? Whose schema is basically being followed in this format of testing and analysis? Consider the following resources (Goodglass & Kaplan, 1972; Jenkins et al., 1975; Eisenson, 1973; Sarno, 1981; Kertesz, 1983).

Karen Twigg

Karen, 9 years 3 months, was referred by Mr. Edward Worjak, an audiologist in a community hospital. He was interested in follow-up audiological services and a determination of Karen's speech, language, and learning abilities. Dr. Caroline Ekelman, speech–language pathologist at Children's Hospital, Carrollton, Georgia will be seeing her. The only information available was the referral note and audiogram sent by Mr. Worjak. Consult the following resources (Northern & Downs, 1978; Keith, 1977; Aram & Nation, 1982; Bangs, 1982; Shriberg & Smith, 1983; Bess & McConnell, 1981).

STUDY QUESTIONS

1.   It is now suggested that the student work with and develop Table 4-4 to gain still greater insight into specific causal factors that can disrupt components of the SLPM, resulting in speech and language disorders. On the table we have provided several minimal, nondetailed examples to demonstrate the use of the table as a way of abstracting essential information about cause–effect relationships. The student should develop the table as a continuing project, adding, deleting, and reinterpreting as he gains more and more sophistication about cause–effect relationships in speech and language disorders. The student should consider all the material and pursue the references presented thus far in this book as a beginning source of pertinent material available in our literature. The table then can serve as a ready reference for reviewing potential cause–effect relationships the diagnostician may see.

Table 4-4. Cause-effect relationships as viewed from the SLPM

Causal factor	Component part affected (can be considered from all aspects)	Normal functions	Resulting disruptions		
			Processes		Products
			Physical	Behavioral correlates	
Cerebrovascular accident	Central language-thought segment	Processes speech and language data for comprehension, integration and formulation; turns auditory data into symbolic, representational form; turns representational data into speech data; overall process of language-cognitive representation	May affect auditory programming, language-cognitive representation, and speech programming	Could affect perception, comprehension, integration, formulation, repetition, and sequencing	Could affect language product on all linguistic levels; could be no language behavior, or what occurs could be use of stereo-typed sounds, words, and phrases; what would be observed depends on site and extent of damage to central language-thought segment
Institutionalization in a nonstimulating environment	Speech and language stimulation	Provides child with input data on all linguistic levels from which he derives language code of his language community	May not affect physical processes and behavioral correlates directly but will not have information to process; processes ultimately affected if deprivation prolonged over critical periods of time during learning of speech and language		Reduced amount of language output; probable that speech product not too involved; that is, phonetic structure, voice, and prosody might be appropriate; language on all linguistic levels affected in terms of quantity and sophistication for age of child; again, depends on degree of deprivation
Cerebrovascular accident: occlusion of prerolandic branch of middle cerebral artery	Central language-thought segment: Broca's area	Involved in behavioral correlate of formulation; turns auditory pattern of language received into motor pattern of language by physical process of speech programming; programs series of muscular activities needed in carrying out speech production	Speech programming affected	Formulation and sequencing	Spontaneous speech nonfluent and lacking some syntax, many phonologic errors; difficulty in transition from one sound to another; in severe form not able to initiate speech
Damage to recurrent laryngeal nerve during thyroidectomy resulting in unilateral recurrent nerve paralysis; adductors and abductors both affected	Speech production segment: vocal folds	Vocal folds vibrate to produce vocal tones	Speech production: phonation	Motor control	Voice hoarse and breathy; may begin to sound better over time (depending on compensation by unaffected vocal fold)

A. The following is only a partial list of "environmental" factors that have been cited as having an influence on speech and language development and use. Place these factors into our scanning mechanism for factors primarily affecting the speech and language environment component (Table 4-1). Search the literature for support and details on these factors and interpret them within the Table 4-4 guidelines. What others might you add? Literature from child growth and development is particularly helpful here (see Sameroff, 1975).

Absence of father	Overprotection
Amount of social contact	Parental age
Bilingualism	Parental aspirations
Birth order	Parental attitudes
Child-rearing practices	Parental rejection
Divorce	Parental standards
Economic deprivation	Peer influence
Educational background	Personality disorders
Emotional deprivation	Poor family constellation
Ethnic background	Poor speech models
Hospitalization	Racial group
Improper teaching methods	Religious conflict
Institutionalization	Sensory deprivation
Lack of reinforcement	Severe discipline
Lack of stimulation	Sibling conflict
Mixed cultural expectations	Siblings talk for child
Multiple births	"Silent" environment
New birth in family	Social class
Number of siblings	Socioeconomic status

B. Below is another partial list of many factors that have been cited as having an influence on speech and language development and usage. Place these factors into our scanning mechanism for factors primarily affecting the speech and language processing component of the SLPM (Table 4-1). Search the literature for support and details on these factors and interpret within Table 4-4 guidelines.

Agenesis of brain structures	Maternal anoxia
Aneurysms	Maternal rubella
Athetosis	Meningitis
Atresia of ear	Mental retardation
Autism	Metabolic disorder
Blood clots	Minimal brain damage
Brain injury	Multiple sclerosis
Breech birth	Neoplasms
Cancer of larynx	Otitis media
Car accidents	Parkinson's disease
Carbon monoxide poisoning	Paralysis
Cerebral palsy	Placenta previa
Cerebral thrombosis	Precipitous birth
Cerebrovascular accident	Prenatal injury
Circulatory disease	Radiation
Cleft lip and palate	Reverse breathing
Contact ulcers	Rh incompatibility
Diseases	Schizophrenia
Drugs	Sensorineural hearing loss
Encephalitis	Short lingual frenum
Endocrine disorder	Skull fracture
Fetal alcohol syndrome	Syphilis
Forceps delivery	Thyroid deficiency
High arched palate	Tongue thrust

Huntington's chorea   Treacher–Collins syndrome
Hyperactivity   Tumors
Intracranial hemorrhage   Uterine trauma
Malocclusion   Vitamin deficiency

2.   Review several case history questionnaires using a similar type of analysis demonstrated in this chapter. The student should determine how the history form has been constructed and what it offers for use in the constituent analysis. Barsch (1968) presents much useful information that assists the diagnostician in case history analysis and interpretation. Since a children's history form was discussed here as an example, we would suggest the student start with an adult case history form for comparative purposes.

Chapter 5

Clinical hypothesis: derivation of cause–effect relationships

The derivation of the clinical hypothesis, done prior to patient contact, is the second step of the diagnostic process as outlined in Figure 3-1. The clinical hypothesis is a formal statement by the diagnostician of the cause–effect relationship he derives from his constituent analysis. He uses his best reasoning abilities to arrive at a statement that offers a logical explanation of the clinical problem.

In the constituent analysis the diagnostician categorized and determined the significance of the constituents. To derive the clinical hypothesis, the diagnostician must now draw together causal constituents and effect constituents and integrate these constituents into cause–effect relationships. He narrows down the number of possible explanations for the clinical problem, forming priorities among the potential cause–effect relationships until he has derived his most likely explanation of the speech and language disorder and its causes.

The derivation of the clinical hypothesis serves several purposes for the diagnostician. Hypothesis statements are attempts to clarify the clinical problem by expressing potential cause–effect relationships. The hypothesis implies a level of understanding rather than a level of knowing. The hypothesis is not a statement of facts, nor is it a "definitive" statement; it is a tentative statement of understanding.

The hypothesis also offers a tentative solution to the speech and language problem. The hypothesis is inferential and predictive; it has a forward reference in that it expresses a relationship that requires further examination. In this sense the clinical hypothesis predicts that an individual has a disorder that would not be resolved without assistance. Hubbell (1981) reinforces the role of prediction in diagnosis.

> If I had to define assessment, evaluation, diagnosis, and similar terms in one word, that word would be *prediction*. During initial assessment the goal is to decide whether or not the child demonstrates a language disorder. The importance of this decision is in the prediction it carries with it. If it is decided that a particular child does not demonstrate significant language impairment, we are really predicting that the child will develop language normally without intervention. Conversely, recommending intervention implies the prediction that the child either will not improve in language skill without help, or at least that such development will be behind schedule. . . While often implicit, prediction is the core of assessment. (Hubbell, 1981, pp. 133–134)

The role of hypothesis formulation is to derive a dynamic cause–effect relationship used for exploring the patient's problem, remembering the complex interactions between speech and language disorders and their potential causes. In general, the clinical hypothesis provides a thrust and an organization for the completion of the diagnostic process. Therefore the hypothesis is always under scrutiny, and in the practical world of diagnosis it may change during the diagnostic process. It undergoes modification as more insight is gained into the clinical problem. Hypothesis derivation, as expressed by Schultz (1973), is a continuous recycling process as more data are gained about the patient.

Three tasks are required of the diagnostician. *First*, he derives the clinical hypothesis by examining and ordering the various relationships that exist between causes and effects, thereby developing a hierarchy of probable cause–effect explanations. *Second*, he states the clinical hypothesis as a cause–effect relationship, considering the most likely hypothesis as well as alternative hypotheses. *Third*, he evaluates the quality of the hypothesis, formalizing this process by presenting the arguments for his position.

As pointed out in the constituent analysis, the steps of the diagnostic process must be adaptable to varying amounts of information. This is also true of developing the clinical hypothesis. We are presenting this step as taking place prior to patient contact; however, during the diagnostic session new information will be obtained that requires the diagnostician to constantly reevaluate his original hypothesis. Reformulations take place frequently, from minor modifications of the hypothesis to completely new derivations.

In order to perform the tasks for deriving the clinical hypothesis the diagnostician relies on three fundamental sources of information. First, he has the patient information from his constituent analysis. Second, be returns to his funds of knowledge, particularly those that emphasize cause–effect relationships. Third, he relies on his knowledge of problem solving and his ability to reason logically.

DERIVES THE CLINICAL HYPOTHESIS

From his mental operations the diagnostician draws together relevant cause–effect relationships, develops new relationships through his ability to infer cause from effect and effect from cause, and identifies missing pieces of information needed to verify his expressed relationships.

Examines the relationships among causes and effects

The diagnostician examines the inventory of constituents, looking for links between causal factors and disordered speech and language. When the diagnostician examines the relationship among his cause and effect constituents, he goes through a process of aggregation and delimitation. He wants to identify those that have a past and a current effect on the speech and language disorder. The process of aggregation requires integrating all the constituents that in some way make up the patient as a human being. The process of delimitation is like a progressive approximation toward those constituents bearing the most significance for explaining the cause–effect relationships.

For example, if a series of constituents about physical growth and development reveal that all motor milestones are within normal limits, the chances are that the diagnostician will rule out retarded physical development as a potential explanatory factor. On the other hand, the diagnostician must ask himself if he has sufficient information about physical growth and development to rule it out as a causal factor. The information he has may be limited, may be wrong, or may be inaccurately reported.

Suppose we have examined a set of product constituents and have tentatively concluded that Lucia has either a prosody or a severe phonologic disorder. The strength of these conclusions rests with the interpretation of the constituents as examined in relation to each other; it may not be an either/or situation. Lucia's deviant phonologic formulation may make her so unintelligible that she has developed a number of starts and stops to get her parents to understand her. Add to this her age; she is not quite 4 years old—an age when speech and language use may not be easy for a child. Her speech is filled with whole-word and phrase repetitions. Thus, what may be occurring is not a prosody disorder but normal nonfluencies exacerbated by a significant deviation in the use of the phonologic system. Her parents may be reacting more to the nonfluencies as the basis for the unintelligibility than to the sound deviations. To add further to the mix, the parents were told by Lucia's pediatrician "not to worry about the way she produces speech sounds; that's normal for her age." Therefore the diagnostician's interpretation of constituents as a group changes the clinical probabilities he might draw about cause–effect relationships.

All the cause–effect relationships examined are potential explanations for the patient's speech and language disorder, whether they are revealed in the constituent analysis or the diagnostician develops them from his inferential strategies. To derive the "best" clinical hypotheses the diagnostician must be skilled in problem solving. Because so little is known about cause–effect relationships for speech and language disorders, and because at times there is so little information available about patients, diagnosticians often work inferentially, (see for example Hubbell, 1981). The diagnostician must recognize the strengths and weaknesses of the inferences he makes, using his deductive and inductive reasoning abilities in the most logical way for deriving appropriate hypotheses. For example, he may have discovered in his analysis that Trisha, referred for a "speech disorder," had serious chronic bouts of otitis media from the age of 8 to 20 months. His analysis leads him to suspect that associated with otitis media were significant temporary hearing losses, even though this was not reported. From his knowledge and inferential reasoning he might develop a relationship between the bouts of otitis media, the hearing losses, and a presumed phonologic disorder. That is, a causal constituent has led him to a particular language product effect—an explanation he could arrive at only by using his knowledge and inferential strategy. In his diagnosis he has to "fill in" this relationship if it becomes his clinical hypothesis. Knowing that this hypothesis was derived inferentially should keep the diagnostician cautious and conservative about the diagnosis he makes from it.

SLPM schema for examining and deriving cause–effect relationships

It is vital to patient management that the diagnostician appreciate and understand the range and complexity of cause–effect interactions. Rather than search for a cause of each specific disorder he sees, the diagnostician must expect an interaction of causal factors. He needs to explain how the causal factors interacted to produce the disorder that he is currently seeing. Most speech and language disorders are not direct cause–effect relationships; by the time the diagnostician sees the patient, multiple factors must be accounted for. The diagnostician needs a perspective that addresses questions such as, How did this disorder come to be? What went wrong? When did it happen? How long did it last? How severe was it? Was anything done about it? What is going on now?

One of the major stumbling blocks to developing mutual professional understanding of cause–effect relationships is the diverse levels of abstraction used to predict and explain causality. For example, different diagnosticians all noting Trisha's inability to produce speech sounds requiring the use of the tongue might ascribe the following causes: she cannot move her tongue; her tongue muscles are not functioning properly; her genioglossus and styloglossus muscles are impaired in their functioning; she has paralysis of tongue musculature. All of these causal explanations refer to the same behavior, Trisha's lack of tongue movements to produce sounds. What may be noted here is that the observer's level of information and point of view can influence the way in which he abstracts.

Perkins and Curlee (1969) have discussed levels of abstraction. They note that no one level of abstraction is necessarily any more "correct" than another; the preference for a level of abstraction should be determined by its relevance to the stated questions. They suggest that for speech–language pathology the behavioral level may be most appropriate since the questions asked in diagnosis of speech and language disorders are too complex to be answered at any other level of abstraction. We would agree with Perkins and Curlee (1969) that the behavioral level may be very appropriate in many instances; however, it is not the only level that will explain satisfactorily all the complex cause–effect relationships seen in speech and language disorders. More complex views of cause–effect relationships that go beyond the behavioral level of abstraction are needed by the diagnostician (Sameroff, 1975; Duffy, Watt, & Duffy, 1981). What is important is that the diagnostician be able to explain the cause–effect relationships he develops, including the level of abstraction he chose for explaining causality.

Since the constituent analysis was performed within the SLPM framework, this same orientation can be used to derive the clinical hypothesis. Within the SLPM framework in Chapter 2 we developed a consistent schema that allowed the diagnostician (1) to classify speech and language disorders on three levels, (2) to scan the range of potential causal factors that may affect the patient's speech and language environment and/or processing system.

In this chapter we will further develop the SLPM perspective for examining and deriving clinical hypotheses. From the SLPM the diagnostician examines his cause–effect relationships in terms of speech and language products affected, behavioral correlates, and physical processes disrupted. Causal factors are viewed in terms of their effect on the speech and language environment and the speech and language processing system. In essence, the diagnostician places the patient into the SLPM; in each diagnosis the patient becomes a *mini slpm*.

The SLPM also provides the diagnostician with his basis for drawing inferences about the constituents when supporting information is not available. From this orientation the diagnostician may infer certain causal factors for the speech and language characteristics that have been revealed, or he may infer certain speech and language product disorders from available causal information. His power of inferential reasoning becomes a major tool for deriving his clinical hypothesis—sometimes the entire basis of the clinical hypothesis.

The diagnostician must develop perspectives that allow him to interpret the complexities of the cause–effect interactions—perspectives emphasizing that

1. Cause–effect relationships are multidimensional, complex, and dynamic, not static and unidimensional;
2. Contemporary disorders seen are a reflection of all that has come before.

To do this the SLPM schema for deriving clinical hypotheses develops three major perspectives, as represented in Figure 5-1. They are the *causal factor perspective, directness perspective,* and *timing perspective.* Using this diagram the diagnostician can focus on the multidimensional interactions that occur over time.

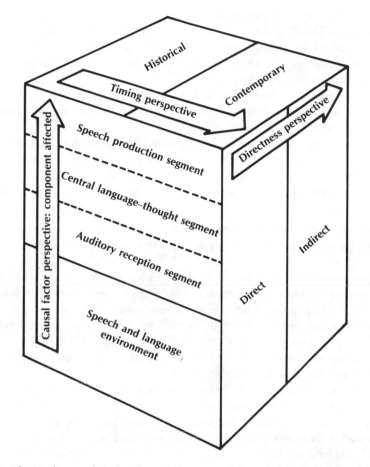

Figure 5-1. Three-dimensional schema for causal factors of speech and language disorders. Causal factors are plotted according to time, directness, and component affected by causal factor.

Causal factor perspective

Earlier, we developed a scanning mechanism (Table 4-1) that classified causal factors as (1) primarily affecting the speech and language environment and (2) primarily affecting the speech and language processing system. This scanning mechanism is the first dimension of our causal factor perspective (see Chapter 4). When he is trying to answer cause–effect questions, the diagnostician can use the SLPM scanning mechanism for causal factors to determine how the factors uncovered may have primarily affected the speech and language environment and/or primarily affected the speech and language processing system.

The use of this SLPM-based scanning mechanism for deriving clinical hypotheses has several distinct advantages.

1. The causal factors are not considered as specific etiologic categories. They are superordinate categories and serve as a search mechanism for any number of specific causal factors that could affect the speech and language environment and/or the speech and language processing system. Therefore the categories are flexible and open-ended.

2. The emphasis of the scanning mechanism is on what is affected rather than on the causal factor. Therefore the diagnostician is not impelled to learn long lists of etiologic factors. Instead, he searches for any factors or determinants that may help explain the speech and language disorder. The focus is on the interaction of causal factors with the components of the SLPM.
3. The traditional functional–organic dichotomy is deemphasized. Even though the scanning mechanism is built around environmental and physical processing factors, the intent is to discover cause–effect interactions.
4. The scanning mechanism provides a useful and flexible aid for the diagnostician for hypothesizing, analyzing, and interpreting dynamic cause–effect relationships rather than proposing static etiologies for speech and language disorders. It should force the diagnostician to consider a wide range of potential causal factors, thus reducing the myopia of each diagnostician's causal biases.

Now we expand this causal factor perspective to consider two other important dimensions, the *multiple nature of causation* and *chains of cause–effect interactions.*

• *Multiple nature of causation.* We in the speech and language disorder field have a problem common to other behavioral sciences, that of attempting to explain complex behavior with simple answers. What frequently results is a search for the cause of a speech and language disorder, particularly at the macro level, rather than undertaking the more complex task of recognizing multiple causation and interactions. Much of the thrust behind "differential diagnosis," as so often used in speech pathology, emanated from or resulted in this search for *the* cause (Myklebust, 1954).

Perhaps it has been easier to look for a specific cause of a speech and language disorder than it has been to look for the multiplicity of factors that may account for the sequelae of behavior that truly confront us. For example, we may be able to relate directly Noel's cleft palate to his resonance and phonetic structure disorder; but does it account for all of his speech and language abilities? There may be other factors in Noel's history that have to be considered in a multiple causation hypothesis. In children born with cleft palates the literature cites other factors as potentially causal, some of which have more clinical and research support than others. In Noel's case we would want to consider hearing loss (Nation, 1970), dental and occlusal deviations (Starr, 1971), hospitalization (Nation, 1970), and other psychosocial and cognitive factors (Goodstein, 1968; Fox, Lynch, & Brookshire, 1978). Besides these primary causal considerations, the diagnostician would also consider other experiences Noel has encountered, many of which may have nothing to do with the fact that he was born with a cleft palate. For instance, Noel resides within a certain family constellation and a certain sociocultural setting, all of which contribute to the speech and language input he receives. These multiple causal factors and their interactions account for the differences diagnosticians see among patients defined as the same "problem type," in this example, cleft palate.

It is only from attempting to identify the multiple-sided nature of causation that diagnosticians can obtain fuller understanding of the presented disorder, leading to more effective remedial plans. Thus, in his consideration of cause–effect relationships the diagnostician should be searching for causes, not *the* cause. As Kessler (1966) has stated:

> ... all behavior, whether normal or abnormal is overdetermined; no single act can be explained in terms of one determinant or one variable. ... Diagnostic formulations are likely to be in paragraph form, rather than in single terms, describing both the strengths and the problems of the child and postulating the major contributing factors, usually several in number. (p. 87)

Analyze this patient from a multiple causation view. Fred was born after a prolonged labor; he weighed 8 pounds and 14 ounces. Bruises were apparent on his head, and he was slow to begin breathing. At 6 months of age a medical diagnosis of cerebral palsy was made. Now, at 6 years of age, he speaks in unintelligible "one-word" responses and seems to comprehend little of what is said to him. His hearing has been tested; he responded at 500, 1,000, and 2,000 Hz at 50 dB HL. His IQ score obtained from the Cattell (1947) was 50.

• *Chains of cause–effect interactions.* One cause often causes a second cause, which causes yet another cause, and so on. Causal factors are frequently seen as a part of a chain, or series, of cause–effect relationships. We often see confusion in placing a causal factor within its relative position in a series of cause–effect relationships. As Kessler (1971) has pointed out, the behavioral outcome does not always reveal which cause came first.

Diagnosticians sometimes find themselves tracking down a chain of original causation. For example, the cause for Philip's inability to elevate his tongue may be muscular paralysis; the cause for the paralysis may have been fetal anoxia; the cause of fetal anoxia may have been maternal toxemia; the cause of maternal toxemia may have been poor nutritional health of the mother; the mother's poor nutritional health may have been caused by an inadequate income. In such a chain of cause–effect relationships it may not be possible, practical, or useful to arrive at the ultimate causation. The diagnostician's concern is in recognizing the relationships among all these causes, some currently operating and some of only historical significance. Which causes, in such a series of cause–effect relationships, are of importance to the diagnostician? Can we ever truly arrive at the ultimate causation, and even if we do, what difference does it make? These are issues that the diagnostician must face in searching out the complexities of chains of cause–effect interactions.

What might the series, or chain, of cause–effect interactions be in the following patient? Ed, 3 years of age, has virtually no comprehension or formulation of language. His only output is an occasional use of jargon sound sequences seldom used in a communication situation. His history reveals an alcoholic, syphilitic mother (both conditions present during her pregnancy with Ed). When he was born, Ed was jaundiced and required an immediate blood transfusion. He remained hospitalized for over 2 months; on several occasions he almost died. He was removed from his home at 1 year of age because of parental neglect. At that time he weighed only 16 pounds. He is now is a state institution for the retarded. When he was admitted, the diagnosis was profound mental retardation.

Directness perspective

Any given causal factor may have both *direct* and *indirect* effects on speech and language learning and use. Consider, for example, the causal factor of Down's syndrome or other genetic factors known to cause significant mental retardation. While the mental retardation accompanying Down's syndrome may be seen to be directly responsible for much of the language delay presented, this same causal factor, Down's syndrome, may also account for other less direct influences on a child's language. For example, a parent's inability to accept such a child may result in limited verbal interaction between the parent and child. The child may be provided with little opportunity for sensorimotor exploration and learning in his environment. Thus the causal factor of Down's syndrome may both directly contribute to reduced language learning and indirectly influence the amount of speech and language input provided.

In another example the causal factor of chronic otitis media would directly affect the auditory reception segment of the speech and language processing component, affecting the physical process of auditory acceptance–transduction and the behavioral correlate of sensation. This direct disruption, if severe enough, could also result in significant perception, comprehension, integration, and formulation difficulties by limiting the auditory information needed by other physical processes. Thus, otitis media as a disease has a direct, primary effect on the auditory reception segment as well as indirectly affecting other segments of the processing system. Still another indirect effect of the disease is on the speech and language input provided by the mother. If the child is not responsive to auditory stimulation, the mother might unconsciously reduce the amount of talking she does to the child, completely unaware that she has done so.

Similarly, causal factors more directly affecting the amount and type of speech and language input may have an indirect effect on the processing system. An extreme example is seen in the reported cases of the so-called feral children (Lenneberg, 1967) who, after several years of living with wolves and presumably being exposed to no speech and language stimulation, were unable to learn to talk beyond a very basic level. Here the absence of speech and language input apparently led to an inability to process speech and language at a later age. A less extreme example of a similar effect is the reported results on speech and language development of children living in institutions (Brodbeck & Irwin, 1946; Goldfarb, 1945–1946; Mussen et al., 1969).

Thus, mere specification of a causal factor does not ensure the directness or potency of its effect on the individual. The point here is that a particular causal factor does not always have a known, invariant effect on an individual. Rather, in one instance a factor may be direct *or* indirect in its effect, while in another instance it may be *both* direct and indirect.

Consider this patient from a direct–indirect causal view. Robert, 5 years old, has a significant phonologic disorder. He primarily uses vowel sounds, although the phonemes /p,b,t and d/ are heard with some frequency. His history reveals mildly slow physical development, visual acuity that borders on legal blindness that was not discovered until he was 2 years of age, and a bilingual background—his parents speak English, but his grandparents who live with the family generally speak German. After his visual problem was discovered, his mother seldom left him alone; she became quite anxious and fearful of what might happen to him.

Timing perspective

The variable effect of time is a major perspective through which causal factors must be interpreted. It is one thing to propose a direct cause–effect relationship that specifies what causal factor might have resulted in the onset of a speech and language disorder, however, a question of equal priority is how the disorder developed. A speech and language disorder does not come into existence and develop in a unidimensional manner. From the time of onset to the time of diagnosis, many influences have come to bear on the patient's use of speech and language.

Diagnosticians need to view causal factors in terms of when they happened, how severe they were, how long they persisted, and what has been done about them. Timing considerations are our way of maintaining a "developmental viewpoint" about speech and language disorders. What is seen when a patient appears is a result of interactions over time. Some of these interactions have been positive, for example, the mother who might increase her verbal stimulation to a child who is retarded. Others are negative influences, for example, the mother who rejects her child who has a cleft lip and palate, thus spending little time with him. Sameroff (1975) makes this point concerning developmental adaptation to early "causal factors."

> Developmental outcomes must be interpreted as the products of a child's characteristics, his material environment and the cognitive levels and values of his social milieu. Where the social environment fosters rigidity, stereotyping, and concreteness in thought and behavior, early deviancies can become resistant to the normal restructuring implicit in development. Where flexibility, openness, and adaptability are fundamental characteristics of the environment, early problems are dissipated as the child advances in his construction and organization of both his cognitive and social world. (Sameroff, 1975, p. 291)

Some exceptions to this point could be raised. Certain disorders seem more direct and unidimensional, for example, the adult who sustains brain injury resulting in a language disorder (aphasia). This language disorder is a direct concomitant of a causal factor—brain damage. However, by the time the diagnostician sees this patient for diagnosis and treatment he is no longer seeing a direct effect. True, the basic language disorder is because of the brain damage, but by now there will be other dimensions to consider regarding the aphasic's language usage. The spouse may reject the aphasic and not provide speech and language interaction. The patient may be so depressed that he withdraws and refuses to communicate. These are some of the potential concomitants that may be seen; again, they make the diagnostician's causal interpretation of the patient's disorder multidimensional rather than unidimensional. Thus, even when the cause–effect relationship seems direct, the diagnostician must always remember that timing considerations can affect the speech and language disorder he eventually sees.

Basic to our timing perspective is a time continuum, ranging from the distant past to contemporary events. From this time continuum we discuss causal factors as historical causation and contemporary causation. Viewing causation as historical or contemporary allows us to interpret causation in two important senses: causation as historical events that have affected speech and language and causation as seen in current input and processing deviations.

- *Historical causation.* Historical causation refers to any past events that have affected either the speech and language environment component or the speech and language processing component, and it essentially demonstrates the interactions between causal factors and the components of the SLPM over time.

Plotting causal factors from a timing perspective forces the diagnostician to consider the *time of occurrence* of any causal factor. For example, maternal rubella in the first trimester produces a more generalized and devastating effect on the central nervous system of the embryo than in later pregnancy. A moderate sensorineural hearing loss acquired at 8 years of age will not have the same effect on speech and language that it would if acquired at 11 months of age. Similarly, the addition of a new sibling may characteristically create feelings for a 2-year-old that are not experienced by an 8-year-old.

Plotting historical causal factors from a timing perspective also allows the diagnostician to examine causal interactions over time, highlighting multiple causation, chains of cause–effect interactions, and direct–indirect effects of causal factors. For example, while a child may have been born with a cleft lip and palate, his structural and psychological condition at 5 years of age is quite different. At birth the child may have a cleft palate (biological makeup–structural defect) that "causes" repeated middle ear infections (diseases) as well as repeated hospitalizations (experiential restrictions) during the early language-learning years. Not only has he probably had numerous surgical and therapeutic procedures but also time to develop an attitude about himself and his condition (psychological–emotional mechanisms). Therefore in considering causal variables diagnosticians are concerned not only with occurrences that clearly are past history such as pre-, peri-, and postnatal factors but also occurrences that, while part of the patient's history, may continue. For example, chronic medical conditions, emotional instability, and many other dimensions of the patient's life style may be ongoing influences.

To visually represent the use of the timing perspective in interaction with the causal factor perspective we have prepared Figure 5-2 for study. The causal constituent analysis can be explored in this fashion to derive clinical hypothesis.

• *Contemporary causation.* Contemporary causation in our timing perspective is concerned with the patient in the here and now. As well as knowing and understanding historical causation we also want a clear understanding of the patient's current status. In addressing contemporary causation the diagnostician searches for the presently existing input and processing deviations that may account for the observed speech and language disorder. The presumption, of course, is that contemporary causation may have its basis in historical causation. For example, a current hearing loss, disrupting physical processing, may well have been present for some time.

Contemporary causation emphasizes disrupted physical processes and behavioral correlates as causal factors, which may explain the disordered product. For example, a disruption in speech programming (physical process) or sequencing (behavioral correlate) could be cited as the contemporary causation for a child's phonologic disorder. Or paralysis of the tongue (historical and contemporary cause) prevents the articulation process (physical process as a contemporary cause) from taking place and is observed in poor motor control (behavioral correlate as a contemporary cause). This poor motor control results in many phonetic structure errors (speech product disorder). Thus, poor motor control, a behavioral correlate, can be cited as the contemporary cause of the phonetic structure disorder.

We could even go so far as to say that a child's comprehension, integration, and formulation problems (behavioral correlates) are the contemporary causes for his language product disorder. In some ways this is a departure from frequent diagnostic practice. Sensation, perception, sequencing, and motor control (behavioral correlates on the SLPM) often are cited as causes for speech and language disorders; however, seldom would comprehension, integration, or formulation be considered as causes, contemporary or otherwise. We do not really advocate the use of comprehension as a cause but do want to make the point that current processing deficits measured as behavioral correlates can be profitably considered as contemporary causation.

Distinguishing contemporary causation in our timing perspective is vital to the diagnostician for the following reasons.

1. It more closely ties what is going on currently with the speech and language disorder.
2. The speech and language disorder cannot be accounted for just on the basis of historical causation.

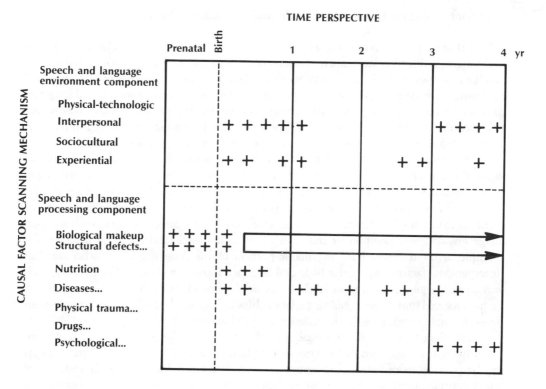

Figure 5-2. Plotting causal factors of hypothetical patient: Celeste, 4 years of age, was born with bilateral cleft of primary and secondary palates. A study of speech and language disorders of children with cleft lip and palate will assist in interpreting this figure. A + = an adverse condition suggested as being present within a 3-month time period.

3. At times, even though historical causation has been relevant for understanding the speech and language disorder, it is no longer particularly relevant for management.

4. Contemporary causation may be available for change, whereas historical causation may not.

Bertheva, 5 years of age, has a moderate sensorineural hearing loss present since she was 3 years of age. Develop a summary cause–effect statement from our historical–contemporary time perspective.

Viewing causation for speech and language disorders from the causal factor, directness, and timing perspectives gives diagnosticians a more complete picture of the complex, dynamic basis for cause–effect relationships. The diagnostician will arrive at much better solutions to his diagnostic problems by taking this complex route through causation than by using lists of causal factors or etiologic classification systems as his means of explaining how a speech and language disorder came to be. In something as complex as speech and language behavior diagnosticians cannot expect to arrive at a static, stable picture of causation. Instead, they must appreciate the complexities of interactions that take place over time.

Impact of causal factors on speech and language behavior

Now that we have presented the various perspectives toward our causal schema for speech and language disorders we want to demonstrate generally the impact that causal factors can have on speech and language processing and behavior. Through our examples we intend to illustrate the complex, dynamic interactions that go on to create a speech and language disorder. Our purpose is to provide a means for analysis and interpretation of the cause–effect relationships of importance to the diagnostician, not to discuss specific causal factors.

Figure 5-3 represents a set of basic interactions that can exist between causal factors and components of the SLPM. From this figure the diagnostician can draw any number of example cause–effect relationships. The timing perspective in Figure 5-3 is represented simply by a two-dimensional arrow; its purpose is to focus the diagnostician's attention on the fact that these multidimensional causal interactions are always occurring over time.

Interaction 1 implies that there is an adverse causal factor affecting the speech and language environment component that can result in a speech and language disorder. For example, a child exposed for the major portion of his time to parents who are deaf (interpersonal factor) may receive little oral language input stimulation. The child's speech and language product will most likely be reduced, dependent on how much stimulation he has received from other significant relationships in his speech and language environment (interpersonal factor). Thus, in this interaction the characteristics of the speech and language product reflect the quantity and quality of the speech and language input stimulation.

Recall that we suggested that environmental factors be analyzed in terms of their effects on the parameters of speech and language input. After the diagnostician has identified any potential causal factors, he must explain how the factor exerted its influence on the quantity and quality of the input, which parameters have been affected, and how this might account for the observed speech and language disorder.

For example, twinning may present a situation where the primary companionship is each other. Each child's predominant phonologic and syntactic input may come from the other twin rather than from more mature older siblings or parents. However, these twins may be given adequate opportunity for sensorimotor stimulation and exploration that contributes to their semantic development. Thus, twinning as a "causal factor" may differentially affect the speech and language input parameters, not necessarily reducing input "across the board." In another set of twins there may be other siblings or playmates close to their age, providing them with normal speech and language input on all levels. Therefore a particular factor identified (in this example, twinning) does not have an automatic influence on the speech and language input. Instead, the influence depends on the particular multidimensional environmental context created.

While research has begun to describe the linguistic characteristics of the normal child's speech and language environment, the questions of quality, quantity, source, and timing of speech and language input remain largely untouched. How do competing environmental stimuli affect the language learner's ability to receive speech and language input? How direct must the stimulation be for the learner to profit from its information? Must the language learner be actively involved in receiving, manipulating, and reformulating the language input, or may he be a passive observer of the speech and language scene? A basic question yet unanswered is how much stimulation is enough and under what conditions. Is "one-shot" exposure sufficient for a child to have gained from the language experience, or is repeated presentation necessary? What do we know about the differential effects of various sources of language input? Is one source, possibly the mother, a more potent language

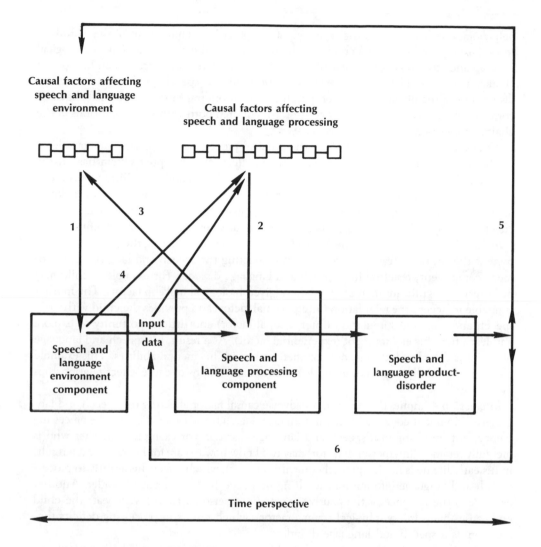

Figure 5-3. Schematic of basic causal interactions

provider than other sources? What contribution, if any, do the radio and television make to language learning? What is the appropriate timing of speech and language stimulation, and how do the requirements change over time? Is one form of stimulation more effective at one age than at another or more appropriate for providing data for one level of language than for another?

Interaction 2 implies that there is a adverse causal factor affecting physical processing that can result in a speech and language disorder. For example, an adult who sustains brain injury (physical trauma and accident factor) to the central language–thought segment may present a language disorder termed aphasia. The specific characteristics of his language disorder will be related to the location and severity of the brain injury. Thus, in Interaction 2 the speech and language disorder is reflective of the disrupted physical processes and behavioral correlates within the segments of the processing component of the SLPM. A second example could be of a child born with damage to the cerebellum (given biological makeup and structural defect factors). Viewed as a direct relationship, this child's speech characteristics would be reflective of disruptions in the speech production segment— disruptions of the physical process of speech coordination–transmission and the behavioral correlates of sequencing and motor control. (In children born with such conditions entire chains of cause–effect interactions are seen.)

Whenever causal factors that affect the physical processing component are considered by the diagnostician, he is concerned with the effects the disrupted system has on the patient's ability to derive information from input stimulation and his abilitiy to formulate and produce messages. In management considerations the diagnostician will want to know if he can alter the way in which the patient processes the speech and language data to effect better speech and language behavior (contemporary causation viewpoint).

Interaction 3 implies that there is an adverse causal factor affecting the processing component that in turn creates an adverse factor affecting the speech and language environment component, resulting in a speech and language disorder. For example, a child may be born with significant mental retardation (given biological makeup factor). The mother is unable to accept the retardation (interpersonal factor) and provides the child with little speech and language stimulation (interpersonal factor) and little opportunity to explore and learn from his environment (experiential factor). As a result, his speech and language behavior is disordered, that is, not commensurate with his mental abilities. This example also provides an illustration of multiple causation and chains of cause–effect relationships over time.

Interaction 4 implies that there is an adverse causal factor affecting the speech and language environment component that in turn creates an adverse factor affecting the processing component, resulting in a speech and language disorder. For example, a mother who is mentally retarded (interpersonal factor) may not know how to care for her child. As a result, in his early life he is not fed properly (nutrition factor), which affects his abilitiy to process speech and language information, resulting in a speech and language disorder. Another example is the instance of the abusive parent (interpersonal factor) who beats the child and causes brain injury (physical trauma factor), which results in processing deficits that are seen as a speech and language disorder.

Interaction 5 implies that the speech and language output product (whether normal or disordered) creates an adverse factor affecting the speech and language environment component, resulting in a speech and language disorder. For example, a child may be mentally retarded and yet developing speech and language within his abilities (normal speech and language product), but his parents cannot accept the level of development (interpersonal factor) and begin to put excessive demands (interpersonal factor) on the child for "better" speech and language. As a result, the child withdraws (psychological–emotional mechanism factor) from interpersonal communication, using less speech and language than before. In this example we reintroduced Interaction 4 to complete the series of cause–effect relationships.

Interaction 6 implies that the speech and language output product (whether normal or disordered) serves as input data to the speaker creating an adverse factor affecting the processing component, resulting in a speech and language disorder. For example, an adult male coach has a normally high pitch (normal speech output product) but does not like the way it sounds; it does not fit his self-image (psychological–emotional mechanism factor). In order to project a "masculine image" he lowers his pitch (disordered speech process), which results in contact ulcers on the vocal folds (physical trauma factor), resulting in a more pervasive voice disorder.

These are the six basic interactions demonstrated in Figure 5-3. Any number of other interactions can be illustrated by following the arrows in the directions indicated as many times as needed to explain the multiple, serial, direct–indirect interactions that may have occurred in the development of the speech and language disorder. All six of the basic interactions or any combination of the six over time could apply to a patient being seen. For example, a child born with a cleft lip and palate (given biological makeup and structural defect factors) will encounter other causal factors as a result of this condition and its treatment. During his early life he may have difficulty feeding (nutrition factor). He will certainly undergo surgery (experiential and physical trauma factors), perhaps require orthodontia (physical trauma factor), may have a number of x-ray studies done (irradiation factor), undoubtedly sustain middle ear infections (disease factor), and be treated for them (physical trauma and drugs factor). Later in life he may be seen for speech and language diagnosis and treatment (interpersonal factors). All these factors in interaction would seem to be enough to result in a speech and language disorder even though many of them are rehabilitation procedures utilized to prevent such a disorder. However, with this child the diagnostician may also see a mother who is rejecting, guilty, and overprotective (interpersonal factor), who does not stimulate the child verbally (interpersonal factor), who will not let him out of her sight (experiential factor), and who does not have the income to care for the child properly (sociocultural and physical–technologic factors). At the same time the father may blame the mother for the birth of this child (interpersonal factor), begin to drink excessively (interpersonal factor), abuse both the mother and child (interpersonal and psychological–emotional mechanism factors), and finally leave the home for parts unknown (interpersonal and experiential factors). The child may have a severe reaction to his own disordered speech (disordered speech product) and develop feelings of insecurity, anxiety, and worthlessness (psychological–emotional mechanisms), and then give up trying to make his speech sound any better. This example would seem to take into account all the basic causal interactions and then some.

Develops a hierarchy of probable cause–effect explanations

From his examination of cause–effect relationships the diagnostician hopes to arrive at some conclusions that potentially explain the patient's clinical problem. The chances are there will be more than a single relationship revealed, and the diagnostician will then develop a hierarchy, a set of priorities, for explaining the speech and language disorder. If, for instance, the integration of the constituents indicates that Aiko has severely delayed language on all linguistic levels but no causal information has been provided, the diagnostician will have to recall and research the most likely causes for severe language delay in children and order his set of explanations accordingly. He might infer a number of causal factors: mental retardation, childhood aphasia, or deafness. From a disrupted processing viewpoint he might infer language–thought representation or speech production. Or he might infer that Aiko just arrived from Japan and has not had enough exposure to the English language.

The diagnostician rules in and out the various interactions until he arrives at a set of relationships he feels will explain the speech and language disorder. This set is ordered in terms of the diagnostician's reasoning that one expressed relationship explains the disorder better than another. The more closely related the explanation is to the time of onset of the disorder and of expected disruptions in speech and language processing, the more likely it may be as a potential explanation.

In developing his set of probable explanations the diagnostician may put at the top of his list a cause–effect relationship that has less information from the constituent analysis than another; however, it may be more theoretically secure because of the diagnostician's inferential strategy. His explanation for the disorder may be better, more appropriately computed, than the explanation offered by the constituents. Or the diagnostician may develop a relationship that has led him to different explanations than those provided by the referral source or the parent in the statement of the problem on the case history questionnaire. There will be many such statements of the problem offered that are not theoretically secure, particularly as they relate to causal factors, for example, when a parent states that "Chloe does not talk because she doesn't eat right." Even if he hypothesizes a different causal route, the diagnostician still has to account for these other statements and referrals in his overall planning. At times he derives not only his own clinical hypothesis but also poses clinical hypotheses ordering the cause–effect relationship in the way it is viewed by the referral source or the parents.

For example, suppose that the constituent analysis has indicated that Ellen has disordered phonetic structure. When she produces the /s, z, ∫ , and dʒ / phonemes, they are distorted by lateral emission of air. The only causal constituents that were available came from the mother's statement. Mrs. Wirley felt that Ellen's speech problem was due to her inattentiveness. "When I tried to show Ellen how to say the sounds, Ellen wouldn't pay attention and do it." Now this constituent might be important to the overall analysis of Ellen's problem; however, it is not very secure theoretically as a causal factor and could not be placed at the top of the diagnostician's list of potential explanations. Instead, his inferential strategy may lead him to consider a different set of explanations: (1) disrupted articulation process—a contemporary causal explanation; (2) maturation—Ellen is not ready to produce these sounds; (3) dental deviations—malocclusion; and (4) mislearning—She is now maintaining these sound productions through habit strength. These may be only some of the inferences the diagnostician makes for this example, which represents only one possible ordering of the explanations. How the set is ordered depends on the strength and support for each cause–effect relationship expressed, including the one presented by Mrs. Wirley.

Any inappropriate referrals and associated problems should be revealed during this hypothesis task if not before. The diagnostician should discover them when he examines the relationships between causes and effects. Associated problems that are not causally related cannot be integrated into a cause–effect relationship. At times a patient will be seen who has a significant history of emotional difficulty, but the emotional difficulties are not responsible for the speech and language disorder; nor is the speech and language disorder necessarily related to the emotional difficulty. Patients who are seen with stuttering behavior sometimes represent this complex relationship. The diagnostician has to sort out the relationship of the stuttering behavior to the patient's personality, his emotional difficulties. Each problem may need to be explored and treated, but not necessarily by the speech–language pathologist. The diagnostician must be aware when he examines cause–effect relationships that not all the problem areas he views in a given patient will have causal relationships, even though they may have an effect on the patient's overall communicative interaction—his adjustment to life.

Thus, throughout this first task the diagnostician is looking for the *most to the least likely potential explanations*, his own explanation perhaps being more likely than the explanations offered by others. At times the diagnostician may develop his list of priorities based on the preponderance of the information he has available, whereas at other times he must rely more heavily on his inferential strategies. Sometimes his inferences take precedence over the specific information available. In either instance he must provide his reasoning for the explanations he is offering. As a result of his ability to derive potential clinical hypotheses, the diagnostician arrives at a set of explanations ordered in a most likely to least likely hierarchy.

STATES THE CLINICAL HYPOTHESIS AS A CAUSE–EFFECT RELATIONSHIP

Now that the cause–effect relationships have been derived, the diagnostician's second task at this step is to formally state his most likely clinical hypothesis and propose alternative hypotheses, explanations that were not considered as the most probable hypothesis but that could become a more likely hypothesis before the diagnostic process is completed.

Statement of the most likely clinical hypothesis

From the first task where he ordered the list of potential cause–effect relationships, the diagnostician selects the most likely to him and formally states this as his clinical hypothesis—stated as clearly as possible to reveal the potential solution to the clinical problem. It is important to remember that, unlike the researcher, the diagnostician is not stating a hypothesis that he wishes to prove or disprove. Instead, the clinical hypothesis is conceived of as a working hypothesis, a guide to his clinical design.

We want to make it clear to the student that this formal statement of the clinical hypothesis is the diagnostician's working hypothesis. It is not generally used in a discussion with parents or other professionals, nor does it appear in reports as "the statement of the problem." It is the diagnostician's diagnostic guide. At times, however, when he is talking to a parent he might say, "I'm thinking about approaching Denise's problem this way." Or to a professional referral source he might say, "It appears to me that Bonnie's stuttering might really be normal nonfluencies." These types of discussions are statement of the diagnostician's hypotheses to other sources, but they are qualitatively different from the formal statement and are used quite differently.

Even though it is a working hypothesis, the hypothesis is a statement of probability. In his formally stated hypothesis the diagnostician is inferring that the stated disorder is related to the stated causal factor. Thus, the wording of the hypothesis is of prime importance. The statement gives direct evidence for the diagnostician's level of understanding and security about the clinical problem. The following two sample hypotheses reflect, through their wording, different levels of security between the stated disorder and its cause: (1) Herbert has a language disorder related to mental retardation that appears to be secondary to brain injury sustained at birth. (2) Herbert has a language disorder due to mental retardation that was caused by the brain injury he sustained at birth.

Furthermore, the way in which the hypothesis is worded will imply various interpretations of the stated cause–effect relationship. The hypothesis statement can be modified according to severity as denoted by "mild," "moderate," and "severe." In addition, it can be ordered chronologically according to time of onset as expressed by the terms "congenital," "acquired," "prenatal," "developmental," and "recurrent." Even the general ordering of several causal factors embedded within the hypothesis has implications as to their "direct" or "indirect" importance as determiners of a particular speech disorder.

What is the difference in the causal emphasis placed on these two hypotheses? (1) Anthony has a voice disorder resulting from vocal abuse that caused contact ulcers. (2) Anthony has a voice disorder related to the presence of contact ulcers that stemmed from constant vocal abuse. Will these two hypotheses signal any differences in your approach to the diagnosis or to your possible management of the problem?

Of special importance to the diagnostician is the level of abstraction at which he states his hypothesis. If a hypothesis is too abstract, it becomes open–ended; everything is possible: "Pequetti has a speech disorder due to many causes." If it is too specific, it becomes subject to greater error; too little is possible: "John produces the /m, n, and ŋ / phonemes without appropriate nasal resonance due to hypertrophied adenoids that are blocking the nasopharynx." All clinical hypotheses cannot be expressed as specific, concrete causes and effects. The diagnostician seldom has enough prior information to allow for such specificity, although he tends to know more about specific effects (behaviors) than causes. More often the hypothesis is stated abstractly, expressing a general relationship among the cause–effect factors under consideration. Further empirical testing is usually required before the hypothesis can be stated in specific terms.

Regardless of the level of abstraction, however, the diagnostician's statement of his clinical hypothesis should express a relationship that assists him in designing the diagnostic session. The broader, more abstract the hypothesis, the more open-ended the design; the narrower, less abstract the hypothesis, the more specific the design. For example, if a hypothesis is stated as "Linda cannot say her /l, r, t, d, and n/ sounds because she can't elevate her tongue due to an extremely short lingual frenum," and this is a true hypothesis, the remainder of the diagnostic process is rather clearly specified.

For every patient seen a hypothesis can be stated—even if at a high level of abstraction. The diagnostician must learn how to state his hypothesis at the most useful level of abstraction warranted by the information and still offer a potential solution to the clinical problem. He can build security into his clinical hypothesis by stating it at various levels of abstraction; that is, he can create a series of hypotheses around the same cause–effect relationship. Within this series of hypotheses he hopes to find the true hypothesis. For example, from the same information about a patient the following series of clinical hypotheses might be derived—stated from the least to the most specific.

1. Rufus has a language disorder related to a hearing loss.
2. Rufus has a language disorder related to an auditory processing deficit caused by a sensorineural hearing loss.
3. Rufus has a language disorder characterized by both comprehension and formulation disruptions related to an auditory perceptual problem that is secondary to an auditory processing deficit, due to a sensorineural hearing loss resulting from eighth nerve damage.
4. Rufus has a language comprehension and formulation disorder primarily on the phonologic level related to his inability to process (discriminate) the phonemes of his language. This processing deficit is related to his sensorineural hearing loss that was caused by eighth nerve damage.

This series of hypothesis statements reflects several levels of understanding the diagnostician has about the information available to him. The first hypothesis might be chosen because it is more open-ended; the diagnostician would design a more comprehensive diagnosis. However, he may feel secure with his derivation and go for the fourth hypothesis, thereby designing a more specific diagnosis. Part of this task—stating the hypothesis—is related to the diagnostician's comfort level. That is, how comfortable is he with his understanding of the information, with his ability to use his professional knowledge at the risky inferential level?

Proposes alternative hypotheses

If there are indications from his derivation task of more than one potential cause–effect relationship, the diagnostician must now propose his alternative hypothesis. There will be as many alternative hypothesis as warranted by the cause–effect relationships revealed during the constituent analysis and the hypothesis derivation tasks. One source of a potential alternative hypotheses arises when the diagnostician's derivation does not match the statement of the problem presented by others. Earlier we presented an example patient, Ellen, whose mother felt she had sound errors because of inattentiveness. On the other hand, the diagnostician may have derived a clinical hypothesis that pointed strongly to a malocclusion as responsible for the sound distortions, and he stated this formally as his clinical hypothesis. Now he can state an alternative hypothesis more in line with the mother's concern; even if he believes this not to be at all likely, he is stating it to fulfill certain purposes of diagnosis. Thus, he may state an alternative hypothesis as "Ellen has sound distortions because she is inattentive to methods of teaching her how to produce them." In his design he would then determine if Ellen could be attentive and learn the production of these phonemes. He would then be able to discuss this consideration with the mother during the interpretive conference.

Alternative hypotheses express different cause–effect relationships and purposes than stated in the primary hypothesis, the original clinical hypothesis. The following examples illustrate this.

1. Alterations of the causal factor:
   a. Lamar has a language disorder related to mental retardation.
   b. Lamar has a language disorder related to brain injury.

2. Alterations of the speech and language disorder:
   a. Bertha has a language disorder related to cerebral palsy.
   b. Bertha has an articulation disorder related to cerebral palsy.
   c. Bertha has a prosody disorder related to cerebral palsy.

3. Alterations of both the causal factor and the speech and language disorder:
   a. Ed has a language disorder (aphasia) due to a cerebrovascular accident.
   b. Ed has a phonetic structure disorder related to an unspecified neurologic disease.
   c. Ed has a voice disorder related to Huntington's chorea.

These alternative hypotheses are ordered by the diagnostician, following the original hypothesis in terms of probability of correctness from most to least likely. This ordering provides him with his probability estimate. His original hypothesis is his best, followed in decreasing order of probability by each of the alternative hypotheses ordered from 1 to *n* alternatives. Of course, the diagnostician anticipates his original hypothesis to be the "true" hypothesis, but if not, his hope is that the "true" hypothesis is embedded within his alternatives. As he proceeds with his diagnosis, his order of probability may change, his third alternative becoming the most likely, and his original hypothesis becoming his least likely. Alternative hypotheses must be incorporated into the design of the diagnosis along with the original hypothesis. Therefore they, too, must be stated with clarity, express a potential solution to the clinical problem, and be worded at an appropriate level of abstraction.

A final alternative hypothesis must be proposed by the diagnostician. He always proposes that the patient may have no speech and language problem and states the alternative, the "null" clinical hypothesis: "Andrea has no speech and language disorder." Whenever the diagnostician states a possible clinical hypothesis: "Kay has a speech and language disorder related to——" he automatically states the alternative: "Kay has no speech and language disorder." This alternative is particularly important since all speech and language disorders are comparative—compared to normal speech and language development and usage. The alternative hypotheses keep the diagnostician on track, that is, to focus on the distinctions between speech and language variations versus disorders. It also assists in viewing certain causal factors, and one that comes immediately to mind is mental retardation. The diagnostician must know that mental retardation can slow down a child's use of speech and language, but this slowdown may well be normal within the degree of mental retardation. So the alternative hypothesis of no speech and language disorder applies. A strange way of putting this is "There may be a cause—but no effect."

EVALUATES THE QUALITY OF THE HYPOTHESIS

The diagnostician's third task in developing the clinical hypothesis is to make an evaluation of the quality of the hypothesis he has stated. This task formally explicates why and how the particular hypothesis is offered and examines the strength of the hypothesis. The diagnostician must account for why he has derived one hypothesis rather than another. Even though we are presenting this quality evaluation as the third task in developing the hypothesis, it should be apparent that this task also runs throughout the second step of the diagnostic process.

When he evaluates the quality of his hypothesis, the diagnostician is concerned about both the specification of his hypothesis and the support he can offer for it, that is, the arguments he might present to defend his hypothesis. To do this he must have guidelines and criteria for evaluating the quality of his hypothesis.

In specifying his hypothesis the diagnostician strives for absolute clarity of statement. He provides an unambiguous statement that includes formal propositions and specifications for testing them. In our discussion of the previous task, points were made about clarity of terms, levels of abstraction, and ways of expressing the cause–effect relationships.

Ringel (1972) suggests that the diagnostician evaluate his clinical hypothesis in terms of the following two questions: (1) Is it clearly stated and pertinent to the solution of the problem? (2) Does it reflect an adequate understanding of the problem or an objective attitude? Other questions might be asked: (3) What is the strength of the relationship expressed in the hypothesis? (4) What are the factual versus inferential aspects of the hypothesis? (5) Are the relationships expressed in the hypothesis available for testing? (6) What are the sources of error in the hypothesis? (7) What support is available for this hypothesis versus alternative hypotheses?

Another way of evaluating the clinical hypothesis with emphasis on the causal relationship comes from Duffy et al. (1981). They state:

> The basic goal of science is to establish relationships among variables which *describe, explain,* and *predict*. A relationship which fulfills all these requirements is generally called *causal*. Several general, interrelated conditions must be met before a relationship between two

variables can be called causal. These conditions may be labelled *spatial contiguity, temporal priority, covariance,* and *necessary connection.* (p. 475)

Spatial contiguity implies that the cause and effect must be together in physical space and the units of analysis are specified. Temporal priority reveals that the cause is sufficient to explain the effect and comes before the effect in time. Covariance indicates that if you vary either the cause or the effect you anticipate corresponding changes in the other. Necessary connection requires that an appropriate rationale exists for hypothesizing the cause–effect relationship. It assumes that there is an appropriate rationale for the hypothesis, a basis for the connection between the cause and the effect.

The diagnostician responds to these evaluative questions and concepts by presenting his arguments both in support of and in opposition to the hypothesis he has derived. For the practicing diagnostician this might be in the form of the mental process he goes through prior to the diagnostic session. In some settings staff participation may be required. In these settings the diagnostician may have to prepare a more formalized presentation. This is likely in settings where staffings form the basis of diagnosis, and it is a practice we require of students in training. When supporting his hypothesis, the diagnostician presents his documentation, his arguments; he shows the evolution of the problem from his fund of knowledge and from the literature that supports it. The diagnostician's supportive arguments come from his constituent analysis and hypothesis derivation, which reflect his reasoning abilities. Any errors he has made are reflected in the quality of the hypothesis he has derived.

In teaching this task, we require the student to develop a formal written support paper emphasizing documentation from the literature since at this stage in their career they seldom have extensive clinical experience from which to draw; their professional fund of knowledge is limited.

As a way of demonstrating this last task, several hypotheses are stated here, and comments are made regarding their quality. The student should delve into these examples further. Are our comments about quality relevant? Should we have approached them differently? Is further information needed to continue the evaluation?

1. *Odvar has a language disorder due to unknown causes.* Even though clearly stated, little specific information is provided in this hypothesis. It is highly abstract and provides little information as a potential solution to the clinical problem. Some level of the language product must be affected—pragmatic, semantic, syntactic, phonologic, or perhaps all of them. The diagnostician does not know if comprehension, integration, formulation, or all are involved. Nothing is known of causal factors. The diagnostician would have to design his diagnosis primarily from inference for this hypothesis; his inferential abilities would be the sole basis for causal factors. This hypothesis reflects that the diagnostician either had little information to go on or else did not feel secure about his interpretation of available information.

2. *Gregory has a language disorder on all linguistic levels related to an emotional disturbance.* More specificity is introduced into this hypothesis. We know that the language product is affected on all levels; however, we do not know whether comprehension, integration, or formulation is affected. Severity might be inferred, since all levels are affected; however, it would help to specify this. The major weakness of this hypothesis is in the statement of causation. The causal factor lacks clarity; it is highly abstract and ambiguous. What does "emotional disturbance" mean? What support can the diagnostician offer that an emotional disturbance is related to the language disorder? How has the necessary connection condition been met? This hypothesis may not reflect an objective and adequate understanding of the problem. An alternative hypothesis may

have been more likely. The interactions between emotional problems and language disorders are difficult, at best, to discern and secure. Which comes first? Perhaps in Gregory's case the language disorder was apparent early in development and created subsequent frustration that led to significant episodes of depression. If all levels of language are affected, the probability of resultant emotional problems is a potential. For further evaluation of this hypothesis, refer to our earlier discussions about associated problems.

3. *Nancy has a formulation disorder primarily affecting syntactic development related to her learning abilities. Nancy has been classified as an educable mentally retarded child with an IQ of 75.* This hypothesis is stated clearly and provides some rather specific information. The diagnostician has stated that the language disorder is formulation of syntax. The disorder is expressed as both a behavioral correlate and product disorder. A specific relationship has been expressed that provides a potential solution to the problem. In his design the diagnostician might focus on syntax to determine what might be necessary to increase Nancy's ability to formulate better syntactic structures. The hypothesis also specifies the causal factor; presumably it means Nancy has learning problems because she is an educable retarded child with an IQ of 75. This relationship provides a source of error in this hypothesis, perhaps a lack of adequate understanding of the problem. We have to assume here than Nancy has not developed syntax because of learning problems. Is this typical of a child with an IQ of 75? Perhaps an alternative hypothesis would be better: "Nancy has syntactic development commensurate with her mental age." Or perhaps there is another causal factor interacting with her mental abilities that may be a better explanation for the language disorder. There are other aspects of this hypothesis that need clarification.

4. *Joyce has a severe language comprehension, integration, and formulation disorder on all linguistic levels due to mental retardation that is secondary to central nervous system dysfunction resulting from brain injury. Joyce sustained a severe blow to the left temporal cortex when she was 3 years old.* Evaluate the quality of this hypothesis. Consider carefully the interactions of causal factors; what is implied, and what must be inferred.

SUMMARY

The derivation of the clinical hypothesis stems from the diagnostician's examination and integration of the cause–effect relationships revealed in the constituent analysis. In stating the clinical hypothesis, the diagnostician delineates the speech and language disorder he expects to see and its probable cause. The hypothesis is a working hypothesis that expresses a potential solution to the clinical problem. Once the clinical hypothesis and any alternatives are stated, they are evaluated for their clarity and relevance to the clinical problem, serving to organize and design the remainder of the diagnostic process.

In developing his clinical hypothesis, the diagnostician performs three tasks.

1. *He derives the clinical hypothesis.* He performs this by drawing relationships between causes and effects, using the perspective provided by the SLPM. The SLPM schema for interpreting dynamic, complex, multidimensional cause–effect relationships emphasizes three perspectives:

   a. Causal factor perspective considering the causal scanning mechanism, multiple nature of causation, and chains of cause–effect interactions;
   b. Directness perspective considering the many direct and indirect effects of causal factors;

    c. Timing perspective emphasizing the historical and contemporary nature of causation, incorporating the other two perspectives.

He presents his integration of relationships as a hierarchy of most to least likely cause–effect explanations for the clinical problem.

    2. *He states the clinical hypothesis as a cause–effect relationship.* This task is the formal statement of the most probable cause–effect relationship as revealed in the preceding task. In addition, he also offers alternative hypotheses—those he considers as less likely to explain the clinical problem. He always proposes the null hypothesis—that no speech and language disorder exists.

    3. *He evaluates the quality of the hypothesis.* Here the diagnostician presents his evaluation of the specification and support for his hypothesis. He addresses the clarity of his statement and presents his arguments in support of his hypothesis, including those factors that might weaken as well as strengthen his position.

    Now that this step of the diagnostic process is completed, the diagnostician is one step closer to fulfilling the goals of diagnosis. He then turns his attention to designing the diagnosis, selecting and developing the clinical tools for testing the hypothesis.

KATHERINE COMPARDO
Derivation of the clinical hypothesis

    Again, we turn to our patient example, Katherine Compardo, to demonstrate how the diagnostician derives his clinical hypothesis. At this point we will assume that the constituent analysis from the previous step has been completed and documented where necessary. Therefore we now know which categories of constituents are significant for drawing out important cause–effect relationships. In this demonstration, once again, we do not present all of the details that would go into the derivation of Katherine Compardo's clinical hypothesis. Our intent is to demonstrate how the task works; the student should explore this derivation in greater depth. In Table 5-1, we explore some of the relationships revealed in the constituent analysis, and then present a hierarchical ordering of these relationships, from most to least likely.

    Table 5-1 is constructed to reveal how the cause–effect relationships were derived within the SLPM framework. The lefthand column presents conclusions that have effect significance, and the righthand column presents conclusions that have causal significance. Through the use of arrows, where relevant, we show the direction of inference that might occur in deriving the cause–effect relationship.

States and evaluates the clinical hypothesis

    With Katherine we exemplify the last two tasks of Step 2 of the diagnostic process. First we state the clinical hypothesis and an alternative; then we evaluate the quality of the hypothesis and present a brief support paper.

    From the list of potential cause–effect relationships the most likely relationship is stated as a formal clinical hypothesis. The first relationship expressed in Table 5-1 was "Childhood aphasia—cause and effect implied."

Statement of the clinical hypothesis

    Katherine Compardo has congenital childhood aphasia and apraxia characterized by language integration and formulation disruptions observed on all language product levels, thus implicating the physical processes of language–thought representation and speech programming. The cause inferred for this disorder is implied in the terms "aphasia" and "apraxia"—central nervous system dysfunction (more specifically a disruption of certain parts of the central language–thought segment).

Statement of an alternative hypothesis

    Katherine Compardo has congenital apraxia of speech that has greatly limited her use of all levels of language. The causal relationship is implied in the term "apraxia"—disruption of the central language–thought segment (in this hypothesis more specific to the speech programming process).

Table 5-1. Derivation of the clinical hypothesis—examining and integrating selected, significant constituents about Katherine Compardo

Effect significance	Causal significance
	Speech and language environment component
	The general environmental background does not offer much information that may be causal; rather, it suggests a relatively normal environment and family structure, providing adequate speech and language input stimulation.
	Speech and language processing component
	There is little direct information to support any causal factors affecting the processing component. Pregnancy and birth history and immediate postnatal period are reported as normal. Age of mother at this last birth and the three children in close succession might be relevant but highly inferential.
	Would Katherine's borderline, slow physical development be indicative of any causal factor? Slow mental and cognitive development?
	Central language segment
Language product	→ *Integration and formulation: language–cognitive representation*
We have a good bit of information that supports a disorder of language. Katherine has been very slow in the onset and development of all aspects of the language product. Language usage is characterized by a minimal vocabulary; few two-word combinations are used, thus both syntax and semantics are delayed. She also tends to prefer gestures over the use of the speech she has. Might this be because she is unintelligible? Or do we have reason to question as well the pragmatic level of speech and language usage.	Formulation is disrupted as evidenced by the speech and language product, thus inferring that language–cognitive representation is disrupted. Unless, of course, the reason for the defective product is in the speech production segment.
The constituents indicate that the → phonologic level is also delayed or deviant. Katherine makes most sounds incorrectly. She should have many correct sounds by this age.	*Formulation: speech programming*
	→ *Perception: auditory programming*
	There is some information here. Questions can be raised about auditory programming on the basis of her speech and language behavior. Perhaps her problem with speech sounds relates to problems of auditory programming—a disruption of some aspects of the behavioral correlate of perception—perhaps sequencing and discrimination of speech sounds are disrupted.
Language product	← *Comprehension: language–cognitive representation*
	Comprehension is reportedly intact. May want to question this conclusion. If comprehension of language is present at age level, it would be difficult to conclude that a perceptual problem—a disrupted auditory programming process—could account for Katherine's deviant language product, unless auditory programming acts differently at the semantic and syntactic levels than at the phonologic level. She reportedly does not imitate speech, although she does understand it.

Table 5-1. Derivation of the clinical hypothesis—examining and integrating selected, significant constituents about Katherine Compardo—cont'd

Effect significance	Causal significance
	Speech production segment
Speech product	➤ *All behavioral correlates and physical processes*
But are her sound errors more a speech product deviation than a phonologic deviation?	It would seem that if these processes were affected, we might have received reports of greater difficulties in the speech musculature—the behavioral correlate of motor control. We do have a few comments regarding Katherine's difficulty with the tongue and mouth when she talks. "When she talks" is a significant aspect of this constituent. If we were to see a motor control problem, it would most likely be seen at times other than when she talks.
There is no information about prosody or sound patterns. This would be helpful if we had it. The only clue is the late development of two-word combinations. Could this be evidence for difficulty putting sounds or words together?	
	Auditory reception segment
	Some confusion from the constituents, but it seems most likely that hearing is intact; the processes up to auditory programming will not provide much secure information for causal factors.

POINT: Katherine's information does not point to clearly established causal factors for the significantly delayed speech and language. The diagnostician may want to emphasize contemporary causation—behavioral correlates and physical processes—rather than infer a special causal factor when he formally states his hypothesis. We will not take this approach totally but will express a causal factor.

The hierarchy of cause–effect relationships from most to least likely for Katherine Compardo is stated quite broadly as follows:

1. Childhood aphasia—cause–effect implied
2. Childhood apraxia—cause–effect implied
3. Dysarthria—cause–effect implied
4. Language disorder related to auditory processing deficits
5. Language disorder related to mental retardation

The students should now try their hand at stating their hypothesis for Katherine Compardo or stating various alternatives as reflected by the cause–effect relationships established earlier. They also should evaluate the quality of the specification of the above hypotheses.

Development of a support paper

We present only a relatively brief support paper for Katherine Compardo. The student can study this position paper and add more evaluative details. Our intent is to exemplify the task, not present it in detail. We develop our position paper in the following way. First, we present viewpoints on the concept of childhood aphasia and apraxia. Following this, we demonstrate briefly how Katherine's constituent analysis supports our position stated in the hypothesis.

There is not complete agreement in the literature regarding the condition so often refered to as childhood aphasia or developmental aphasia (Aram & Nation, 1982; Wyke, 1978). When early attention was brought to this condition by Myklebust (1954), the current concepts of adult aphasia were simply transferred to children. Thus, "aphasic children" were either receptive, expressive, or global aphasics. Since then, more attempts have been made to differentiate the language characteristics seen in this group of nonverbal children. However, there is still a primary differentiation into two essential types of childhood aphasias (Eisenson, 1972; Morely, 1972; Rapin & Wilson, 1978) or combinations of them. Adding to this classification difficulty, the concept of childhood apraxia was introduced into the childhood aphasia schema. As in adults, questions exist about whether apraxia is a component of "expressive aphasia,," or if it can occur in isolation (Aram & Nation, 1982; Guyette & Diedrich, 1981).

Examining Katherine's hypothesis in light of some of this information lends support to the position that she has childhood aphasia and apraxia characterized by language integration and formulation difficulties on all lingusitic levels. Katherine is a "nonverbal" child who does not present any significant sign of mental retardation, emotional disorder, hearing loss, or physical problem. These signs are in keeping with both Eisenson's (1972), Morley's (1972), and Stark & Tallal's (1981) criteria defining aphasia in children in almost this way. The characteristics presented in Morley (1972) fit Katherine: a severe delay in the onset of speech, little or no vocal play or babbling, and one or two isolated words used during the first 2 to 3 years of life. As well, she indicates that the aphasic child is emotionally stable and has normal hearing, intelligence, and social interests—all of which seem to be the case with Katherine.

The interpretation of Katherine's ability to comprehend language is crucial to this hypothesis. Does the literature support a diagnosis of aphasia that is characterized primarily by language formulation difficulties but leaves comprehension intact? We have already mentioned the dichotomy of types of childhood aphasia that have been offered in the literature. Morley's description would add that if comprehension was at age level, then the developmental aphasia would be considered as predominantly expressive. Eisenson concurs that this circumstance can occur; however, he might consider this type of child, one who comprehends but does not speak, as congenitally apraxic. He indicates that this includes only a small number of nonverbal children. See also how Aram & Nation (1982) and Stark & Tallal (1981) treat the relationship between comprehension and expressive deficits. We conclude that Katherine is one of these, a child who comprehends but is basically nonverbal. Her sound development, "makes most sounds incorrectly" and the reported "difficulty moving her tongue and mouth when she talks," provides added evidence for apraxia.

All in all, Katherine Compardo appears to fit Eisenson's concept of congenital oral apraxia, which is synonymous with Morley's developmental expressive aphasia with accompanying articulatory apraxia. Katherine understands spoken language but has failed to develop formulated language appropriate for her age. She has a significant cluster of other characteristics that support this hypothesis: She responds to sounds and noises and comprehends spoken language, even though there was little early babbling, cooing, and vocal play, and she still does not imitate speech. She uses gesture for communication, although we do not know how highly developed her gesture system is. Her speech output is quite limited; she primarily uses single-syllable words composed of front consonant plus vowel combinations.

As mentioned, this support paper is intended to be a brief demonstration. Students should now review the criteria discussed for evaluating the quality of a hypothesis and develop a more extensive support position for Katherine Compardo, either using the hypothesis presented here, an alternative hypothesis, or their own derived hypothesis. Keep in mind that the support position can consider many aspects of the potential problem, including how the disorder may have come about, what effects it will continue to have on the patient, and what management considerations might be proposed if the hypothesis is true. The position paper is an interpretation of the hypothesis, which is, in effect, a testing out of the hypothesis to determine its clinical validity.

PATIENT PROJECTS

The student should return to the patient projects introduced in Chapter 4 and derive clinical hypotheses for each of them. Making use of the devices presented in this chapter will help to clarify the process, and will add to the student's funds of knowledge and clinical problem-solving skills.

STUDY QUESTIONS

In Chapter 4 you were asked to classify two sets of causal factors into the causal factor scanning mechanism: (1) those primarily affecting the speech and language environment, and (2) those primarily affecting speech and language processing. These same factors (see Chapter 4 Study Question 1) should be examined and interpreted in light of the six types of interactions presented in Figure 5-3.

Chapter 6

Clinical design: development of the measurement plan

The third step of the diagnostic process, done prior to patient contact, follows logically from the constituent analysis and the development of the clinical hypothesis. This step involves the overall planning of the diagnostic sessions for testing the clinical hypothesis. By the time he reaches the third step of the diagnostic process, the diagnostician has a firm grip on the potential clinical problem he will see. Now he must focus on methodology; he must design his diagnostic session. To complete this third step we have specified three tasks. First, the diagnostician plans for systematic observation and measurement of the clinical hypothesis. Second, he selects the specific tools he wants to use to fit his measurement plan. Third, he develops an overall testing strategy for efficiently carrying out his plan while optimizing data collection.

PLANS FOR SYSTEMATIC OBSERVATION AND MEASUREMENT

The constituent analysis and the clinical hypothesis direct the diagnostician's planning of the diagnostic design. His intent is to gather data to verify his hypothesis or, as the case may be, to discover alternative cause–effect relationships. If, for example, a prosody disorder characterized by sound repetitions and prolongations is hypothesized, the diagnostician's plan will take quite a different form than if a severe language problem is hypothesized. Similarly, if the hypothesis points to motor control problems as probable causal factors, he will plan his diagnostic time differently than if sensation problems are hypothesized.

Uses the SLPM as a measurement framework

As well as providing the diagnostician with a conceptual framework for viewing and measuring normal and disordered speech and language, the SLPM provides a measurement framework for establishing cause–effect relationships. The SLPM can guide and direct the measurement strategies the diagnostician utilizes for determining when speech and language are disordered and why they are disordered.

In using the SLPM the diagnostician must learn how to *systematically elicit, observe,* and *measure* the data needed. He must attain these major skills. The diagnostician must learn how to direct his observations. He must separate what he can observe from what he can only partially observe, and from what is not directly observable by him. He must learn what strategies to use to elicit the behaviors he wants to observe. He must become highly skilled at designing tasks—developing *measurement strategies*—that reveal relevant information about the patient's ability to use speech and language. The behaviors he elicits may be as simple as the raising of a finger in response to hearing a sound or as complex as the many verbal responses patient's make to questions asked. In some instances, the diagnostician may choose equipment to assist him in making his observations and measurements.

The diagnostician's major measurement tool, however, remains his own skill as a *systematic observer*. Through his knowledge, experience, and training, the diagnostician becomes a *"calibrated instrument."* He is his own best friend and worst enemy when it comes to making appropriate observations of the information needed to isolate his patient's speech and language disorder. His observations will be only as good as his developed skill level.

The environmental component and planning

When the diagnostician attempts to discover something about the patient's environment, he is primarily measuring information that is, at best, only *partially observable* to him. The speech and language stimulation the patient received in the past cannot be observed directly. Instead, measurements of this *historical speech and language environment* usually take the form of a report of past events. The diagnostician asks for information from various sources—from a parent, social worker, referring physician, or the patient himself. The diagnostician must not confuse this information with direct observation of the environment, but rather he should take this information for what it is. It is partially observable information based on an informant's perception and recall of past events, not even necessarily the past as reality. The diagnostician can only assume that the informant has observed the historical speech and language environment. From the information he obtains about the historical speech and language environment the diagnostician draws inferences, that is, makes interpretations about how the information obtained relates to the patient's current speech and language disorder. Gathering data here serves basically as "causal testing."

In addition to the historical speech and language environment the diagnostician himself creates an *immediate speech and language environment* through the tasks he presents and his own interpersonal characteristics. The diagnostician can *directly observe and control* the immediate speech and language environment. That is, he can specify the speech and language stimulus, the sounds, words, and sentences he presents to the patient to elicit certain responses. He also can control the context of the diagnostic setting, the room size, the clothes he wears, the objects and materials he uses.

Through the use of the speech and language environment component of the SLPM, the diagnostician focuses on the speech and language input within the multidimensional environmental context. The diagnostician measures the partially observable historical environment and controls the observable immediate environment. From his observations he interprets the role the speech and language environment has played in the patient's speech and language disorder.

The processing component and planning

The basic schema provided by the speech and language processing component directs the diagnostician's measurements and observations toward any physical bases for his patient's speech and language disorder. Gathering data here is important for understanding causation. The SLPM states that various behavioral correlates (reflective of speech and language use) occur as a result of a series of interrelated physical processes within rather well-defined anatomic boundaries. Therefore the diagnostician directs his measurements to the three aspects presented: *anatomy, physical processes,* and *behavioral correlates.*

For the most part, the physical bases for speech and language cannot be observed directly. There are some notable exceptions. The diagnostician can directly observe certain peripheral structures of the ear and the speech mechanism (the outer ear, the teeth, the tongue, etc.). Other structures are partially observable through the use of instrumental aids. Brain structures can be viewed via radiographic procedures such as the CT scan. In postmortem examination, brain structures can be observed directly to determine if lesions exist that could have accounted for the disorder present prior to death.

In the case of physical processes few of these can be observed directly or even with instrumental aids. Certain movements of the speech mechanism during speech can be observed, but this is a limited view of physical processing. Instead, the diagnostician infers disrupted physical processes based on behaviors he can observe. His source of information comes from behaviors that can be reported by the patient or behaviors observed directly by the diagnostician. When a patient speaks, the diagnostician is able to learn something about the patient's ability to create, formulate, and produce a message by observing the speech and language behavior. Similarly, when a patient responds in some way to a language stimulus, the diagnostician can make observations of the response and then make a statement about the patient's ability to receive, comprehend and integrate a language stimulus.

The diagnostician measures these *externalized behaviors*—correlates to the physical processes. The behavioral correlates represent different stages of physical processing where the diagnostician can "ask for" and then observe the response. Therefore each of the behavioral correlates can be defined by specifying tasks for its measurement.

The behavioral correlates of sensation, perception, comprehension, and integration can be measured from either a verbal or nonverbal response. For example, if we asked a patient, "Is your name Brenda Star?" and she responded correctly, "Yes, it is," we would be able to measure her spoken response and infer that comprehension of the stimulus was present. However, in diagnosis we often rely on *secondary* nonverbal responses to obtain information about the behavioral correlates of sensation, perception, comprehension, and integration. If a spoken response is not wanted, not possible, or deviant, the diagnostician will use other avenues for obtaining a response such as pointing, finger raising, or carrying out commands.

The diagnostician interested in measuring sensation may ask the patient to raise his finger when he hears a tone. Perception may be measured by asking the patient to nod his head yes or no when asked if two sounds presented are alike or different. There are many tasks that have been devised to assist the diagnostician in measuring the behavioral correlates of sensation and perception, particularly the testing techniques devised by audiologists. These measures are taken by presenting stimuli to the patient and asking him to report his auditory experience: "I hear the sound, I hear the differences between those sounds, I've heard that sound before, those are the same."

Similarly, to measure comprehension the diagnostician observes a verbal or nonverbal response to the stimulus. What he measures is the appropriateness of the response in relationship to the stimulus. Comprehension may be measured by asking a patient to physically carry out a command. For example, if we said to an aphasic patient, "Go to the door" and he got up from his chair and opened the window, the diagnostician would judge the aphasic's comprehension as being less than adequate. But this particular response may well have shown some degree of comprehension, as the behavior that occurred seems to relate tangentially to the command. Other tasks could be developed to allow the diagnostician to know if the patient knows the difference between "Laura hit Arick" and "Arick hit Laura," a task for syntactic comprehension.

Diagnosticians need more sophisticated tasks that measure comprehension at the various linguistic levels to determine if the patient's difficulty in understanding is because of phonologic, syntactic, or semantic elements of the message. And, in children's language disorders there is a significant need for measures that give an estimate of how well a child understands in comparison to how well he formulates language.

Measurement of comprehension is receiving greater attention. In the aphasia literature more emphasis is being placed on comprehension and its measurement at various linguistic levels (e.g., Shewan & Canter, 1971; Lesser, 1978; Boller, Kim & Mack, 1977; Spence, 1983). In the literature on child language disorders more tasks are being developed for observing the emergence of comprehension abilities as they relate to formulation and production (Bloom, 1974; Ingram, 1974; Menyuk, 1974; Chapman, 1974, 1978; Chapman & Miller, 1975, 1980).

Integration may be assessed from a number of different avenues. If the diagnostician is interested in more general cognitive ability, he may administer various cognitive tests, such as the Uzgiris and Hunt Scales (1975) or the Bayley Scales of Infant Development (Bayley, 1969). For evaluating how well a patient relates what he has comprehended to his past experience, the diagnostician may employ one of the few tools available which attempts to do this, (e.g., Baker & Leland, 1959; Weschler, 1974; Blank, Rose, & Berlin, 1978). Partially due to the limited number of tools available, however, he more often must rely upon systematic observation of his patient's interpersonal or unstructured use of language.

The behavioral correlates of formulation, repetition, sequencing, and motor control generally require observation of a verbal response. There are exceptions. For example, when the diagnostician observes the diadochokinetic rate of the tongue in nonspeech activities, he is making an observation of motor control. However, keep in mind that this nonspeech activity is not a direct observation of motor control during the speech actualization process. The tasks the diagnostician designs for measuring these behavioral correlates should specify the type of verbal response to be observed. He may ask the patient to name pictures, repeat sentences, talk about what is happening in a picture, prolong a vowel sound, produce a sequence of phonemes, or sing the musical scale.

Diagnosticians thus set up tasks that allow measurement of externalized behaviors reflecting physical processes. The SLPM attempts, throughout the speech and language processing component, to relate behavioral correlates to the anatomic and physical processing bases for that behavior. From his observations the diagnostician can seek the physical basis for the observed behavior.

Objections are frequently raised about viewing processes in a way that makes them seem to be isolated events occurring only at a given anatomic level (Duchan, 1983). These objections are justifiably raised. They help prevent oversimplified views of speech and language processing as discrete, discontinuous steps rather than a continuous interrelated processing system. Even though anatomic and processing boundaries are presented on the SLPM and processing is discussed this way, the speech and language processing component must be viewed as an interacting, continuous processing system; a disruption in one segment will have an effect on the processes in other segments. Finally, diagnosticians see speech and language disorders that reflect differential disruptions in the auditory reception, central language–thought, and speech production segments. Disorders may sound similar but stem from different disrupted physical bases. We believe that the SLPM aids in sorting out and measuring the complicated physical basis for the disorders observed.

The product component and planning

The speech and language product provides the diagnostician with the *most accessible behavior for direct measurement*. As a spoken response, the product can be observed for two basic purposes: first, as a set of parameters for determining if the patient's speech and language behavior is normal or disordered. Second, the product can be observed as behaviors that reflect speech and language processes. The speech product most directly reflects the physical processes within the speech production segment, and the language product most directly reflects the physical processes within the central language segment (see Figure 2-4). Thus, the diagnostician can observe the parameters of the speech and language product to provide information rather directly about the behavioral correlates of formulation, repetition, sequencing, and motor control. At the same time the diagnostician should not lose sight of the fact that the patient's spoken response can also provide information and insight into the patient's ability to sense, perceive, comprehend, and integrate speech and language. Thus, the speech and language product component of the SLPM is perhaps the diagnostician's most powerful measurement tool. What the speech and language product does for the diagnostician depends on his *diagnostic intent*—what he wants to measure and why he is measuring it.

With this in mind the speech and language product component was designed to provide a specific set of parameters to which the diagnostician can direct his observations and measurements. He can direct his attention to all the parameters, the entire spoken response, or to a parameter of basic concern. For each parameter he can specify how he will observe and measure the speech and language his patient produces.

The diagnostician can measure the physical characteristics of the acoustic product. Through instrumental analysis he can analyze the acoustic waveform, specifying the frequency, intensity, spectral, and durational characteristics of the acoustic product. This form of measurement is particularly useful where exact, specific physical data is wanted; for example, when the following diagnostic question is asked, "What are the format characteristics of Howard's hypernasality?" Because the measurements are typically made through refined instrumentation, human error and judgment are minimized. Use of physical measurement allows exactness of measurement that is readily quantifiable and gives high observer agreement.

Several difficulties, however, are associated with utilizing physical measurement in many clinical situations. Frequently the instrumentation required is expensive, bulky, and time consuming, thus reducing the ease and flexibility with which it may be adapted to nonpredictable clinical situations. Furthermore, while instruments give data, they usually do not provide judgments. Yet most diagnostic problems require judgment; for example, does Howard's /s/ fall within the range of acceptable production of the English phoneme /s/? Is Mr. Hardie's voice quality excessively breathy?

Although measurements of the physical characteristics of the acoustic product are sometimes made by the diagnostician, his most frequent method of observation resides in his knowledge and skill as a "listener." His eyes and ears take in information that he uses to make auditory and visual analyses and comparisons to judge if speech and language are disordered.

The diagnostician designs diagnostic tasks to elicit speech and language responses, and his formal knowledge of the details of the speech and language products directs the specific measurements he makes. His interest may be in describing parameters of language to determine if his client has a disorder of syntax, semantics, or phonology. Or he may design tasks to address questions such as, "Is Mr. Moore's /r/ phoneme, voice quality, pitch, or rate within normal limits?"

Since the diagnostician "carries" this method of observation with him, it provides maximum flexibility and efficiency in terms of cost, equipment, and ease of administration. However, considerable measurement error may be introduced into his observations, since they are dependent on the training and skill of the specific diagnostician. If the diagnostician has not learned to differentiate between phonetic variations, he may not "hear" or be able to record the difference between his patient's lingual and lateral productions of the /s/ sound. If the diagnostician has not experienced hypernasality versus hyponasality, he is going to have difficulty identifying and specifically describing the distinctions he hears in the resonance product. Or two diagnosticians with different skill levels may not agree on the amount of hoarseness heard in the patient's vocal tone.

An inferential measurement strategy

The diagnostician's behavioral observations do not always specify cause–effect relationships. More often the information needed by the diagnostician for measurement of cause–effect relationships will be only partially observable to him. Therefore he must plan to observe cause–effect relationships on the basis of inference, the inferential measurement strategy.

The essence of the inferential measurement strategy is to say something about an event that is not fully understood, based on whatever observations and theoretical understanding one has of the event. It is the *problem-solving level of measurement*. For the diagnostician involved in investigating the nature and causes of speech and language disorders it becomes one of his most crucial measurement strategies.

The SLPM assists the diagnostician in developing the use of the inferential measurement strategy by addressing the *interface*, the relationships and interactions, among the physical and behavioral aspects of speech and language. This interface is represented by the three components of the SLPM.

From the information he plans to gather and the observations he will make within each component of the SLPM, the diagnostician addresses his cause–effect relationships. Each patient can be thought of as a *mini-SLPM*. The patient's environmental background can be studied; his anatomy and physical processing systems can be investigated; and the speech and language product can be observed. From the data he gathers the diagnostician can draw his inferences about what the disorder is, what has caused it, and what he might propose for remediation.

The diagnostician's use of inferential measurement strategy can be represented by demonstrating the directional route the inference takes as seen in the following examples. If the diagnostician plans to see a child with a significant disorder on the phonologic level, he might decide on the following directional route for his inferential strategy.

Language product ⟶ Physical process ⟶ Speech and language environment

This strategy represents his approach to studying the cause–effect hypothesis. Following the preceding inferential strategy, the diagnostician would first aim to investigate information that might be indicative of a disrupted physical process for phonologic formulation. Then he would investigate the child's speech and language environment. In this example, if the diagnostician found nothing to signal a processing disruption but did discover that the child's mother spoke with a similar speech pattern, he would probably conclude that the child's phonologic disorder (effect) was related to the speech and language stimulation (cause) provided by his mother.

Or, in another example, the diagnostician may find that his patient's responses to auditory tasks were faulty; the patient could not hear the sounds; he could not discriminate between sounds. Depending on the responses observed, the diagnostician may hypothesize impaired anatomy of the hearing mechanism and suggest that the patient has an auditory processing disorder, disruption of the physical processes within the auditory reception segment. The inferential measurement strategy might look like this:

Behavioral correlates ———————> Physical basis ———————> Physical basis
(sensation, perception)   (anatomy)   (auditory processing)

Or, in still another example, if the diagnostician hypothesizes faulty vocal tone, he will want to know why and how it was produced. He knows that vocal tone is related to the speech actualization subprocess of phonation. Therefore his first level of investigation might be into the process of phonation, including an investigation of the condition and function of the laryngeal mechanisms. However, the nature of the vocal tone disorder could lead the diagnostician to infer other physical processing disorders from which he may hypothesize certain anatomic disruptions. This inferential strategy might look like this:

Speech product ———————> Speech actualization subprocess ———————> Other physical
(vocal tone)   (phonation)   process/anatomy
                                                                          (e.g., speech
                                                                   coordination–transmission)

Designing the diagnosis to relate the observed speech product to its physical basis allows the diagnostician to test cause–effect relationships, thereby aiding in his understanding of causal factors and planning for patient management. Any number of these diagrams, singly or in combination, could be used to demonstrate how inferences are made among the components of the SLPM. Thus, a most important aspect of the SLPM for the diagnostician is that it has been designed to help specify and measure cause–effect relationships. The SLPM helps the diagnostician measure all aspects of speech and language, not only the product but also the underlying processes and the input stimulation that may help to explain the speech and language disorders heard.

Operationalizes the clinical hypothesis

In planning his clinical design with the SLPM as his measurement framework the diagnostician must first determine if his hypothesis is testable. Can he measure the relationships expressed in the hypothesis? If not, he must go back to the drawing board and derive a more testable hypothesis. He must determine what information may be easily obtained and what may be more difficult to measure. In general, the easiest to measure are the characteristics of the disorder, the variations in the speech and language product. Planning for the causal factors generally presents more difficulties than does planning for the speech and language behavior; that is, language products are easier to measure than brain injury.

As part of his planning the diagnostician considers his various alternative hypotheses, including the null hypothesis of no problem. These alternative hypotheses reflect cause–effect uncertainties on the part of the diagnostician; he must design his diagnosis to reduce these uncertainties, to determine which hypothesis may be the "best fit." One way he can facilitate the reduction of uncertainties is by planning systematic measurements that rule in and out several probabilities simultaneously. For example, he may be working from a hypothesis that states that Annie Mae has a language disorder only on the phonologic level and an alternative hypothesis that states the semantic level is disordered as well. He could plan measures that let him observe Annie Mae's use of phonology through a naming task, a task that would also estimate her vocabulary usage. If she was able to name the items but with many phonologic errors, strength is gained for a phonologic disorder and for ruling out the hypothesized semantic disorder. When the diagnostician finishes, he wants to be able to state how strong his conclusions are; he hopes to have reached the most likely probability. Thus, the diagnosis should be designed to systematically and simultaneously observe as many aspects of the alternative hypotheses as possible.

Hypotheses based on a high degree of inference require extreme care in planning. These hypotheses have far more missing information than hypotheses derived from specific, clear information. An inferential hypothesis is more subject to error than one based on more factual data. This is more often the case in designing for causal considerations than for the speech and language characteristics. But in some instances it may be otherwise. For example, we referred in the last chapter to a child, Trisha, referred with a history of repeated otitis media. No information was available other than "speech disorder" for developing an effect hypothesis. The diagnostician inferred a phonologic variation, a product inference based on a potential cause. Without any factual support for this effect aspect of the hypothesis, the diagnostician must carefully design his approach for testing and verifying this highly inferential cause–effect relationship.

When conducting the previous two steps, the diagnostician often finds the information available incomplete and unclear, which raises many questions needing follow-up. The diagnostician carefully selects his tools to learn more about these questionable areas. For example, a physician may have reported that "Rachel was the product of a difficult labor." The diagnostician may question what "difficult" means and the effect of that labor on Rachel, exploring this information in the interview with the parent. Or a parent may have reported that "Patty is hard to manage." The diagnostician may both want to question the parents further about this problem and to observe Patty's manageability for himself. In short, all that is known about the patient, the information received and the diagnostician's study of that information in the first two steps, is used to help him operationalize his diagnostic design.

Task specification

A major part of the planning done at this stage is task specification. Let us say that the diagnostician has hypothesized a semantic disorder for Sandra. He may specify tasks to measure the extent of her vocabulary, her use of nouns having varying degrees of abstraction, or tasks to evaluate the semantic relations signaled by her utterances. Or if he has hypothesized an auditory processing deficit as responsible for Nathan's comprehension disorder, he may specify various types of auditory measurements from audiometric tests to tests of auditory comprehension.

Depending on his hypothesis, the diagnostician may specify processing tasks more than product tasks. If he hypothesized a disruption of the articulation process as responsible for the phonetic errors, he may devise many tasks for measuring the functions of the articulators. Or if he is more interested in the phonetic product, he may devise many tasks measuring phonetic structure in as many contexts as possible and spend less time with the articulation process. The diagnostician has many degrees of freedom available to him for task specification as long as his tasks solve the problem and allow him to propose appropriate management plans.

What would be the level of task specification for the product in this "hypothesis"? "Mr. Theisen cannot talk because his larynx was recently removed." How much detail would you want or expect to obtain about the speech product? What would be the purpose of task specification for this diagnosis?

As a part of the task specification, the diagnostician is concerned about measures that give estimates of the severity of the problem and estimates of prognosis. Tools that have built-in severity and prognostic guides would be useful. Both of these aspects of diagnosis are difficult to plan since so few measurements are available to provide reliable estimates. More often the diagnostician's clinical experience guides his judgments about the severity of the disorder and prognosis for change.

Patient characteristics

Sometimes it must seem that our interest is a cause–effect relationship instead of a specific patient. We hope, in making our points about the purpose and process of diagnosis, we have not forsaken patient concern; it is the patient with all his personal characteristics in whom we are interested. When we plan our diagnosis, we ultimately must design it around the specific needs and abilities of the patient. An aphasic who is extremely depressed will not respond adequately to the measures we plan unless we first work through the depression. A child who is running around the room will not "point to the shoe" until we get him controlled. A child who will not talk cannot be expected to name the items on our language test until we are able to establish much better rapport. The examples of particular patient needs, abilities, and behaviors that must be met are endless.

In his planning the diagnostician must consider what type, level, and range of tasks the patient will respond to; what stimuli will be motivating enough to permit observable responses. The diagnostician must control all the variables that enter into the diagnostic session; he must plan for them.

The diagnostician must consider many patient characteristics when he is developing his overall plan for systematic observation: age, sex, type of disorder, cause of the problem, personality, emotionality, physical disabilities, affect, need to communicate, parental attitudes, motivation, interests, cultural background, ability to attend, and level of concern— a few, among many. His plans for systematic observation must be considered within the abilities of the patient. If he does not plan for the individual characteristics of his patients, his best laid plans may be spoiled.

The following are summary statements derived from several informants' remarks about their child's "personality adjustment." How might you use this information to plan your systematic observation? A hypothesis is provided for each child.

1. *Edward Moore, aged 6 years, 3 months, stutters because of an emotionally unstable family background.*

Summary statement: Ed was described by Mr. Moore as an active, healthy boy who eats and sleeps well. He plays mainly with his brothers and sisters and "gets along as well as kids ever get along." He is shy with adults and somewhat reluctant to talk to them. Mr. Moore considers Ed "as easy to discipline, even though he requires a lot of it. He tries to be too much like his older brother, who is a real problem."

2. *Jacqueline Smith, aged 5 years, 5 months, has a severe language disorder related to slow mental development.*

Summary statement: As reported by Mrs. Dana Faith, Jacqueline's foster mother, Jacqueline is a happy child who gets along well with both children and adults. At times Mrs. Faith has found it difficult to discipline Jacqueline, while at other times she responds immediately. Mrs. Faith noted that Jacqueline "seems inconsistent in behaving and seems to act on impulse." She seems to have diffiulty concentrating, especially on directed work such as learning the alphabet, although at times "she seems to think deeply and remembers well."

3. *Mimi Wetherbee, aged 4 years, 9 months, has a severe articulation–resonation problem related to her cleft palate condition.*

Summary statement: As reported by her mother, Mrs. Leslie Wetherbee, Mimi usually plays with other children her age and gets along with both children and adults. She does not have difficulty concentrating and enjoys having books read to her. She is an active girl who likes being outdoors and doing things with her father. However, she is cooperative with other adults only when "properly motivated" and not when "pushed." Mimi's playmates are teasing her about her speech. She reacts by ignoring them and leaving their presence, but Mrs. Wetherbee feels Mimi is hurt by the teasing.

SELECTS TOOLS FOR MEASUREMENT

Next, the diagnostician asks himself, "Now that I have an overall plan, what tools or techniques will allow me to take my measurements?" The selection of tools to fit the plan is a critical task for designing the diagnosis. We have all had diagnostic failures because of poor selection of tools. Did failure occur because the tool was inappropriate for the patient—the child was too young? Did failure occur because the tool was inappropriate for the hypothesis—an articulation test was chosen for a language disorder? Did failure occur because the tool was too complicated—too many behaviors were sampled? Did failure occur because the administration procedures were unfamiliar—too little practice with the tool? Careful selection of tools based on the clinical hypothesis, the characteristics of the patient, and the diagnostician's skill level will reduce the number of assessment failures. In this task the diagnostician retrieves tools for the specific patient, that is, he tailor-makes his diagnostic design.

Commands knowledge of infinite tools

A major information base needed for completing this third step of the diagnostic process is knowledge about the tools and tests available for designing the diagnosis. The number of tools available to the diagnostician to assist him in systematic measurement is, perhaps, infinite—what has been and what will be. All of these tools, no matter how developed, were and are intended to provide information about some aspect of speech and language disorders and their causes. Some of the tools were developed from very practical bases, others highly theoretical. They have come from many sources: schools, clinics, researchers, teachers, and commercial publishers, to name a few. They come in many forms: some highly structured, others very unstructured, some highly objective, and others very subjective. Many are also specified by type: language, articulation, speech mechanism, screening, hearing, interview, and perceptual–motor. They also are scored and interpreted in a variety of ways.

From all of them the diagnostician must be able to select the tools needed to fulfill his measurement design. He must be familiar with a wide range of tools and know how to use them, that is, what they will and will not do for him. He must know what the tools are designed to do and evaluate their usefulness in gaining the information he wants. Since new testing tools are being made available with great frequency, the diagnostician must also be able to evaluate and incorporate these into his diagnostic practice.

To be able to utilize all these tool resources, the diagnostician needs an orientation for learning about and selecting from the vast possibilities available. Our intent here is to point up some categories of tools, to suggest criteria for evaluating the adequacy of tools, and then to present a "tool-retrieval system" for use in selection.

Categories of tools

There have been various attempts to classify diagnostic tools into dichotomous categories such as standardized–nonstandardized, subjective–objective, formal–informal, and structured–unstructured. These classifications have seldom been satisfactory and at times have promoted false reliance on tools described as standardized, structured, and objective. At this time we will not attempt to present an encompassing classification of the tools and techniques potentially useful to the diagnostician. Instead, we will first present some rather arbitrary categories of sources, forms, and types of tools. Later, we discuss a more systematic means of organizing available tools.

Diagnostic tools may be organized into five categories; however, any specific tool might be found in any number of the categories. The five categories discussed are the interview, commercial tools, experimental tools, setting protocols, and guided observation.

• *The interview.* The interview, unlike many other techniques, does not have a circumscribed use in the diagnostic process. There is no single approach to interviewing; rather, there are many approaches depending on the interviewer's purposes (Bingham & Moore, 1941; Fenlason, 1952, Garrett, 1972; Molyneaux & Lane, 1982; Richardson et al., 1965; Stevenson, 1971; Sullivan, 1954; Webster, 1977).

Often in the diagnosis of speech and language disorders the concept of the interview is approached from a narrow perspective, that is, a verbal exchange between a parent and a diagnostician for gaining the parent's impressions of their child's speech and language disorder. However, the interview in its more general sense is a tool that can be used with any person who can provide information about the patient's speech and language disorder, including the patients themselves. Even paper and pencil tasks can be viewed as forms of interviews. For example, when the parent fills out a case history questionnaire prior to the diagnostic session, information is being exchanged between the parent and the diagnostician.

For the purposes of this book, we want to confine our view of the interview to the information exchange that takes place during the diagnostic session with the patient or anyone who accompanies him. The interview is used to gain information and insights about the patient from whomever is interviewed—the parents, spouse, social worker, the patient, or any other interested person. The use of pencil and paper tasks might be incorporated into the interview techniques, but it is seen primarily as a verbal exchange of information. We will introduce our basic concepts about the interview at this step of the diagnostic process; however, because we formally view the interview as data collection, the next step of the diagnostic process, we augment interview information there.

The information obtained from an interview depends on the purposes of the interview. If much patient information was available prior to the diagnostic session, the diagnostician might design the interview around management concerns. If little information was available, the interview might become the primary source of data about the specifics of the disorder and thus have a constituent analysis intent. Or the interview may be primarily designed to discover causal factors that were unclear, thus having primarily a hypothesis development intent. Each interview, therefore, is designed for specific purposes, assisting the diagnostician in completing any of the diagnostic tasks at any of the steps and at any time during the diagnostic process.

The interview can be used to gain both verbally reported and extraverbal observed data. Verbally reported data is that information given us in words by the informant. In gaining such information, however, we need to keep in mind the possible discrepancy between the information that the diagnostician wants to learn, the information that the informant wants to tell, and the information of real importance to understanding the true nature of the speech and language problem.

Three interrelated processes are operating when gaining verbally reported data: *amplification, clarification,* and *verification.* If the information offered is insufficient or irrelevant, there is a need to amplify. An increase in quantity of data may help increase the validity and reliability of the information. Many of the diagnostician's questions are of an amplification type. There is a need to clarify if the information offered is vague, ambiguous, or inconsistent. Ideally, a question should be worded in a way that limits the degree of ambiguity of any possible response. By doing so, there is a subsequent increase in specificity—the diagnostician gets at the details he seeks. There is a need to verify if the information offered seems unreliable. The diagnostician should be aware of inconsistencies in behaviors or verbal responses that suggest unreliability. If he suspects that the informant is offering inaccurate information, he must try to determine if these are conscious or unconscious distortions. This helps assess the informant's awareness and understanding of the problem.

All three intents—amplification, clarification, and verification—can be embedded in a single question. A question might be asked primarily to expand (amplify) information from the patient history form. If the response is not clear or accurate, a question or statement to clarify or verify the response is provided, for example, "What do you mean by——?" or "Then, what you are saying is —— ."

In addition to the verbal data obtained in the interview the diagnostician also gains information from extraverbal observations. He may assess the gestalt of the interview, considering what is said as well as what is not said. For example, why is there no mention of the child's relationship with the father? The diagnostician will want to note gaps in information as well as recurrent references or themes that emerge. He may be particularly alert to inconsistencies between what the informant says and how he appears to feel about what he says. For example, if the informant's words indicate concern but his voice and manner indicate indifference, the diagnostician might question the reliability of the information that is being offered. Why is the informant distorting the information? If a parent, is he trying to defend his ability to raise children or mask his fear that the child may have a serious problem?

The diagnostician may wonder what he may do with such subjective, nonexplicit observations. Such information may be particularly usefull in learning the informant's real concerns and feelings about the information he is giving. Such observations also may cue topics where discussion may be very fruitful. Finally, observing the informant's extralinguistic behavior may provide a foundation for understanding that person, which would be particularly helpful when interpreting the results of the diagnosis and planning management.

Togehter, verbally reported data and extraverbal observations may serve to fill in missing constituents, to support or reject the clinical hypothesis, and to assess the informant's understanding, insight, and concern relating to the patient's problem.

• *Commercial tools.* At first glance this may seem an illogical category, and it is. However, we want to draw the student's attention to the wide range of tools available through the commercial publishing houses. Commercial sources of tools are more prevalent today than in the past. Perhaps it is a sign of coming of age in our profession that we now have tools available for purchase and no longer need to rely on developing our own for each patient we see. There is a great surge in commercially published tools. Monthly, new tools are marketed, each vying for a place in the diagnostician's testing repertoire. Many of these tools are outgrowths of techniques first used experimentally or clinically.

Tools are commercial only in the sense that they are available for a price. Beyond that, this category of tools has little in common. Some tools are highly original; others are thinly disguised adaptations of information readily available. Some give impressive normative data; others give none. Some obtain credible validity and reliability, while others do not address these concerns. Some tools require elaborate or official training procedures before their use is authorized; others can be used by anyone who can read and follow instructions.

Many of the available tools have been designed to measure some aspect of a specific "problem type" (tests of articulation, aphasia, language) or to measure some rather specified level of speech and language behavior (morphology, speech sounds, syntax, nonfluencies); still others have been designed to measure certain defined "processes" (comprehension, sensation, perception, diadochokinesis, phonation). Other tools are available that are more appropriate to causal testing or for other related dimensions, some of which are the primary province of other professionals, some the province of the speech–language pathologist, for example, auditory tests, perceptual–motor tests, intelligence tests, personality tests, and projective tests. Psychology, psychiatry, neurology, education, and other professions have all contributed commercial tools useful in the diagnosis of speech and language disorders.

• *Experimental tools.* The research literature offers another source of useful tools and procedures that can be adapted by the diagnostician. These tools come in all types and forms and measure many different aspects of speech and language disorders and their causes. The experimenter has developed his tool to systematically measure some aspect of his hypothesis, a situation not unlike the diagnostician confronted with a range of clinical hypotheses; therefore these tools and procedures are usually relatively objective. However, at times they may not be as reliable nor as valid as the experimenter had hoped. Many of the tools now commercially available for diagnosis were originally developed out of research projects (Carrow, 1968; Lee, 1970; MacDonald & Blott, 1974; Vignolo & DeRenzi, 1962; Wiig & Semel, 1976). If not commercially available, some of the tools have been presented in the literature with suggestions for their diagnostic use (Nation, 1972).

- **Setting protocols.** There are all types of forms of tools that have been constructed by personnel working within specific work settings. Settings may develop their own "private label" test for aphasia, articulation, stuttering, and so on. For example, in most settings a format can be found directing the speech mechanism examination, a format for observing and analyzing stuttering behaviors, and a format for observing parameters of voice. Many tools such as these do not strictly fall into a test format and seldom achieve commercial publishing status; they are setting protocols. For example, the pragmatics protocol developed by Prutting (1982) and presented in Chapter 2 represents such a tool.

   Other setting protocol tools are highly structured; they are first developed for clinical use to fit a specific need of the diagnostician, then they may be used in experimentation, and ultimately, may end up as commercial tools. The Minnesota Test for Differential Diagnosis of Aphasia by Schuell (1965) basically took this route as did the Illinois Test of Psycholinguistic Abilities (Kirk, McCarthy, & Kirk, 1968). Tests like this were originally devised to fill diagnostic and research needs in certain work settings when no tools were available.

   From work settings, then, comes a primary source of tools for diagnosis. Tools derived from this source often are our most practical, applicable tools even when the standardization data may be limited. There is much to be said for tools that have a professional's clinical experience guiding their construction. These tools have been designed specifically for disordered populations. They often may be more applicable than tools worked out on normal populations. Some of these tools gain wide distribution through the clinical literature— articles that discuss certain types of disorders and how to test for and treat them.

- **Guided observations.** We have specified a final tool category for diagnostic design. For want of a better term we have called this category guided observations. This category encompasses all the observations the diagnostician wants to make that do not fall under the rubric of a test or a specific observational form. These are the tasks frequently referred to as unstructured, general, or informal observations. We prefer to think that all our observations are guided—that structure is present in the observations made of the activities and behaviors of the patient. The patient's behaviors may not be structured, but the diagnostician's observations should be. Observations are planned and thus constitute a tool of diagnosis. All tools are primarily techniques for structuring and guiding our systematic observations. Thus, every activity that occurs in the diagnosis serves as a source of data to be observed; no source of information should go unobserved or be wasted.

   At times the stimuli presented are rigorously controlled; at other times, they are controlled only in a very general sense. For example, when a patient is asked to sit down, stand up, or hop, skip, and jump, the diagnostician has controlled his stimuli to specify a response. He may want to observe the patient's motor abilities and/or his ability to follow directions. If the plan is to obtain as much spontaneous speech as naturalistically as possible, the diagnostician's stimulus specification may be more general; that is, the diagnostician bases his conversational stimuli on the patient's spontaneous conversation. But the diagnostician's observations of this conversation may be highly planned and structured to obtain specific speech and language data. If the diagnostician wants to tap the patient's use of past or future tenses, he may need to introduce topics happening in the past or future. This use of planned communicative interaction between patient and diagnostician in many instances becomes his only tool, developed from and based on guided observations. Even when considerable data from more specific tests are available, the diagnostician will use guided observations of these spontaneous situations to gain additional data about the patient's abilities. Diagnostic design is often a balance between responses to structured tools and responses obtained in a more naturalistic activity.

Some diagnosticians develop observation forms to guide them during the diagnosis, structuring the observation form differently depending on the hypothesis and the personal characteristics of the patient. These observational protocols are useful for designing the diagnostic session; they guide the diagnostician in recalling all the things he may want to note during the time he is with the patient.

The five categories of tools discussed provide the diagnostician with an infinite variety of tools to use, from stringing beads to a highly formalized tool such as the Goldman–Fristoe–Woodcock Test of Auditory Discrimination (Goldman et al., 1970). Many tools are designed to elicit only a specified set of behaviors. For example, most articulation (phonetic structure) tools sample the patient's sound production within a specific context, usually at the beginning, middle, and end of a word. Rating scales for judging voice and stuttering behaviors provide the diagnostician with a systematic method for observing and recording when and how much a certain behavioral characteristic may be present. Other tools sample more than a single level of behavior. For example, some tests of language measure many language products and processes such as the Boston Diagnostic Aphasia Examination (Goodglass & Kaplan, 1972) and the Tests of Language Development (Newcomer et al., 1977, 1982).

Adequacy of tools

As well as knowing what tools are available for use, the diagnostician must be able to evaluate their measurement adequacy (Darley, 1979). He must determine how well each tool selected assists him in his skill of systematic observation, that is, how much precision he gains from its use.

More and more reliance is being placed on the so-called objective, standardized test for making clinical decisions; for example, when tests and test scores are used as formulas for determining which children are eligible for learning disability services. Scores are often being used in place of the diagnostician's descriptive data and clinical judgments. Objectivity in testing and interpretation is playing a greater role in diagnostic design. While objectivity is essential in evaluating the adequacy of a diagnostic tool, determining adequacy still rests with the diagnostician: Did the tool do the job for him? For example, if the diagnostician used a well-standardized test for measuring a child's phonologic errors but the items on the test did not sample this specific child's primary errors, it was not adequate for the child. As a tool, no matter how extensive its standardization, it has failed. The diagnostician must remember it is not the tool that is ultimately important; it is his use of the technique to obtain appropriate information. Even though tools are essential to the diagnostician, an accurate diagnosis of speech and language problems is the diagnostician's success, not the success of a tool, a test, or any set of tools. **Testing is not diagnosis.**

A part of the researcher's concern is the precision with which he measures the responses he wants. The same is true of the diagnostician. He must know when his tools provide him with adequate, accurate, reliable, and valid information. If the diagnostician is to design and control his diagnoses to reduce error and bias and to gain precision of measurement, he must develop an appropriate awareness and respect for measurement criteria—for objectivity.

It is not our intent to provide a detailed discussion of measurement theory, although we do believe it is an essential component of a diagnostician's knowledge. Instead, we will briefly discuss certain concepts that must be considered by the diagnostician in his design of the diagnosis. Our intent is to develop an awareness and a motivation for evaluating the tools selected. Salvia and Ysseldyke (1981) can be consulted for more information.

The diagnostician must have criteria for evaluating the adequacy of the tools he considers. The criteria discussed are validity, reliability, and standardization. These criteria arise from measurement theory, criteria often applied to something called a "test," but it can be applied to any tool. Even when a tool does not have data reported on these criteria, it is not necessarily eliminated from diagnostic usefulness. Questions arising from these criteria can be applied: Does the tool do the job intended by the diagnostician? Is the tool consistent? If repeated, will similar results occur? Does the tool provide comparative data, intra- and intergroup comparisons?

* *Validity.* Validity is of primary concern in tool construction (Messick, 1980), but it is often one of the most overlooked criteria in terms of supporting research. In its basic form, validity states that the tool is designed to measure or sample what is intended—the behavior of interest. The diagnostician would not first choose a test of phonetic structure if he hypothesized a prosody disorder. Often, validity is assumed; a statement is made that the tool has face validity, another way of saying that it is supposed to be obvious that the tool measures what was intended. For example, if we were interested in measuring syntax, we might develop a tool that asks a patient to produce verb forms, thus concluding that the tool has face validity; it generates a response about one level of syntax. Using such a tool, the diagnostician is asked to accept the rationale, the face validity, on which the tool was based. Validity in this broad sense only serves the diagnostician's general purposes for measuring dimensions of the cause–effect relationship. That is, he selects tools that appear valid for his use. He asks, "Does the tool measure a specific disordered behavior? Does the tool measure some aspect of the causal factor?"

However, even if a tool has face validity, it cannot be assumed that it differentiates among various populations. The Northwestern Syntax Screening Test (Lee, 1969) is an example of such a tool. In a study of its internal consistency, Ratusnik and Koeningsknecht (1975) revealed that although the test gave consistent results, it failed to differentiate among the clinical groups studied as well as among the clinical and normal groups. There were variable findings regarding the receptive and expressive portions of the test. Therefore the diagnostician could not use this tool and assume that it provides him with complete information about a child's language disorder. Likewise, McCauley and Swisher (1982) discuss difficulties in the use of the Northwestern Syntax Screening Test for identifying language disordered children.

Validity criteria, however, are more complex. Tools can be evaluated in terms of various types of validity: concurrent, predictive, content, and construct validity. Each of these types of validity tells the diagnostician something different about the tools he may be using, although all are bound tightly together.

When the diagnostician is choosing between two tools that were designed to measure the same thing, he is concerned with *concurrent validity.* Are the tools equivalent to one another, and will they provide him with equally adequate information? Any number of tools may be available to measure a selected aspect of speech and language performance. A question that must be asked is, "How equivalent are the tools for measuring that performance?" Is Test A for syntactic formulation equal to Test B? Do they tell us the same thing? The evidence seems fairly clear that we would not always obtain the same information with different tools. Little has been done experimentally to determine test equivalency.

Nation and Corlew (1974) pointed out that naming items in aphasia tests are not equivalent, and an article by Needham and Swisher (1972) shows that measures of auditory comprehension in aphasic patients measure that behavioral correlate differently. Thus, when selecting tools, diagnosticians must always remain aware that the tools used are only estimates of performance and may vary depending on the tool used.

When the diagnostician chooses a specific tool in hopes that he can generalize about other aspects of behavior, he is concerned with *predictive validity*. Can he estimate how intelligible a child might be on the basis of a tool that measures single-sound production in words? Will this tool be predictive of what errors the child might make in spontaneous speech production? The diagnostician is interested in predicting more general behavior from the data obtained in a specific circumstance.

When the diagnostician is choosing a tool to provide a representative sample of a specific behavior, he is concerned with *content validity*. Are the items used and the behavioral responses required representative of that class of behaviors? Should he use an articulation test that samples individual phonemes in the context of words, or should he use a test that samples syllables as the basic unit of speech? Beyond this the diagnostician should ask if the items selected provide a range of responses from easy to hard, from early to late, from concrete to abstract?

When the diagnostician is choosing between tools designed to obtain information about the same disorder, he is concerned also with *construct validity* (see concurrent validity). If his interest is in the rationale, the theory on which the tool was based, his concern is construct validity. Should he choose the Western Aphasia Battery (Kertesz, 1982) or the Porch Index of Communicative Ability (Porch, 1967)? Choices like these are especially difficult to make, since many similar tools developed from different theories have experimental literature that support them as appropriately designed tools; that is, each has construct validity. Construct validity takes into account the theory by which a test was constructed. If the theory is strong, experimentally supported, the test may be strong. But if the test is constructed on incomplete or inadequate theory, the test will be weak.

* **Reliability.** Once responses have been obtained, the diagnostician wants to know if they can be relied upon. Are they reflective of true responses? Or has the diagnostician obtained spurious results? Tools that are objective, provide standard instructions for stimulation, and provide standard procedures for scoring responses have a good chance of being reliable as long as the patient is responding in a typical way. Reliability, therefore, focuses on two primary concerns. First, the diagnostician needs to be concerned with the consistency of the responses offered by the patient. Would he perform the same if given the test a second time—*test–retest reliability*? Second, the diagnostician needs to be concerned with scoring consistency. Scoring reliability is frequently evaluated by *interjudge* and *intrajudge* reliability. Two diagnosticians following the same scoring protocols must achieve similar results before interjudge reliability of a tool can be established. Intrajudge reliability is established when the same diagnostician scores the tool the same at different times. Diagnosticians should occasionally check themselves for scoring consistency to prevent scoring biases from creeping into their analyses.

* **Standardization.** The number of tools for diagnosis of speech and language disorders that have achieved standardization status is very small (Darley, 1979; McCauley & Swisher, 1982; Bright & Matkin, 1983). Although more objective tools with reported reliability and validity estimates are available, there are few with normative data based on large

representative samples. According to Weiner and Hoock (1973), there are probably no tools exempt from serious criticism. Thus, even though the diagnostician has more objective tools to select from with some "normative" data, he cannot use the normative data uncritically. To do so may result in inappropriate analysis and interpretation.

Another aspect of standardization of importance is the construction of stimulus items. For any tool to be useful the diagnostician must know if the items are appropriate to the patient (see discussion of content validity). The items in a standardized tool should obtain a range of responses. Age is an important consideration. Standardized tools that measure developmental data must present items applicable to various ages. At the early years, for some language measures, this may mean items selected at 3- to 6-month intervals. As well, pass–fail criteria for each item, or groups of items, by the standardization population should be available. Diagnosticians will need this information to make comparisons with their patient.

Most tools that are standardized have been developed using what is termed a "normal" population. This practice can, in a sense, reduce the usability of a tool with a disordered population, at least until "normative" data is available on the disordered population. Knowing that a patient has a disorder of speech and language requires the diagnostician to view performance in light of the abnormality rather than simply normative comparisons. A standardized tool appropriate for a normal 4-year-old child may be highly inappropriate for a 4-year-old child with a severe reduction of language abilities related to central language processing disruptions. What are needed, as well, are standardized objective tools that allow the patient to perform in the presence of his special disability. For example, most language comprehension tools present both an auditory stimulus, "point to transportation," and the visual representation of the auditory stimulus. If the patient has a visual or auditory impairment, standard presentation of this tool could become inappropriate. The diagnostician would have to find alternative ways of providing the stimulation. Thus, alterations in instructions are sometimes necessary when using objective standardized tools. Of course, any alterations must be accounted for in the analysis and interpretation of the results.

• *Clinical adequacy.* There are few, if any, tools that do meet all the measurement criteria discussed. These adequacy criteria are difficult, if not impossible, to meet, if for no other reason than the fact that the time and expense involved in standardization on large representative populations are frequently prohibitive. These adequacy criteria should be regarded as guides to the development of tools for diagnosis, and test makers should work toward achieving these goals and clearly report in their test manuals which goals are not yet achieved. Until adequacy information is completely supplied for each tool, the diagnostician will have to carefully evaluate the tools he selects when designing his diagnosis. He can develop a level of confidence in their use based on his analysis of their objectivity and construct validity. He can also rely on his professional experience to determine if a selected tool helps him interpret the speech and language problem, that is, to determine if the tool is *clinically adequate.* This issue is exemplified by what is considered to be an assessment crisis for "non-mainstream speakers." Vaughn-Cooke (1983) highlighted this crisis by examining seven assessment alternatives for minority children. Following her evaluation Vaughn-Cooke (1983) concluded that assessment approaches for these children revealed a rather dismal, yet accurate picture and she calls for solutions in the form of valid, reliable assessment tools.

The diagnostician must be a careful reader of the literature, sharpening his knowledge about tool construction. He can study the rationale, the theoretical constructs by which the tool was designed. He can ask himself if the tool seems reasonable in light of what he knows about the behaviors being tested. He can look carefully at the operation of the technique—how it samples behavior. Is it sampled in a systematic, standard manner, or does it seem loosely constructed or haphazard?

Thus, the diagnostician selecting tools for designing his diagnosis should evaluate all tools critically. Darley (1979) is an extremely useful resource for tool evaluation, and his comments about tests are equally relevant.

> Some test makers have done superior work in selecting and refining items, testing for reliability, occasionally determining validity, and preparing materials that are attractive and durable. But we recognize that we may be overimpressed by the simple fact that a test has been put into print.... The more aware we become of the complexity of the human beings with whom we work, the more the tests we use lose credibility. We find that available tests are necessarily restrictive.... So clinicians are presented here with an array of techniques, variable with regard to merit and usefulness—but not *all* the techniques available. They will want to maintain a liaison between the literature and the clinic and make translations of their own into clinical procedures. With a sufficient grasp of the areas being assessed, they can be creative and go beyond the limits of the formal tests here reviewed. (p. v)

This does not mean that he will select only tools that have been standardized or that are always absolutely objective; it only means that he will judiciously select tools for the individual diagnosis, knowing what each tool is capable of providing for him. More investigation is occurring to determine how well certain tests differentiate normal from disordered individuals, mostly in child language disorders. Aram and Nation (1975) used a battery of tests to differentiate children based on their comprehension, repetition, and formulation abilities at three language levels. Differential patterns of behavior did emerge based on the tests used. More recent examples of investigations of test adequacy are found in McCauley and Swisher (1982), Demetras, A. Matkin, and Swisher (1982), and Bright and N. Matkin (1983).

Works from a tool-retrieval system: The SLPM

Darley (1964) states that the diagnostician has only two basic tools at his disposal, the test and the history. He goes on to specify a test as a stimuli presented to patients to elicit some form of response—a sample of behavior. In line with this perspective we maintain that the diagnostician has only a single measurement method available to him—systematic observation. All tools, regardless of how structured, of what type, or in what form, are techniques designed to elicit responses that are to be systematically observed.

However, before he can select tools for systematic observation, the diagnostician needs a way to organize and retrieve the many available tools—a *tool-retrieval system*. The earlier categories of tools we presented are not a particularly helpful method of organization. As an alternative, the diagnostician might choose to organize his tools according to the traditional problem-type classification system, that is, tools for articulation disorders, voice disorders, and so forth (Darley, 1979). Although the problem-type classification has served professionally over the years, it has serious drawbacks that we feel limit its usefulness for organizing and retrieving tools.

A more logical retrieval system would be one tied closely to the purposes of diagnosis and the SLPM framework. Just as the diagnostician can view and classify speech and language disorders and their causes from the SLPM perspective, so also can he view and classify the tools needed to diagnose these disorders and their causes. A tool-retrieval system based on the SLPM focuses more on what a tool does than on what a tool is called. Using the SLPM, the diagnostician is free to study tools in relationship to his clinical hypothesis rather than simply relying on the stated purpose of theoretical orientation of a given tool.

Components

Tools can be organized around the three components of the model. There are many tools available that directly measure some detail of the speech and language product component. These tools are designed to provide detailed information about the characteristics of the speech and language variation to determine if, in fact, it is disordered. Any tool that allows the diagnostician to systematically observe some detail of the speech and language product could be an appropriate tool to include in the diagnostician's design, dependent on the effect to be measured. Some tools are better than others for the type and amount of information offered; some provide more detailed data than others.

The following four tests for phonology and/or phonetic structure give varying amounts and quality of information: the Assessment of Phonological Processes (Hodson, 1980); the Deep Test of Articulation (McDonald, 1964); the Arizona Articulatory Proficiency Scale (Fudala, 1970); and Natural Process Analysis (Shriberg & Kwiatkowski, 1980). Which might you use with 8-year-old Hildegarde who has /r, ɔ˞, l, and l̩/ errors?

The speech and language processing component is far more difficult to measure. As previously discussed, it is measured primarily through speech and language products and behavioral correlates. The diagnostician obtains a measure of some behavior that he understands to be correlated with physical processes. Thus, this component is measured primarily through inference. The tools used to measure the speech and language product are often the same as those used to draw inferences about physical processes. At other times behavioral correlates are measured, for example, gestures that tell the diagnostician about certain physical processes. The inference is made that if the behavior is intact, so is the underlying process. Designing tools for this component requires careful consideration of the inferential measurement strategy discussed earlier. Almost any tool provides some degree of information about physical processing.

What physical processes might you be "testing" if you used the following tools in your diagnosis of 49-year-old Mr. Moore: the "Rainbow Passage" (Fairbanks, 1960) and production of /a/ at three different pitch levels?

Tools to tap the speech and language environment component are used primarily to discover causal factors. Most of these tools are restrospective, trying to discover past occurrences that may be causally related to the current speech and language disorder. Case history questionnaires and direct interviews are the tools most commonly used. Of course, the diagnostician can look at the current environment of the patient by "visiting" him in his various environmental circumstances: at home, on the job, at school.

What series of questions might you devise to discover if 3-year-old Ed had and is receiving enough speech and language stimulation to compensate for his mild bilateral hearing loss, which is suspected of being responsible for his delay in language development?

Appendix III presents a listing of many tools available for use by the diagnostician for designing his diagnosis within the SLPM framework. Instructions for use of the appendix are provided there. It is suggested to the diagnostician that this appendix be expanded and adapted to his specific needs in his work setting. Aram and Nation (1982) have used this system in child language disorders. Also, Owens, Haney, Eiesow, Dooley, and Kelly (1983) have developed a matrix system for viewing language levels of a selected set of language assessment tools.

Causal factors

When the diagnostician designs his diagnosis to gain support for his causal hypothesis, he must recognize his causal testing limitations. There are some causal factors the diagnostician can design and test for; for example, if hearing loss has been hypothesized as the basis for the speech and language disorder (auditory testing), if a short lingual frenum has been hypothesized (speech mechanism testing), or if a lack of speech and language stimulation has been hypothesized (interview testing). There are other causal factors the diagnostician can only partially design and test for; for example, if mental retardation has been hypothesized, if inadequate velopharyngeal closure has been hypothesized, or if neurological dysfunction has been hypothesized. In many such instances the ultimate design and testing for causal factors must be left up to other specialists. For example, if neurological dysfunction has been hypothesized, it will be the neurologist who will make the final causal diagnosis; if it is mental retardation, it will probably be the psychologist or the educator; if emotional disturbance is hypothesized, it will be the psychologist or psychiatrist.

Because of the nature and complexities of causal factors, the diagnostician has few tools that he can use to direcly test the causal factor. Generally, the tools the diagnostician uses in his design measure certain behaviors that provide support for potential causes but do not provide direct, demonstrable proof. Beyond the case history analysis and the interview, the diagnostician can select and use certain tools that provide information about visual abilities, hearing status, motor performance, social development, psychological status, emotional status, and mental abilities. These tools, along with guided observations that focus on extraverbal behaviors accompanying interpersonal communication, provide information about the patient's overall areas of functioning that could be causally or coincidentally related to the speech and language disorder.

Guided observation may provide one of the few avenues the speech–language pathologist has for gaining data pertinent to causal factors. Observations of a child's play behavior may provide much information about the child's level of intellectual and cognitive ability. The diagnostician may present a child with a certain selection of things to do such as doll furniture, dolls, and doll clothing (stimulus control) and observe how the child explores, plays with, and develops relationships among the sets of materials he has been given. Observing the child who demonstrates excessive motor activity, is unable to attend, is in leg braces, drools constantly, is highly emotional, or seems frightened; and the adult who appears with a right hemiplegia, is depressed, and walks into things are among the many observations that may lend evidence supporting certain causal factors that have been hypothesized.

There are questions that sometimes arise about the professional qualifications necessary for using certain tools, particularly if the tools are "borrowed" from another professional discipline. The use of some tools by the speech–language pathologist as "causal tests" raises few questions, for example, the Bruininks–Oseretsky Tests of Motor Proficiency (Bruininks, 1978; Doll, 1965), whereas others may raise considerable questions, the Bender-Gestalt Test for Young Children (Koppitz, 1964). Still others are generally considered out of bounds, for example, the Wechsler Intelligence Scale for Children—Revised (1974).

However, in this age of interdisciplinary and transdisciplinary education and work settings, lines of demarcation for test use are sometimes fuzzy. There are tools that are used across various professional groups, depending on the level of training and how the information from the tool is to be used and interpreted. The most frequently cited examples are intelligence and personality tests, generally considered as part of the psychologist's armamentarium. Can the speech–language pathologist justifiably select and use some of these tools to gain information about causal factors? Many of these tools are used in our experimental literature. As we grow and develop as professionals with greater interdisciplinary interests, there may be less concern over who uses what test and more concern over why the test is being used by the professional. For example, many tools being used to assess language and communication in infancy and early childhood (e.g., the Hedrick et al. Sequenced Inventory of Communication Development, 1975) follow developmental assessment of children as long pursued in pediatric medicine and psychology (e.g., Gesell and Amatruda's Development Diagnosis, revised by Knoblock & Pasamanick, 1974).

From the tools he uses the diagnostician may have arrived at strong inferences about causal factors and then must rely on other professionals to verify his causal hypothesis. When these causal circumstances exist, referrals to other specialists are needed to complete the design and testing for the causal aspect of the hypothesis, so referral becomes another tool for diagnostic design. But the diagnostician has to know what other specialists do if he is to make informed referrals. The diagnostician must know what he wants, how to get it, what it means when he gets it, and what it does for him. The ability to state, "I need a neurologic examination" is not enough to obtain needed answers to diagnostic questions. The diagnostician must understand the nature and intent of a neurologic examination—what information it will and will not provide that is pertinent to the patient being diagnosed. Diagnosticians have an obligation to understand some of the basic tools used by other specialists. For example, the diagnostician who refers for medical information should know the essentials of what may be done by the physician. His first consideration should be referral to a physician who understands speech and language disorders. However, depending on the causal factors of concern, different specialists will be called on. In voice disorders the otolaryngologist will be important; for children with language disorders the pediatrician or pediatric neurologist may be called on; for dysarthria due to any number of causes the neurologist or physical medicine and rehabilitation specialists will be important. Each of these specialists generally approaches the patient in a similar fashion. A general examination is done, followed by special tests for isolating causal factors for the speech and language disorder or, from their point of view, the medical or physical problems the patient may have.

As well as providing information about causal factors, certain tools used primarily by other professions also can provide significant data about speech and language. This is very evident in intelligence tests that require verbal performance. We (Aram & Nation, 1971) did an analysis of speech and language items on a number of frequently used intelligence tests using an earlier version of the SLPM as a framework for the analysis. It became quite clear from the analysis that a child with a significant deficit in speech and language would be greatly penalized by many of these tools because of their heavy verbal loadings. Having information like this assists the diagnostician in both making referrals and interpreting data he receives. Thus, knowing tools that other specialists use is one way of making intelligent referrals, of using referrals as tools of diagnosis.

In Appendix III a number of tools that are considered primarily causal tools or tools for associated behaviors are listed. Some of these are used by diagnosticians of speech and language disorders; others are not. Salvia and Ysseldyke (1981) is an excellent resource for tools that we consider as causal and related measures, and Lezak (1976) provides information on tools used in neuropsychological assessment.

In summary, knowing the conceptual orientation to the SLPM gives the diagnostician the knowledge needed to develop a tool-retrieval system for diagnostic design, regardless of the type of patient, the type of speech and language disorder seen, its specific characteristics, and the many causal factors that may have been or are interacting with the speech and language disorder. The SLPM not only gives the diagnostician a frame of reference for selecting the tools appropriate to his hypothesis, but it also allows him to "plug in" new tools as they are developed. Relating tools to the conceptual framework of the SLPM forces him to question what a tool does for him. With this approach to design and selection of tools, the diagnostician can expose himself to a wide range of tests and procedures, develop his skill in using the tool when needed for a given diagnosis, and evaluate the effectiveness of the tool, thereby having available an inventory of tools for future reference.

Retrieves tools

Once the diagnostician has worked out his plan for systematic observation, he must select the specific tools by which he will carry out that plan. We have discussed the infinite number of tools available to the diagnostician, developed a tool-retrieval system through a SLPM organization, presented a selected list of available tools in Appendix III, suggested a series of criteria by which tools can be evaluated, and have indicated that the personal characteristics of the patient and the work setting must be considered.

Several other considerations should be mentioned at this time. First, the diagnostician is working under time constraints; he must be able to administer the tools he selects within his time limitations. Therefore, he may select a single tool to measure several things simultaneously. Second, the diagnostician should understand his own limitations—is he familiar with all aspects of the tools he has selected? Third, the diagnostician must consider some rather practical aspects of the tools. Of importance is their portability. Carrying around suitcases of props or heavy equipment simply is not feasible in many work settings. Thus, tools must be physically manageable.

Given this entire set of considerations for retrieving the specific tools needed for testing the cause–effect hypothesis, we proceed to a set of diagnostic situations exemplifying these considerations. These situations are only schematic. They are representative of certain circumstances the diagnostician may confront in his various work settings. The student should develop the overall planning that would go into each of these situations that leads to tool selection. All the tools presented in the examples can be found in Appendix III.

Harriet Nordell, 3 years, 6 months, was referred to a community speech and hearing agency. Hypothesis: "Severe language disorder on all linguistic levels — — "

The diagnostician, Ms. Seligman, has available to her a full range of tools. To observe the language product she first selects a *spontaneous speech and language sample* and the Vocabulary Usage Test (VUT; Nation, 1972). Diagnosticians often rely on a spontaneous speech sample to measure language performance (for example, Lee, 1974; Crystal, Fletcher, & Garman, 1976; Hubbell, 1981; Miller, 1981). All language products can be observed if the patient offers any language output. Since Harriet has a severe language disorder, Ms. Seligman may have difficulty obtaining enough of a sample for analysis or she may obtain all that the child is capable of, from unintelligible vocalizations to one- or two-word responses. The stimuli produced by Ms. Seligman will be crucial to obtaining this sample. Ms. Seligman chose this tool because she has a firm comparative foundation—knowledge about the normal language behavior of children this age. What information, other than the language product, might you obtain with a spontaneous speech sample?

The VUT was selected because it provides information about a specific language product, the semantic level. This tool was chosen based on the stages of language acquisition; semantic items (vocabulary) are seen first in a child's development. Since Harriet has a deficit on all linguistic levels, her best output performance may well be in vocabulary usage. The tool is developmental and objective although not highly standardized. Ms. Seligman also feels she will obtain some other information from this tool that allows her to distinguish between possible comprehension and formulation deficits. The Vocabulary Usage Test requires the child to respond to pictured items from an auditorally presented stimulus.

Ms. Seligman also selected the following tools for Harriet: Sequenced Inventory of Communication Development (Hedrick, Prather, & Tobin, 1973); Arthur Adaptation of the Leiter International Performance Scale (Arthur, 1952). What information do you think she was trying to obtain from these tools? How useful might the Preschool Language Assessment Instrument (Blank, Rose, & Berlin, 1978) be for Harriet?

The spontaneous speech and language sample ranks high among the various techniques selected to observe language products. The diagnostician is likely to obtain more typical responses with this measure than with some of the structured stimulus–response tools that may be available. From his sample the diagnostician performs various analyses on the data for comparison to normal language development (e.g., Crystal, Fletcher, & Garman, 1976; Miller, 1981). However, analysis of the data from this procedure is not easy. It is easier to record a response to a structured stimulus; for example, right or wrong, and from the derived score determine if the patient's performance is above, at, or below the norms than it is to take a spontaneous language sample that, in all likelihood, will have to be tape-recorded, listened to over and over, and then apply analysis procedures to arrive at a description of the child's language behavior. However, the end result of this latter procedure may result in better treatment planning.

The diagnostician must remember that when a child produces language, he also reveals information about his underlying language processes. For example, if the diagnostician presents a stimulus, "Tell me what's happening in this picture," and the child responds, "Boy throw ball," the diagnostician can easily measure the semantic and syntactic levels of the language product. If the response is on target, he knows something about comprehension and formulation.

Ms. Marge Celeste, the kindergarten teacher, asked the speech pathologist, Mr. Jim Thorington, to see Paul Cronise who had just entered her kindergarten class. Ms. Celeste thinks Paul may be retarded. Mr. Thorington formulated the following hypothesis: "Severe language comprehension disruptions."

Mr. Thorington selects the Peabody Picture Vocabulary Test Revised (Dunn & Dunn, 1981) and the Token Test for Children (DiSimoni, 1978). Both of these tools are objective and in the case of the Peabody Picture Vocabulary Test well standardized, although not without criticisms of the standardization (Weiner & Hoock, 1973). Mr. Thorington selects these tools because he wants an objective baseline of Paul's ability to comprehend at the semantic and syntactic levels. Comprehension, a behavioral correlate, has always been difficult to measure. It cannot be observed directly but must be measured by observing certain responses from which the diagnostician infers comprehension abilities. Thus, objective measures as selected by Mr. Thorington are extremely important to use since it is difficult to know from general conversation at what level Paul may be comprehending. For example, how would he know which of the following two stimuli would be appropriate for Paul: "Would you like to color in the coloring book?" and "Did you walk to school today?"

Typical tools of comprehension, such as those selected by Mr. Thorington, ask a patient to point to a choice of pictures that correspond to the auditory stimulus presented or comply with a series of commands. Stimuli may be words, phrases, sentences, and paragraphs. Foil pictures are often used to check for accuracy of response or closeness of response. What is measured in comprehension tasks has been questioned by Waryas and Ruder (1974) and Rees & Shulman (1978). How could these authors' reservations in assessing comprehension be addressed with Paul?

Since Ms. Celeste is concerned about mental retardation, Mr. Thorington hopes the Peabody Picture Vocabulary Test may provide him with useful information. But Mr. Thorington is aware of the use of verbal measures for estimating the intelligence of children with speech and language disorders, particularly in Paul's case since he has hypothesized a severe comprehension deficit. This very issue was addressed by Weiner (1971) who studied the reliability and stability of two measures of intelligence on children with language disorders—the Peabody Picture Vocabulary Test and the Arthur Adaptation of the Leiter International Performance Scale (Arthur, 1952). Further, Aram, Ekelman, & Nation (in press) have found the Leiter to be a good predictor of language, intelligence, and school abilities during adolescence.

From Weiner's information (1971), what might Mr. Thorington expect from his use of the Peabody Picture Vocabulary Test with Paul? If he were to refer Paul for psychological testing, what justifications could he offer for the specification of an intelligence tool to be used?

Evaluate the following tools also selected by Mr. Thorington for Paul: the Illinois Test of Psycholinguistic Abilities (Kirk et al., 1968) and the Flowers-Costello Test of Central Auditory Abilities (Flowers et al., 1970).

Marie Shivers, age 4 years, 9 months, has little language. She is being seen by Mr. Alex Orosz, speech pathologist at University Hospitals, as a part of a comprehensive inpatient workup. Hypothesis: "Severe language comprehension, integration, and formulation disorder related to cerebral dysfunction."

Mr. Orosz selects guided observations of all aspects of general behavior during Marie's daily activities while in the hospital. Mr. Orosz has taken this approach in order to observe behaviors that may signal the presence of cerebral dysfunction as a basis for the lack of speech and language development. He is particularly interested in any direct physical signs such as gait, awkward coordination, and speech-mechanism deviations as well as behaviors that are at times predictive of cerebral dysfunction—signs such as hyperactivity, compulsivity, inability to attend, motor perseveration, emotionality, and variable, inconsistent responses to auditory and visual stimulation. His goal is to assist the team in organizing the most efficient set of tests for isolating the basis of Marie's speech and language disorder. From his findings he will provide recommendations for testing to the other team members.

Mr. Orosz recommended the use of the following tools: the Arthur Adaptation of the Leiter International Performance Scale (Arthur, 1952). Bruininks–Oseretsky Tests of Motor Proficiency (Bruininks, 1978; Doll, 1965), and the Developmental Test of Visual Perception (Frostig, 1964). What does Mr. Orosz hope will be accomplished by the use of these tools?

Dr. Maureen Whitney is seeing her first aphasic patient at Springfield General Hospital. She has a range of aphasia tests accessible to her and appropriate training in their use. The hospital staff, however, has always used the Minnesota Test for Differential Diagnosis of Aphasia (Schuell, 1965) because of its prognostic ability. While Dr. Whitney understands the prognostic implications for using this test, her theoretical orientation to aphasia leads her to other choices of tools. She has been asked to justify her selection of the Boston Diagnostic Aphasia Examination (Goodglass & Kaplan, 1972) for initial diagnostic purposes followed by the Porch Index of Communicative Ability (Porch, 1967) for later objectification and prognostication.

Can you justify Dr. Whitney's approach to selection of tools to fulfill the purposes of diagnosis? Are these tools practical for all settings? In what type of setting might this approach be most useful? How much time would it require to administer the tools? Would Kertesz' Western Aphasia Battery (1982) fulfill the requirements of prognostication?

Prognosis for change of disordered speech and language behavior is a major part of the diagnostician's function. Following his diagnosis, the diagnostician should be able to make tentative judgments about the patient's ability to change if given the maximum therapeutic intervention needed. Aside from his clinical experience with similar patients, the diagnostician has little to guide him in making prognostic statements since only a few tools have been developed that give prognostic information. Notable among them are the Minnesota Test for Differential Diagnosis of Aphasia developed by Schuell (1965).

The diagnostician often relies on *stimulability testing* to determine if a patient can learn, can change his pattern of speech and language given appropriate stimulation (Milisen et al., 1954). Thus any tool or device that demonstrates that a patient can learn to change his behavior has potential for prognostication. Some tools have been developed to assist the diagnostician with specific types of patients. Jacobs et al. (1970) have developed a stimulability test, the Miami Imitative Ability Test, for children whose speech characteristics are related to a cleft palate condition. The cleft palate child's improvement in articulation can be occasionally prognosticated on the basis of results from this test. Aram, Ekelman, & Nation (in press) have identified certain preschool language and cognitive measures that predict abilities during adolescence.

Dr. Ivan Cook is seeing Ms. Leslie Golden, age 28, who was referred for stuttering therapy. There is no doubt in Dr. Cook's mind that she is a stutterer. Thus, he selects tools to determine the type, extent, and severity of her prosody disorder. He wants information that will tell him when she stutters, what type of prosody variations she is exhibiting, how often these occur, and how much they interfere with communication. Thus, this diagnosis is concerned with a contemporary view of the disorder rather than discovering a historical cause–effect relationship.

Other than presenting various types of stimuli to Ms. Golden and organizing his observations of her responses, what can Dr. Cook do to get the information he is looking for? If you were to follow Riley's procedure (1972) using his Stuttering Severity Instrument (SSI), would you be able to characterize the disorder as well as determine its severity? What information would the Southern Illinois University Speech Situations Check List and the Southern Illinois University Behavior Check List, both by Brutten and Shoemaker (1974), provide for systematically obtaining the information that Dr. Cook wants?

In summary, the diagnostician selects tools to assist him in observing relevant information about the cause–effect hypothesis he has formulated. The tools selected must be appropriate to the individual patient. Although standardization and objectivity are important tool criteria, the diagnostician may use a variety of tools to determine the nature and severity of the patient's disorder.

Determines interview questions

If the interview has been selected as a tool to be used in the diagnosis, the diagnostician must plan the format of that interview. While much of what happens in the interview will be dependent on interpersonal factors, the diagnostician should be prepared to enter the interview situation. We suggest, therefore, that the diagnostician consider two fundamental questions in planning the interview: (1) What information does he want? (2) How does he plan to get it?

As with any tool that has been selected for the diagnosis, the interview aims at gaining data to shed more understanding about the clinical hypothesis that was formulated through the constituent analysis. The diagnostician will need to fill in missing data and, in addition, he will need to amplify, clarify, and verify information made available to him. Some of the information he has is insufficient. For example, on the children's speech and language history questionnaire, in response to, "When did he speak his first word," a parent may have written *late*. Here the diagnostician would want to get a more refined idea of what late means. He may be able to pin down a more specific time or gain a better estimate of the time in relation to other events such as birthdays, visits to grandmothers, and so on.

Often the diagnostician will want the informant to amplify information provided prior to the interview. For example, if reference was made to the fact that a child was in "therapy," the diagnostician would want to delineate more clearly the details of that therapy. Was it speech therapy, psychotherapy, or physiotherapy? What were the goals of therapy? What was its duration and frequency?

At other times the diagnostician will need to clarify information that is ambiguous or inconsistent. For example, a teacher may report that "Larry has trouble keeping still in class." The diagnostician will need to determine if "still" refers to Larry's verbal or activity level and what circumstances surround his difficulty "keeping still." At times information from different sources (or even from the same source) is inconsistent and contradictory. A pediatrician may report that Ruth had difficulty being toilet trained, while a parent reports no such problems; or one source may report two siblings and a second source reports three. A mother may report hemorrhaging during pregnancy, while the pediatrician's report states an uneventful pregnancy. In all such situations, further information is needed to reconcile the contradictory information.

Finally, a diagnostician may need to verify information if he questions its reliability or validity. For example, a referring social worker may suggest that family stresses, including a working mother and alcoholic father, are the basis for Victor's speech and language problems. During the interview, the diagnostician will want to explore the nature of these family stresses more thoroughly to determine if in fact the home situation does adversely affect the speech and language environment of the child.

In the following examples determine what missing data needs to be gained and where amplification, clarification, and verification of constituent analysis information are indicated.

1. A physician, Dr. Draeger, reports that 6-year-old Alexander has had a history of chronic otitis media.

2. The only information regarding motor milestones for 10-year-old Sarah is walking at 15 months. She has been described as clumsy by her gym teacher and is doing poorly in reading and spelling in school.

3. An adult patient, Mrs. Rockman, describes her speech and language problem as "difficulty making myself understood."

4. The referring psychologist reported that 4-year-old Tommy's parents are divorced. Tommy lives with his mother and maternal grandmother and 6-year-old sister. The father has visitation rights and spends every other Sunday with Tommy and his daughter.

5. On the children's speech and language history form, Mrs. Rupert checks *yes* to "eating problems," "difficult to manage," and "personality problem" but did not explain or give ages.

Having decided what information he wants, the diagnostician next needs to think through how he plans to get that information. Here he is concerned with framing his questions. Styles of eliciting information differ markedly from a nondirect approach, where the information evolves from considerable dialogue and reflection on the informant's comments—"I see that you are concerned." "You feel uncertain about Jerome's abilities." "Renee's stuttering worries you"—to a direct question–answer exchange characteristic of much political poll taking or consumer interviewing: "Do you have a dog?" "What brands of dog food have you used in the past month?" "Have you ever tried Grow-pup Super Meat?" "Is your income bracket below $10,000, between $10,000 and $25,000, or above $25,000?"

We can view most forms of interview probe questions as falling on an open–closed continuum determined by the degree of structure allowed in the informant's response. Closed questions elicit specific, relatively predictable information; the number of alternative answers or choices in answering is limited. Questions such as "Hold old is Lee?" "When did Jonathan first begin to walk?" "Did Carter ever have any ear infections?" are examples of relatively closed questions. Open questions, at the other end of the continuum, allow for considerable choice and flexibility in the informant's responses. Such questions gain elaborate, less predictable information and are often feeling oriented (Bernstein, 1970; Richardson, et al., 1965). "How does Leigh spend her day?" "How would you describe your husband's problems in speaking?" and "How did you understand the problem as Dr. Bastob explained it to you?" are open-ended questions. Table 6-1 lists a number of types of questions that are arranged in terms of their degree of openness or closedness. There are many variations and additions to these types of questions, and there is nothing sacred or special about the particular list of question types in Table 6-1; rather, these types of questions represent a range often used in the interview.

While some writers recommend that open questions should predominate in the interview (Garrett, 1972; Richardson et al., 1965), we maintain that a range of question types are useful and that the information needed determines the type of question asked. Yes/no, multiple choice, and fill in the blank questions are direct, efficient means of gaining specific, relatively nonequivocal factual information. For example, if the diagnostician wants to know

Table 6-1. Closed-open question continuum

Question type		Examples
Closed end	Yes/no	Did Martin require any oxygen immediately following birth? Did your husband want to come today?
	Multiple choice	Does Emory use his left hand, right hand, or both? Does Mark primarily use speech or gestures?
	Fill in the blank	John is how old? What drugs were used during delivery? Where was your husband's surgery performed?
	Circumscribed amplification	Describe Torry's speech problem. What kinds of things does Kevin play with? How have Mr. Worzella's spirits been since his stroke?
Open end	Take off anywhere	What would you like to talk about today? Is there anything you would like to talk about that we haven't already discussed? I'd like you to try to give me a picture of Sandy as you see her at home.

if there are any siblings in the family, a yes/no question, "Does Ramon have any brothers or sisters?" would gain the information most directly.

In using relatively closed questions, however, the diagnostician needs to guard against presenting prepackaged alternatives and specifying dichotomies when none exist. For example, "Is Sarah toilet trained?" may elicit a simple yes/no response when a range of toilet training can exist—from no control, through degrees of control, to complete control. Asking a parent if they are "relieved or unsettled" by Max's placement in a school for the retarded may in no way match their feelings about the situation. Not all informants are secure enough to disregard the nonapplicable alternatives presented in the interview questions. Thus, in using closed questions, the diagnostician needs to be sure he furthers data collection, not cuts it off or elicits invalid information. His questions should not inhibit spontaneity on the part of the informant or allow the informant to outguess him and give the "correct" rather than the accurate answer. Too many closed questions will make the interview appear rote and prefabricated. The question may make the informants feel that the only information wanted from them is the yes/no, multiple choice, or fill in the blank variety. They may interpret this as disinterest in how they really feel about the problem at hand. The diagnostician should be sure to allow for amplification and self-expression by the informant even when using closed questions. Often, for example, a yes/no question may be followed by a question asking for more information. "Does Shorty have any brothers or sisters?" If answered affirmatively, it may be followed by further fill in the blank questions: "How old are they?" or with circumscribed amplification: "What kinds of things do Shorty and his sister do together?" or "How does his sister respond to Shorty?"

Open-ended questions allow for maximal individual expression on the part of the informant. Such questions tend to let the informant say what is important to him in the way that he wants to express it, thus restricting possible bias or shortsightedness on the part of the diagnostician. The diagnostician cannot predict all that he needs to know; thus he must allow the informant room to say what he wants to say. Open-ended questions, however, are inefficient in gaining specific, nonequivocal information. If the diagnostician wants to know if Kate has had psychological testing, he does not need to go all around the barn to get an answer. A question such as "What have you done about her problem?" may not address the information wanted.

Also, at times, some informants have difficulty responding if some structure is not provided for their response. Some may feel that "there's no place to start" in describing a pervasive problem; others "don't know what to say." Such informants may respond in one or two words to "take off anywhere" questions but not provide much more information to circumscribed amplification questions. In sum, the diagnostician should have a range of question types at his disposal as different information and patients will require different question types. Framing interview questions is not an either/or proposition, rather it is a purposive selection and combination of several question types.

After determining the information needed and framing questions to get that information, the diagnostician will then be ready to launch his questions in the interpersonal context of the actual interview.

Tailor-makes the design

Two practices often occur in non-problem-solving approaches to diagnosis: first, the practice of performing routine diagnoses or using routine tools and second, the practice of performing problem-type diagnoses. Neither of these practices fulfills the orientation developed in this book; however, both can be viewed in relationship to this orientation.

Many speech–language pathologists make the mistake of considering diagnosis to consist of a series of standardized routines, for example, all children with language disorders are given the same invariant set of tools. At times, unfortunately, this is the dictate of the specific work setting. To us, this subverts the diagnostician's basic problem-solving job function. Instead, it forces the diagnostician to rely on tests rather than searching for answers to clinical questions.

An invariant battery of tools for a given disorder or a given causal factor will result in the use of some tools that are inappropriate and will overlook tools that are more appropriate. Reliance on a battery of tools can create the attitude that tools in the battery, which may not reveal much information, should be eliminated. It also creates the attitude that the "new tool" must be added to the battery. No technique should be discontinued as part of the diagnostician's catalog of tools simply because it is useful only for a selected number of patients. Tool selection is based on the diagnostician's judgment of what may be needed for each specific patient.

There are instances where the concept of "routine procedures" may partially apply; for instance, when the diagnostician receives little prior information beyond knowing the age and sex of the patient and that some type of speech and language disorder presumably exists. If the diagnostician is confronted with many of these referrals in his work setting, he may establish what could be called a basic testing plan for beginning his diagnosis. This basic plan would be designed to sample quickly many speech and language behaviors and processes. From this, the diagnostician can isolate the problem area and establish "on-the-spot" hypotheses and then select tools for detailed analysis.

This basic plan can be considered a "screening device." Dependent on the work setting, the diagnostician may devise several of these for different populations of patients. Of course, the most basic procedure is to engage the patient in conversational speech and carefully observe the speech and language product as well as the way the patient responds to the various stimuli provided. If this can be done, the diagnostician is on his way to deriving a clinical hypothesis.

Routine testing, the invariant selection of a tool for all diagnoses, stems from the concept of routine diagnoses. A common example is the routine use of the speech mechanism examination. The assumption apparently underlying this practice is that since we "talk with our mouths," the mouth must be examined. Similarly, we find routine use of audiometric procedures. The same type of assumption is present since we "hear with our ears," they must be examined. Another practice that occurs is based on the dictates of a work setting or a diagnostician. Frequently we hear, "the Illinois Test of Psycholinguistic Abilities (Kirk et al., 1968) is given to all children with language disorders." There is no way from our orientation that we can rationalize an underlying assumption for this practice. It tends to occur most often when a new tool appears that is promoted as a well-standardized tool. An adverse result of this practice is "throwing the baby out with the bathwater." Other tools, previously used, that have been useful are discarded in favor of the new tool. The fad of the "new test" strikes us much the same as the "wayward child."

Again, the use of routine tools may have a place in diagnosis, but they should be selected and used on the basis of the diagnostician's concern about certain dimensions of his hypothesis. Routine tools are helpful in reducing uncertainties the diagnostician may have as expressed in alternative hypotheses, including the null hypothesis. For example, routine speech mechanism examinations and audiometric procedures assist in ruling in or out disruptions in two major segments of the speech and language processing component—the auditory reception segment and the speech production segment. However, there is no reason to assume that in all speech and language disorders there may be either a disrupted speech mechanism or a hearing problem. For example, if a child has highly intelligible, precise, articulated speech, the purpose for performing a speech mechanism examination is questionable. The diagnostician should be able to state the importance of any routine practice in light of each specific hypothesis; it should not be an unthinking selection based on statements like, "we were taught to always give a speech mechanism exam."

The second routine practice, the problem-type diagnosis, is not unlike the routine diagnosis. However, the problem-type diagnosis has more important implications since it stems generally from concern over a specific causal factor. In the problem-type diagnosis the emphasis is on a set of tools selected around the special disability, for example, as in a diagnosis of the cleft palate child, the child with cerebral palsy, the deaf child, or the brain-injured child. If these conditions are hypothesized as the causal basis for the speech and language disorder, then this practice becomes more appropriate. However, the diagnostician should not assume that just because a child has cerebral palsy that the speech and language disorder is related to this physical condition. The child's physical disability may affect only his lower extremities, and the cause of his language disorder may be related to a significant hearing loss. So the diagnostician must not draw one-to-one relationships between certain disabilities and the speech and language disorder. Jumping to these unwarranted conclusions creates unwarranted hypotheses and ultimate failure in diagnosis. Instead, even in those problems where the predicted speech and language disorder may be highly probable, the diagnostician sill develops his hypothesis from all the data and tailor-makes his diagnostic design. He does not want to develop a stereotyped orientation to any specific problem type.

This point can be exemplified in the following two referral statements on the same child: "Darwin is a cleft palate child." "Darwin, who has a cleft palate, stutters." How does this change your thinking about selecting tools to fit the hypothesis?

The point of view that we tailor-make our diagnoses is vital if the diagnostician is to continue to improve with experience. Diagnostic skill is not something that is arrived at by learning a set of required procedures in a rote fashion. The diagnostician must make decisions as to what tools will be most productive of his time and energy. On the one hand, he must not leave out some areas to be tested that are important, and on the other hand, he must not waste time with many unnecessary and time-consuming tools.

DEVELOPS A TESTING STRATEGY

This third task of diagnostic design is a step-by-step thinking through of (1) the order in which the tools selected will be presented to establish the cause–effect hypothesis and (2) the order in which the tools will be presented to elicit the best samples of behavior from the patient. The diagnostician plans his testing strategy to balance the examiner–tool–patient interactions in order to optimize data collection. This advance planning helps reduce the number of diagnostic failures; the diagnostician has thought through possible testing difficulties: If Judy will not talk, the diagnostician has a plan.

In general, but not invariably, the order of tool presentation in the diagnostic session is from the effect to cause, from general to specific, from easy to hard. The diagnostician knows what his tools will do, which are complex, which are simple, which give general information, and which are tasks to obtain specific detailed information. Ordering his tools, the diagnostician obtains the most important information about his clinical hypothesis first, whether it is cause, effect, or both. He can then order the remainder of his tools to get the necessary details for the remainder of his diagnostic specifications.

Ordering the presentation of tools facilitates data collection; the diagnostician knows how he intends to move from one tool to the next, depending on the information he obtains with each tool. Knowing what each tool provides assists the diagnostician in first establishing some baseline of behaviors, which are followed by the next tool; or the next tool could be eliminated if it no longer seems needed. For example, if the diagnostician started out with a spontaneous conversation with Julius and quickly discovered that he understands and engages in dialogue adequately, then the diagnostician could eliminate his tools for comprehension. In this way the diagnostician alternates between causal tools and effect tools as the information accrues until he has verified and specified his cause–effect relationship.

Keeping the patient–tool–examiner interaction in focus facilitates obtaining adequate and representative samples of the patient's behavior, obtaining as many responses as possible within the time limitations. Following the general order from easy to hard can give the patient an early opportunity for successful performance. The harder tasks that he may fail can be presented later at a time when he and the diagnostician have built up a better interpersonal relationship. By then, the patient may be more willing to try difficult tasks and, at the same time, the diagnostician will know more about the manner in which to present the tasks. As the diagnostician and the patient move along in the session, each will gain a better understanding of the other and of the overall purposes behind the tasks. The diagnostician can build in successes to counterbalance the failures the patient may be experiencing.

Most tools are designed to provide easy tasks (basals) before more difficult ones (ceilings). However, there are some tests that present what are considered the more difficult items first (Porch, 1967). Presumably, this is done to counter the usual test procedure of ending with failure on the final test items. The diagnostician must know the order of item presentation and its effect on patient performance. At the same time, the diagnostician's job is to discover the extent of the disorder, and thus he must get samples of disordered behavior and failures as well as adequate performance. The outside world of the patient is not ordered in terms of easy to hard.

SUMMARY

The diagnosis is designed to test the clinical hypothesis that has been formulated from the constituent analysis. To develop such a design, the diagnostician must apply what he knows about speech and language disorders in order to specify what data he wants to obtain. His expertise in measurement tells him how to get the data he wants. He uses various tools drawn from an enormous array of available choices from various sources including the interview, commercial tools, experimental tools, setting protocols, and guided observations. The SLPM framework serves as an organizing system for easy tool retrieval. In addition, the diagnostician applies several criteria for determining the adequacy of tools for selection. These criteria are validity, reliability, standardization, and clinical adequacy.

In designing the diagnosis the diagnostician performs three tasks.

1. He *plans for systematic observation and measurement* of the cause–effect relationships expressed in the clinical hypothesis. He does this by specifying the type of tasks necessary, and considering patient characteristics.

2. He *selects tools for measurement* from his command of a range of choices to fit the plan he has considered in the first task. He tailor-makes the measurement design, considering the criteria for adequacy of tools. He also plans the interview he will undertake.

3. He *develops a testing strategy* with the tools selected to optimize data collection. He plans the order of presentation of his tools and anticipates patient variables in order to obtain the best data within the constraints of the specific diagnosis.

These tasks accomplished, the diagnostician is ready to go to the next step—clinical testing. Finally, the patient becomes a real person to be met.

KATHERINE COMPARDO: CLINICAL DESIGN

We now return to Katherine Compardo, demonstrating in Table 6-2 the first two tasks of designing the diagnosis—planning for systematic observation and selecting tools for measurement. The student is encouraged to develop the information on Table 6-2 to a greater extent.

To aid in determining interview questions refer back to the children's speech, language, and hearing history questionnaire that was available prior to the diagnostic session to determine what additional data we want to get in the interview. Table 6-3 lists examples of the constituents available in Katherine's history and points to areas in which further information is needed. It is suggested that the student continue to evaluate the remainder of Katherine's history questionnaire information in this manner.

Having specified further information needed for Katherine Compardo in the interview, now formulate questions to gain the identified information. Below we have begun to transform this information into specific questions. The reader is encouraged to continue framing questions for the remainder of the information specified in Table 6-3.

Further information needed	*Questions framed*
Where is St. Mary's Street?	Here the diagnostician wants to gain specific location information. He may do this most directly in one of the closed-type questions. "Where is St. Mary's Street?" "What suburb do you live in?" or "Is St. Mary's Street in South Whittier?"
What does this address tell us about the family's lifestyle?	The diagnostician wants descriptive information that helps him understand Katherine's speech and language environment. He can best gain this in a more open question

such as circumscribed amplification: "Tell me about how Katherine functions in your neighborhood. For example, how does she spend her day, where does she play, with whom does she play, and so forth?"

What specifically does Katherine understand?

The diagnostician wants examples that will give him specific information about Katherine's level of understanding. He therefore asks a circumscribed amplification question "Can you give me some examples of situations in which Katherine understands the language used?"

How does Mrs. Compardo judge Katherine's understanding?

The diagnostician wants to verify the mother's observations of Katherine's understanding. He therefore is looking for data that will allow him to judge the validity of her observations. He does not want to offensively question her statement but wants to know how the mother arrived at her conclusions. He therefore wants descriptive data. "How does Katherine let you know she understands what is said to her?" or "Sometimes it's tricky to know if a child understands the words we say to them or gets the message through our gestures or other situational clues. Can you think of any situations in which it was clear to you that Katherine understood what was said to her rather than what she saw?"

Finally, consider the overall testing strategy for Katherine Compardo. Develop a flowchart—how you might proceed from tool to tool, at each step gaining more information about your cause–effect hypothesis. Suppose you are to start with what we have called the hidden object activity. In this activity objects wrapped in loose tissue paper are placed in a paper bag. Katherine is instructed to close her eyes and select one. How would you introduce this activity? What objects would you put in the bag? What type of responses might you want? How would you elicit and facilitate a response that gives you information you need? How many different types of responses would you be able to elicit and observe from this task? Where would you go next?

Table 6-2. Measurement plans and tools selected for Katherine Compardo

Diagnostician's tasks	Planning
Plans for systematic observation	
Cause–effect relationships	
Well specified in the clinical hypothesis	Will need real skill at behavioral observations and presenting stimuli to elicit response for support of the causal hypothesis. Must be careful not to set off unwanted or uncontrollable behaviors.
Based heavily on inference from the constituent analysis	Must fully understand how childhood aphasia and apraxia manifests itself as speech and language behavior.
Expressed in problem-type product, and processing terms	Hypothesis is derived for fomulation; but the problem type would warrant a check of comprehension (see constituent analysis). A lot of inference must go into the plans.
Causal factor not directly observable	What is the difference in behavioral manifestations between children with aphasia and children defined as minimally brain damaged?
	If causal factor appears to be supported, must immediately consider referral as a tool. Best source would be a pediatric neurologist who has experience with this type of child.

Table 6-2. Measurement plans and tools selected for Katherine Compardo—cont'd

Diagnostician's tasks	Planning
Task specification	
Constituent analysis indicates she is not talking	What will Katherine be able to do in the way of specific speech and language tasks?
All language product levels affected	Perhaps best approach would be a sequence of stimulus-response items geared to measure several things simultaneously. Perhaps consider a comprehension-imitation-formulation paradigm.
	Believe effect is most important to verify first. If the hypothesis is on target, the effects should give us support for the causal factor—at least enough to make an informed referral.
	Also, will want to look at any speech and language behaviors that isolate the difference between speech production processes and language formulation processes, particularly speech programming. Behavioral correlates of sequencing and motor control will be important.
Patient characteristics	
Not much to go on here that would make the situation difficult	Being young is our major concern; 27-month-old children, normal or disordered, do not respond that well to directed activities.
Katherine is young	Natural spontaneity with the mother present initially should do the trick. But start out with an "at the table" activity to keep potential overactivity down. Save more active tasks until later.
She has been around adults	
Likes picture books	
Some minimal indication of overactivity	
Selects tools for measurement	The tools are not presented in any order. The selection is mostly task oriented rather than specific, objective tools that are standardized. The student should explore any tools that may be feasible for Katherine and that can be used at this age level with this hypothesized disorder.
	1. Guided observations throughout the diagnostic session: sandbox activity; hidden objects activity; fine and gross motor activities; free play activities; other activities designed to observe Katherine's visual, social, emotional, physical, and communicative behaviors, for example, imitation of gestures.
	2. Sequenced Inventory of Communication Development
	3. Peabody Picture Vocabulary and the Vocabulary Usage Test in a combined comprehension, formulation, imitation task
	4. Naming tasks: Expressive One-Word Picture Vocabulary Test
	5. Speech mechanism observation—direct and indirect tasks—voluntary, automatic, and speech; Screening Test for Developmental Apraxia of Speech *No*
	6. Imitation of sounds, words, and two-word phrases (make use of "here, Daddy, and hi") —is this for stimulus
	7. Direct stimulation for teaching speech responses—emphasis on sequencing
	The student should now tie these tools selected to the plans and task specifications. Consider two factors: (1) what the tool may do for you and (2) why it was selected.

Table 6-3. Determination of information needed in interview

Constituent as reported by mother	Further information needed
I. Identification Address: One St. Mary's Street	Where is St. Mary's Street? What does this address tell us about the family's life-style?
II. Statement of the problem Nothing has been done about it	What does "nothing" mean to the mother? Is "nothing" consistent with her later comments about questioning hearing, convincing herself nothing was wrong, and starting to think otherwise? Have any other family members "done anything" about Katherine's problem?
III. Speech, language, and hearing history Understands everything	What specifically does Katherine understand? How does Mrs. Compardo judge Katherine's understanding?
IV. General development No information reported about toilet training	Has toilet training been started? If so, what progress has been made? If not, is this due to the mother's approach to toilet training or an indication that Katherine is not ready?
V. Medical history No illnesses indicated except chickenpox	Verification of this information is needed. It is unusual for a child with two elementary school-aged siblings not to have had any of the other childhood illnesses? Check colds, earaches, and ear infections.
VI. Behavior Runs around a lot	What are the circumstances surrounding her "running around"? What does "running around" entail? Is this normal activity, purposeless, unrelenting?
VII. Educational history Mother left blank: "Has anyone ever thought she was a slow child."	On the developmental section of the questionnaire, the mother reported: "She seems much slower than my other children." How do you reconcile this inconsistency in information?
VIII. Home and family information—additional information "I have just convinced myself there was nothing wrong, now I have to start thinking otherwise."	Why was the mother trying to convince herself nothing was wrong? What prompted her to feel she must start thinking otherwise?

PATIENT PROJECTS

For each of the patient projects you have studied in chapters 4 and 5 how would you design your diagnosis? To assist in this process we recommend for each of the patients several tools and procedures you might find useful. Our selections have been made on our understanding of a relevant clinical hypothesis for each of the patients.

William Gafford

Standard procedures for voice examination request a determination of voice use in contextual speech, vowel prolongation, pitch range, optimum and habitual pitch, loudness, and overall quality of the voice in various speaking circumstances. Generally profiles and scales of voice parameters are used as a means of recording the information.

Wilson (1979) can be consulted for a voice profile to use with William Gafford. Since vocal tone and voice quality are parameters of speech stemming primarily from the subprocess of phonation, procedures relating overall speech production to voice parameters should be investigated. A careful speech mechanism examination (Appendix IV) would be warranted with Mr. Gafford. Boone (1977) provides overall guidelines and procedures to use for doing a voice examination. A question you must consider in designing your diagnosis is how the causal factor relates to speech actualization resulting in the characteristic voice products exhibited by Mr. Gafford. Aronson (1980) is very helpful in this regard.

Isadore Alexander

We hope that you have arrived at some type of motor speech disorder (neuromuscular speech disorder) as a clinical hypothesis for Mr. Alexander. A motor speech disorder results from some breakdown within the speech production segment. Thus, examination of the processes and resulting behaviors within that segment are warranted for Mr. Alexander. It is necessary for you to work through your procedures to determine the potential neurological basis for the speech disorder. The procedures set forth in Darley, Aronson, and Brown (1975) are crucial to this process. You might also listen to the audiotapes and read the manual provided by Darley, Aronson, and Brown (1975). The "point–place" system used by Rosenbek and LaPointe (1978) is also quite informative. The "assessment and differential diagnosis" section in Berry (1983) is helpful. Intelligibility is a major factor in neuromuscular speech disorders. You might try the intelligibility tool developed by Yorkston and Beukelman (1981) called Assessment of Intelligibility of Dysarthric Speech.

Derek Park

A major complaint expressed regarding Derek Park was his unintelligibility. Therefore a major question needs to be addressed in this assessment: How does his articulation affect his ability to be understood? Careful assessment of articulation in relation to structure and function of the speech mechanism is warranted. A number of procedures have been developed for use with children with cleft lip and palate. Some suggestions for study are (1) the Iowa Pressure Articulation Test; (2) Miami Imitative Abilities Test; (3) repeating selected consonant–vowel (cv) combinations, words, and sentences that contain no nasal sounds; and (4) careful assessment of the speech mechanism in relation to Derek's ability to produce speech sounds. Velopharyngeal adequacy in relation to articulation is vital. We would suggest a review of Trost (1981) to consider articulatory compensations related to velopharyngeal closure. Procedures for determining degree of hypernasality, nasal emission, and other resonance phenomenon can be found in Bzoch (1979), Wells (1971), Kuehn (1982), and Cooper et al. (1979).

James E. Matkin

Evaluations of the adult stutterer generally focus upon both a description of the stuttering behavior, potential factors contributing to the fluency disorder and also on the stutterer's perceptions and feelings about himself and his stuttering. The balance between collecting information in these areas varies with different diagnosticians. Some diagnosticians working with patients who stutter may spend little time collecting detailed information about the behaviors manifested. Instead, their concern is with the personal motivations, level of interests, and attitudes the patient has about changing his stuttering behavior. These diagnosticians save data collection of the specifics of the stuttering pattern until therapy begins if they feel they are necessary to do. What is your reaction to this type of diagnosis—a diagnosis that concentrates on management concerns rather than on an analysis of a behavior that is readily evidenced in most adult stutterers?

Alternatively, we maintain that the diagnosis must serve to describe the speech disorder as well as causal factors. Numerous guided observation protocols are available to help the diagnostician organize his observations of the patient's stuttering behavior. Among them consider the following for use with Mr. Matkin: The Iowa Scale of Stuttering Behavior, the Measure of Adaptation of Stuttering and the Measure of Consistency of Stuttering (Johnson, Darley, & Spriestersbach, 1963); the Stuttering Severity Instrument (Riley, 1972); and the Southern Illinois University Speech Situations Check List (Brutten & Shoemaker, 1974). In addition, the diagnostician may wish to consult Bloodstein (1981), Conture (1982), Brutten and Shoemaker (1967), Dalton and Hardcastle (1977), and Hood (1978) for further guides to describing Mr. Matkin's speech problem. What are the advantages of approaching causal factors from a contemporary versus a historical view?

Marie Abadie

Since Marie Abadie was seen by a speech–language pathologist while an inpatient at Kankakee General Hospital and the Hospital discharge summaries are available, the diagnostician already has considerable data pertaining to both the description of the language disorder and the causal basis. The referring speech–language pathologist, Dr. Mayfield, has reported a series of findings including those based on parts of the Boston Diagnostic Aphasia Examination (BDAF; Goodglass & Kaplan, 1972) and the Minnesota Test for Differential Diagnosis of Aphasia (Schuell, 1965). Since several weeks have intervened since Mrs. Abadie was last tested, we suggest that the BDAE be readministered for comparative purposes and to determine recovery level and rate. Although comprehension problems were not reported, we include the Auditory Comprehension Test for Sentences (Shewan 1980) and the Token Test (DeRenzi & Vignolo, 1962) to provide more sensitive measures of syntactic comprehension. Further, we are interested in how well Mrs. Abadie communicates in realistic settings and thus select the test of Communicative Abilities in Daily Living (Holland, 1980). Finally we include the Apraxia Battery for Adults (Dabul, 1979) to better describe any apraxic components in Mrs. Abadie's speech. How might Darley's (1982) information on "purposes of language appraisal" in aphasia assist in your testing decisions?

Karen Twigg

The referring audiologist has confirmed the presence of a sensorineural hearing loss as one primary causal factor. Our goal in the diagnosis with Karen is to document the articulation disorder which we know is present, identify a potential language disorder and further assess the language-based learning problems that she presents. We have selected the following tools for these purposes: the Goldman–Fristoe Test of Articulation (Goldman & Fristoe, 1969), will serve as our primary formal measure of articulation. The Token Test for Children (DiSimoni, 1978) and the Peabody Picture Vocabulary Test–Revised (Dunn & Dunn, 1981) have been chosen to measure language comprehension, and the Expressive One-Word Picture Vocabulary Test (Gardner, 1979) and the Grammatic Closure Subtest of the Illinois Test of Psycholinguistic Abilities (Kirk, McCarthy, & Kirk, 1968) will provide formal measures of expressive language. A spontaneous speech and language measure also will be elicited and analyzed according to procedures outlined in Miller (1981). Finally the Woodcock–Johnson Psycho-Educational Battery: Cognitive Abilities and Academic Achievement Subtests (Woodcock & Johnson, 1977) will be used as an objective measure of cognitive level and reading, written language, and mathematics achievement.

STUDY QUESTIONS

1. Weiner and Hoock (1973), Darley (1979), and McCauley and Swisher, (1982) have all addressed the issue of standardization of tools used in diagnosis. Each presents a series of criteria and criticisms that can be used by the diagnostician to evaluate the adequacy of the tools he selects. Compare the criteria used by these authors and apply them to the following tools: Auditory Discrimination Test (Wepman, 1958); the Fisher–Logemann Test of Articulation Competence (Fisher & Logemann, 1971); and the Assessment of Children's Language Comprehension (Foster et al., 1973).
2. The student can explore available tools by reviewing the following books that discuss tests for diagnosis: Emerick and Hatten, 1979; Sanders, 1979; Darley, 1979; and Salvia and Ysseldyke, 1981.
3. Often diagnosticians consider instrumentation as belonging in the speech and hearing scientist's laboratory. How many of the instruments discussed by Hanley and Peters (1971) could be used by the diagnostician to gain important information about their patient? As a project, we feel the student diagnostician would benefit from developing a chart that indicates the type of instrumentation that measures the physical characteristics of the speech and language product.
4. With so many potential tools available from the experimental literature, it would be helpful to have a "central" listing of applicable tools. For example, Johnson and Bommarito (1971) and Johnson (1976) have developed a collection of tests and measurements in child development that appeared in the experimental literature. The student might begin a project similar to this for his personal use in designing diagnoses. As a start, the student might wish to review the past 5 years of the *Journal of Speech and Hearing Research* to locate experimental tools which may have diagnostic applicability.
5. Leonard, Prutting, Perozzi, and Berkley (1978) have addressed the use of nonstandard tools in diagnosis. Use their appendix to assist in the construction of nonstandard tools for use in one or more of the patient projects.
6. Wiig and Semel (1976, 1980) have presented multiple tools and procedures to assess various dimensions of language and learning. Review their assessment procedures and code them in terms of SLPM processes that appear to be assessed by the procedures.

Chapter 7

Clinical testing: collection of the data

After his considerable preparation in the previous three steps, the diagnostician now meets his patient and collects data to test his clinical hypothesis. In this fourth step he will be required to actualize what he has planned and prepared. He will now implement his diagnostic design. He will present his tools, elicit responses, and observe and record the responses. As well, he must demonstrate his professional skill in working with people to gain the information he needs to help them with their concerns. At this step, the clinical scientist blends into a clinical artist.

The diagnostician and patient complex are not automatons, gaining and giving data in a completely preprogrammed manner; rather, both are human. Interpersonal considerations thus become a significant new dimension to data collection, a dimension that pervades the diagnostic session. Here the diagnostician needs to draw from his knowledge about people and about himself. He particularly needs this understanding in special testing situations such as with the "difficult child" and the "overwhelmed adult."

From his diagnostic design and his knowledge about how to implement that design in an interpersonal setting, the diagnostician performs three tasks to complete clinical data collection.

1. He prepares for the diagnostic session, arranging the physical space and materials and then meets the patient.
2. He collects his data through the use of interviewing and testing.
3. He closes the diagnostic session, determining when he has sufficient information to provide for appropriate management plans.

PREPARES FOR THE DIAGNOSTIC SESSION

In preparing for the diagnosis, the diagnostician must attend to the physical arrangements for the session and to the initial contact with the patient.

Physical arrangements

The diagnostician should select and arrange his room, materials, and forms to be ready for the session. The furniture should be appropriate to the patient's age; doors should be wide enough for wheelchairs; materials should be arranged in order of use and hidden from view if necessary; all equipment being used should be in working order; simple things such as opening windows on hot days, and turning on the lights should all be remembered. There are innumerable details about the physical arrangements that could be discussed. Many are specific to the work setting—what is available in terms of rooms, furniture, and materials. However, there is one major consideration regardless of the circumstances. The diagnostician should prepare and arrange the physical environment to be as conducive to eliciting cooperation and responsiveness as possible. Thus, when the patient arrives in the diagnostician's room, his physical comfort should be attended to; taking off coats, arranging seating, commenting on the conditions of the physical setting if needed, pointing out toilet facilities, and so forth. However, being concerned about interpersonal interactions generally overcomes any limitations imposed by a poor physical environment, and we have yet to see carpeting on the floor and expensive furniture substituting for professional skill in personal interaction and systematic observation.

Initial patient contact

The diagnostician must decide how he is going to introduce himself to the patient. This initial contact is essential to the further establishment of interpersonal–professional relations. Depending on the setting, the patient may be sent to the diagnostician's office or the diagnostician will go to the waiting room to greet the patient. With adults, the usual introductions are sufficient, providing information about who you are, where you will be taking them, and some information about what you will be doing and how long it may take. Giving information about the general features of the diagnostic session allows the patient to develop a grasp of what it all may mean and what part he may be playing. Molyneaux and Lane (1982) provide useful information about these initial contacts.

Children are quite another matter. If the child has already established separation from his parents, he may go readily with the diagnostician. A procedure that is helpful is to allow the child to approach the diagnostician. While talking to the parent, glance at the child, smiling at him, and letting him see that his parent thinks you are safe. This often arouses his natural curiosity and he may approach you. When this seems likely, the diagnostician can say, "You must be Donald, I'm Jim." From this point, conversation can ensue; the diagnostician can begin to inform the child of what is going to happen, thereby getting him interested in the upcoming proceedings. In medical settings, children often are worried about why they are there. Is it to receive a shot? Are they as sick as other children they have seen in the halls with tubes and wires attached to them? In such instances, reassuring the child that you are a "talking doctor," and that you only will be looking at books and talking will help ally their unspoken fears. Moving to the diagnostic room then may be accomplished with ease. Learning how to interact with young children is the key ingredient.

At other times child–parent separation can be quite problematic. It must be handled with care. How does the diagnostician get a child to come with him to the testing room? Along with the procedures just suggested, the diagnostician should let the parent help. Often the parent is the best solver of a potential separation problem. Take cues from the parent–child interaction; go slow and do not force yourself on the child. The parents often know if the child will go with you, or they will know the things to say to the child so he is willing to go with you.

The parent and child's advice and consent are essential to the diagnostic contract. Should the child go alone or should the parent accompany him? Different professionals take very different approaches to this issue. While some practice routine separation of children from their parents, we feel this practice is ill advised for many preschoolers. Children between the ages of 2 and 5 are in a period of working out their feelings of separateness from their parents, and at this age separation may be a particularly difficult situation for them. Even when some children separate with no problem, there is no assurance that they have not experienced some separation anxiety.

We feel the issue of child–parent separation rests with our purpose—to provide the best help we can for the patient. If a parent can assist in this, then it is appropriate to have the parent present. When a child feels secure about "mommy," he is likely to perform optimally. Likewise, whenever the parent is present, an opportunity for parent–child interaction is available to the diagnostician. Often an interaction must first be established among parent–diagnostician–child before the parent's involvement can be faded. However, there are times when the parent will not allow the child to perform on his own, continually interjecting advice, correction, and help or becoming distraught by the child's performance. In these interfering instances the parents may have to be told directly that thay are not to interfere.

Whether or not to see a child with the parents present or alone thus depends on several factors which the diagnostician must weigh. Of these, the child's age is probably the most crucial. Many preschoolers cannot be separated from their parents in a strange situation and still be expected to perform optimally. On the other hand, elementary and teenaged youth typically perform better or at least more spontaneously when not under a watchful parental eye. While there are always exceptions to these generalizations, age may well be the best clue to whether or not separation should be attempted.

The setting likewise has an important bearing on separation. "Scary" settings, such as craniofacial teams and other medical environments may require parental support, even for older children, while more school-like environments may be easier for a child to adapt to alone. Finally, the presence or absence of an observation mirror may influence the decision. Often the diagnostician as well as the parent may want the parent to observe the session. Many diagnosticians find that if a parent has observed firsthand the tests administered and the child's responses, it becomes easier to explain the test findings and interpret results during the interpretive conference. If this is the case and an observation room is not available, then the parent will have to remain in the room with the child.

COLLECTS THE DATA

The interview and the tools to be used are now administered in as structured, objective, systematic, and efficient a manner as possible. The diagnostician needs many skills to control variables in the immediate clinical testing situation: the patient variables, the setting variables, the tools variables, and the diagnostician variables.

Actually, data collection begins the moment the diagnostician first observes or introduces himself to the patient. As a matter of fact, this initial interaction may provide enough data for the diagnostician to verify that he is on the right track. On the other hand, he may discover he was on the wrong track and immediately must put into effect new plans. For example, if a language disorder was hypothesized for Norma and at the moment she responded to the diagnostician's greeting she blocked on every word she uttered, an obvious change in plans is required. It does not mean that language may not be disordered, only that Norma may both stutter and have a significant language disorder. Probably the diagnostician would study these two products in interaction: Does the stuttering behavior increase as expected language responses increase in complexity?

Throughout the diagnostic session the diagnostician remains alert to all variables that signal needed changes in plans. We do not wish to impart the idea that collection of data is simply the carrying out of the plans arrived at previously. In many instances the diagnostician will discover that a tool previously selected is inappropriate for the patient; thus he must have the ability to switch procedures. Alterations in planning also can occur as a result of information obtained in the interview. Wherever and whenever they occur, the diagnostician must recycle his diagnostic design. The new information is now a part of a new constituent analysis, leading to a reformulation or adjustment of the clinical hypothesis and requiring a redesigning of tools to collect his clinical data.

Interpersonal contact

Needless to say, the many variables considered by the diagnostician when selecting tools are compounded once he begins testing a person. He must manage the chair, table, child, test, parent, and venetian blind all at the same time. He can never anticipate all the potential interactions that take place. Variables will go uncontrolled, get out of hand, not be observed—all while he is trying to go about his business of gathering data.

In implementing the diagnostic design, it is crucial that the diagnostician know how to relate to and adapt his plan to the patients he sees. Many children and adults willingly enter into the diagnostic situation, cooperatively give all the information wanted, and participate enthusiastically in all the procedures planned. Others are there against their will or have fears and behavioral problems that interfere with straightforward collection of data. At times the diagnostician is fighting against the child's short attention span, disinterest, lack of motivation, or lethargy. To be effective he must know how to modify his testing strategy to reinforce the patient to continue responding. With most adults this is a relatively easy matter. The diagnostician can usually explain what is wanted and why the information is needed. With children he can only explain up to a point, and encouragement only goes so far. Children may want to do what is asked, but often their good will gives way to fatigue, boredom, or distraction. How can young children be encouraged to participate? What will bring out their best responses? What can the diagnostician do in the face of a severe behavior problem? How does he handle fear and anxiety? How does he react to the emotionality presented by an aphasic or his spouse? What does he do with the anger expressed by the patient's mother during an interview? Collection of data thus requires an understanding of people, their problems, their concerns, their hopes, their guilt, their anxieties—the whole of what makes them human.

Even though the diagnostician's job is to elicit and observe appropriate responses, the patient does not necessarily know or care about the diagnostician's job—he acts like he is going to act. A child who is out of control does not care if the diagnostician wants him to point to the picture of a cat. During data collection the diagnostician must know how to adjust to the patient. If a child is very active, then the diagnostician must pursue his testing actively; if the child is a plodder, then plod along. Work with the patient, not against him. Backup procedures become essential; change the stimuli presented, ask for reponses in a different manner, rearrange the seating, or, if necessary, go for a walk. Quiet conversation may have to take the place of the structured language test. The diagnostician must be able to change his design if need be. He may not be able to adhere to the tools selected. Unlike the researcher studying a representative sample, he cannot "throw out" his nonrepresentative patient. He must get the best data he can, in whatever way is necessary.

While we usually think of adults as presenting fewer behavioral problems than children, diagnosticians who spend much of their time with adults may feel this to be an overgeneralization. Many of the adults seen for speech and language diagnoses are understandably overwhelmed by their speech, language, and often more pervasive problems. Some have suddenly undergone significant alterations in their lifestyles. One day they are active and the next day because of a cerebrovascular accident they have been reduced to an invalid and a haltingly communicative, partial person. Others have just undergone surgery as a lifesaving procedure and are flooded with concern over their health and disgust, sadness, and anger over their loss. Some come from families that are themselves fearful; others have no families or supportive persons. These adults have lost more than speech and language. All of them may be overwhelmed by their problems and the concomitant effects on their personal, social, and vocational pursuits.

For many of these patients the diagnostician may represent the one professional who has time and interest, who allows them to talk about their concerns, and who has the ability to help them do something about their problems. It is imperative that the diagnostician be sensitive to these needs and adapt his diagnostic design accordingly. In many instances it may be important to acknowledge how concerned the patient is over his health or how hard it must be for him to cope with the new problems. The patient may well need to express his fears and frustrations; he may need to be depressed or cry. He may need to voice his feelings before he can undertake testing. While the diagnostician must be able to offer support and concern, he also must show the patient that his purpose is to help as best he can, to do something about the problem. With these patients it is particularly important to explain what the tools are intended to do and why the information gained is important. Letting the patient know what is happening helps him feel more in control. At all times, however, the diagnostician must not be swept away by compassion, offering more than is warranted. He must remain realistic in his comments, as nothing in the long run is more shattering than unfulfilled hope.

In addition to attending to the adults' feelings about themselves and their problems, the diagnostician may have to modify the presentation of tools to facilitate their ability to respond. Distraught or disoriented patients must be given time to respond. At times the instructions may be given too fast, and when a response does not come immediately the diagnostician may think the patient does not understand and proceed to another item. Adults can be frustrated by this; their responses worsen, and yet they may not be able or willing to tell you that you are doing something wrong. For example, latency of response is common in the aphasic and must be accounted for when testing with a formal tool or in conversation. Too much stimulation, too fast, can result in an emotional reaction—the only means by which the aphasic can handle the situation. These patients are adults; the diagnostician is an adult—a common ground for an interpersonal interaction.

The interpersonal aspect of data collection is far more difficult to learn that the skill of administering a specific diagnostic tool. The information that provided the data base for assisting the diagnostician comes from many sources. Information about communicative interaction is essential, as discussed in Chapter 1. The diagnostician also uses his broad base of knowledge in child rearing and management, management of the ill and handicapped, child growth and development, human personality, psychological growth and development, learning theory, and many other areas. One of the most important areas of knowledge he needs is self-knowledge—what he is as a person.

Ours is a "talking profession." Our concern is with a person's ability to use speech and language. If diagnosticians are not skilled in relating through communication, how can they be skilled in solving speech and language problems?

Interpersonal–professional relationships

From the moment the patient and the diagnostician meet, they enter into an interpersonal–professional relationship—a contract is formed between the parties. The perceptions the patient has of the diagnostician and vice versa will have an important bearing on the diagnostic process.

The diagnostician may assume that the patient comes in order to achieve greater homeostasis in his daily functioning, greater integration among all the aspects of his life: cognitive, sensorimotor, and interpersonal. He is attempting to achieve a better "gestalt." Since diagnosis is an active and not a passive process, the diagnostician enters into the patient's existence just as the patient enters into the diagnostician's existence. The diagnostician must be aware of the patient's reactions to his "help." As well he must be aware of his own needs to help. The diagnostician must discover the patient; the patient must teach the diagnostician. Both must respect each other, be authentic in what they feel, and be ready to "weather the storms" that may occur; they must arrive at some degree of commitment to each other.

These interpersonal interactions are vital; many patients are lost because something goes amiss in this aspect of the process, even when appropriate test information has been obtained. A good diagnosis relies on the feelings that have resulted as well as the tools that were administered.

The interaction or relationship between the diagnostician and the patient is often blithely called "establishing rapport" and somehow is supposed to magically occur. We all know that rapport is essential to the diagnostic process, but we do not always know how to achieve it. Somehow the diagnostician is expected to be "on" with each patient he sees, no matter what his own day or personal life may be like.

Discovering the primary ingredients for successful interpersonal interactions is difficult. We sometimes hear remarks like "You have to be born with it" or "He really knows how to plan a diagnosis, but he can't relate to the patient." Much work needs to be done in this area before we understand why one diagnostician seldom has difficulty relating to all types of patients, whereas another always seems to have screaming children. Shriberg (1971) conducted a study to determine the effect of the examiner's social behavior on children's articulation test performance. During their interactions with the children, the examiners assumed various social behaviors that were judged to represent real behaviors. Even though Shriberg's main variable of the examiner's social behavior was not significant, further studies like his can be important for discovering interpersonal factors affecting patient performance. Perhaps instead of assuming "artificial" behaviors, real diagnosticians with real behavior should be studied.

Probably most difficult for the diagnostician is understanding himself in the relationship. It is much easier to look toward others as the problem and pretend that whatever we contribute to the relationship is optimal. However, relationships are a two-way street: Diagnosticians have no fewer difficulties than do their patients. The diagnostician needs to know what his anxieties and needs are in the situation, his manner of relating, and the life experiences that have made him respond to people as he does.

Even with considerable self-insight and self-change, there will probably always be some personal characteristics in a diagnostician that are going to be reacted to negatively by some of the patients he sees. He cannot be all things to all people. Furthermore, some characteristics negatively reacted to cannot be changed. For example, the diagnostician may be young rather than old, white rather than black, or male rather than female. Haynes and Oratio (1978) have addressed patient perceptions of speech–language pathologists and Crane and Cooper (1983) related speech–language clinicians' effectiveness to personality profiles.

Our skills as diagnosticians must counteract any negative reactions and impressions, the ultimate basis by which we hope to be judged. Age, however, is often a problem with student diagnosticians who may be perceived as both young and without experience. How can patients respect their skills and opinions? If student diagnosticians demonstrate good skills and maturity, they usually are accepted. At other times the issue needs to be confronted, quite appropriately allowing that in fact the student is in training and is being supervised by a professional who has final responsibility for any decisions made.

In relating to patients, the diagnostician must develop an understanding and acceptance of the patient as well as an understanding and acceptance of himself. The diagnostician must regard his patient as the result of a particular set of life experiences and demonstrate that his aim is to help with any information gained. In some cases, patients may be reluctant to give information as they fear the information will be used against them. For example, all parents do not necessarily have equal levels of concern about their children. In truth, some do not care for their children at all, and the fact that the child demonstrates a speech or language disorder only heightens their dislike for the child. Is this something they could reveal to the diagnostician? Parents view their children as extensions of themselves—as their child is judged, so they may be. If the diagnostician can develop and project the attitude that individuals do the best they can with whatever life has presented them, this attitude will contribute to a feeling of appreciation, understanding, and acceptance.

Few parents of patients are ready to flood the diagnostician with the truths of their life during this initial diagnostic contact. Presumably most patients are ready to give some information but not all information. Patients do not and should not share everything. They may give more information than usual simply because the diagnostician is a professional, and they have come to him for some type of help. The more supportive and accepting the professional, the more likely is the patient to offer whatever may be pertinent to an understanding of the problem. There are, however, instances when a patient reveals too much, using the diagnostician for relief of many anxieties and concerns about his life. Such outpourings may produce tremendous guilt, and the patient may not be able to return to the setting. The diagnostician must therefore be careful of how much he lets the patient reveal.

At the same time the diagnostician must be careful of how much he reveals about himself. For example, should a diagnostician, who has his own stuttering under control, reveal that he is a stutterer to a patient being seen for stuttering? Or should a diagnostician talking to a mother whose child has a significant behavioral problem reveal that his child, too, has a behavioral problem? How much does a diagnostician use his personal life experience as a way of relating to the concerns of his patient? There may be no answers to these questions, but there are cautions to exercise. Suppose, for instance, that the diagnostician with controlled stuttering revealed his experiences with stuttering, including the information that he is now experiencing little or no difficulty with his speech. Will the patient feel he can do the same thing? Will this external motivation bring him to therapy? Or will his lack of success be expressed as hostility toward the diagnostician who has been too successful. Using someone else as a model for motivation at times may create more harm than good. The patient may have only perceived the diagnostician's success at controlling his behavior but not the effort, anxieties, and hard work that went into controlling the behavior.

Work setting

Different work settings require that the diagnostician acquire somewhat different information for developing the skill of interpersonal interaction. The diagnostician in an acute care hospital needs more information about interacting with sick people than does the public school diagnostician, whereas the public school diagnostician needs to know more about interacting with active, healthy children at various age levels. The diagnostician in a children's hospital may concentrate on skills used in working with the sick child, while a diagnostician in a nursing home will concentrate on the special needs of the elderly, invalid population. In each of these settings the diagnostician will need to refine his interpersonal skills with the patient and other professionals. Whatever the setting, the diagnostician must try to gear himself to the particular requirements and personalities of the patient rather than expecting the patient simply to adapt to his personality and his need to collect information.

Pat DiCioccio is employed in an extended care facility where she frequently works with patients who are dying. She contributes the following about the special interpersonal characteristics in this circumstance.

> The patient population in an extended care facility not only includes the invalid geriatric patient, but also the patient with progressive neurological disease who can no longer be managed at home. This patient is often a young to middle-aged adult who is in the severe stages of his disease process. There are diagnostic and therapeutic services that one may offer such a patient; however, it is ultimately important that the diagnostician/clinician first have the necessary interpersonal skills that are essential for interacting with this type of patient. The professional in this setting must develop his own understanding of the disease process and the dying patient. He must evaluate his own thoughts and reactions to the dying patient and the magnitude of the patient's problems, and the impact of his situation must be felt by the clinician. He must be able to deal with his own feelings as well as those of the patient as the diagnostic/therapeutic relationship begins to grow, and he must truly understand what he as a professional can offer. These interpersonal skills one develops in this situation are most important in helping the professional provide appropriate diagnostic and therapeutic services. Interacting honestly, compassionately, and professionally with the dying patient, all three somehow equally balanced, must be the underlying framework for any diagnostic or therapeutic service that is provided. (Personal Communication, 1975).

The interview

Most diagnoses include an interview as one of the tools of diagnosis. It is usually formalized into a distinct task of data collection, and therefore, because of its separateness, we will present information about it as a tool to be administered apart from the remainder of the information on tool administration.

The topic of interviewing often is treated in awe by the student trying to learn it and, perhaps to some extent, by the person trying to teach it. If the student approaches the subject in a practical way, he will discover he "interviews" every day of his life. People interview each other daily; they ask questions for information; they discuss areas of concern;

they ask questions of each other about problems they are having; and they ask questions about feelings, health, and attitudes. This is done using all the methods of interviewing: the direct question, the multiple-choice response, under all types of conditions: friendly, hostile, angry, open, closed, and dozens of others. Thus, our daily personal interactions can serve as the bases for learning to conduct interviews in our job setting. The diagnostician moves from this area of personal general knowledge to the specific interview knowledge needed for diagnosis of speech and language disorders.

Interviewing is a complex skill used by many professionals, each having a special purpose and use for the techniques. But overriding all the special uses of the interview is the basic purpose, to obtain information. There is one basic way of obtaining this information—by asking "questions." Each person develops his interviewing style from this basic method of interviewing and from his own personal characteristics during interpersonal interaction.

In the previous chapter we discussed how the diagnostician plans his interview, considering the areas of information in which he is interested, and how he may frame certain questions to obtain this information. He now approaches the interview as a coalition between himself and the informant; a coalition developed for the purpose of understanding the speech and language problem, what caused it, what can be done about it, who is concerned about it, and who can do something about it. It is important to help the informant see his active role in helping to solve the problem. An interpersonal–professional relationship must be established.

We believe in making it clear to the informant that both of us are in this process together, and that our findings and solutions are dependent on this joint involvement. Approaching the interview as a team usually has an energizing effect, particularly on family members. It helps to eliminate parental expectations of easy cures in which they play no role and removes the professional from an authoritarian position. We like to tell parents that they have the information about their child as they live with him 24 hours a day, and we have the training to help put the pieces of information together.

The skill of interviewing is concerned with the how-to aspects: how to obtain the most pertinent informaton without creating undue anxiety, stress, frustration, helplessness, or other unpleasant feelings in the person being interviewed. The diagnostician must develop skills for interviewing the hostile mother, the defensive father, the denying adult, the unsophisticated child—each an individual. Any diagnostician can develop and ask pertinent questions at some level—this is questioning—but the skill of interviewing comes when he knows how to do this in various ways, with different people, with different ideas and concerns. Most of the time the diagnostician is fortunate; the patient and his family come with a problem they want solved. They usually want to cooperate the best they can during the interview. Thus, the diagnostician gets answers to his questions. However, even with willing informants, difficulties can be encountered, for example, a parent who wants to know why his child has not begun to talk but who is denying slow development or mental retardation as a possible explanation. This parent may give all kinds of accurate information about what he thinks caused it. Parents like this are not simply being hostile or defensive; they are sometimes being protective of themselves and of their child.

The diagnostician must decide how he will record the information offered in the interview. Choices range from tape-recording the entire interview to making no notes at all. Tape-recording the session may inhibit the informant's responses, particularly when the information is emotional or highly personal in nature or if the informant questions the diagnostician's motives in using the information. On the other hand, relying on recall of all the detailed information following the interview is a skill achieved by few diagnosticians.

Most diagnosticians choose a method somewhere in between these two alternatives, developing their own system for recording pertinent information. The diagnostician must be sure, however, that his note taking does not impede the information flow, slow down the discussion, or create a barrier between himself and the patient.

The diagnostician can set the tone for note taking by asking for or being sure that all identification information and certain other factual information are accurately recorded. Usually recording such information in the presence of the informant creates no difficulty, for he knows what is being written down and expects it to be written down. Having set the tone for note taking, the diagnostician, as he proceeds through the interview, can jot down abbreviated notes in the form of key items that will serve as memory jogs at a later time. Letting the informant know enough times early in the interview what was written down (e.g., "You said he received tubes at 18 months and that the one in the left ear fell out a few months later"), can assure the informant that the diagnostician is recording what they say, not judging it.

Another approach used by diagnosticians is to take a few minutes immediately following the interview to write down the salient aspects of the information obtained. Some professionals, social workers in particular, are trained to make detailed "process recordings" following the termination of the interview. Early in his training the student should learn a method of recording in which he can become highly skilled.

When the diagnostician prefers to use a tape recorder, we have found that when the interview is presented as a problem-solving effort between the diagnostician and the informant, permission is generally obtained for use of the recorder. The informant can be instructed to have the recorder stopped if information is being discussed that he prefers not be recorded. Having used this technique over a number of years with student diagnosticians, we have not observed a notable difference between interviews using a recorder and those that do not. Our clinical experience is that the informant quickly disregards the presence of the recorder, particularly if placement of the recorder and microphone are inconspicuous. This approach to recording information is invaluable in teaching the interview process or for experienced diagnosticians to check on their own interviewing skills.

In approaching the interview, the diagnostician will need to attend to three aspects of the "live" interview. He first will need to structure his interview as a part of the total diagnostic session. He then will launch into the interview with the informant. Finally, he will enter the heart of the interview, collecting and recording pertinent information.

Structuring the interview

Interviews are often difficult to conduct within the time limits of the diagnostic session. With adults this can be accomplished by incorporating the interview as part of the clinical testing. The questions asked can be used to obtain more information about the problem, and serve as samples of speech and language behavior as well: how well the patient can comprehend and integrate what is said to him, how well he can hear, how he formulates language, and how well he produces it through the speech-production mechanism. Communicative interaction with adult patients often becomes the basis for obtaining interview and clinical data simultaneously; at times no further specific clinical tools are needed.

With children, however, interviewing becomes more problematic. Generally, the diagnostician wants to interview the parent or whoever brings the child prior to testing the child. The question immediately arises as to what to do with the child. If the interview is conducted in the presence of the child, how will this affect what the diagnostician asks or how the parent may respond? Will the child feel ignored if he is not attended to during this time? In many situations there may be no satisfactory answer to these questions; but since the major purpose of the diagnosis is to see the child, the interview must not take up all the time available.

Interviewing the child's parents takes on a different structure depending on the work setting, the diagnostician's philosophy about interviewing, and separation plans. Some professionals advocate seeing the parent for a separately scheduled interview session, followed by a second testing session with the child. If the setting and parents are such that multiple diagnostic visits are possible, this method of seeing the parents and child on different visits often is ideal. When the child arrives, all the attention is his, and the problem of what to do with him during the interview is circumvented. In addition, seeing the parents prior to the child's visit allows the parents to prepare themselves as well as the child for what to expect when the child is tested. Other professionals advocate using a team approach: one interviewing the parent while another sees the child. Such an approach is often used in multidiscipline settings as well as in training centers. In yet other settings a playroom may be provided for the child staffed by a student, an aide, or someone who attends to and possibly makes observations of the child.

These latter two approaches, however, necessitate separation. If separation is not accomplished and the child remains in the interview room, some diagnosticians set up a play corner for the child that distracts him while the interview is being conducted. There are instances, however, when the child stays on his mother's lap and is present throughout the interview. In such situations the diagnostician must guide the interview so that questions and answers are limited to what can appropriately be said in the child's presence. The diagnostician can indicate this directly to the parent, for example, "Let's try to discuss Darwin's problem in such a way that he does not feel uncomfortable about what we say." Similarly, the diagnostician needs to let the child know what they are talking about. He may say, for example, "Your mother is going to be telling me about things you have been doing, so that I know more about you. We will be talking for a short while, and then you and I will have a chance to talk together." At other times, the diagnostician is confronted with a child who cannot be separated and who dominates the interview by his behavior. Probably every diagnostician at some time in his career has had a child dismantle his office or shriek throughout an attempted interview. At such times the only alternative may be a telephone conversation with the parent following the diagnosis or a conference scheduled for a later day.

In the following example situations decide how you would structure the interview within the total diagnostic session. What modifications might be necessary? How can the interview be arranged to gain the best data possible? What impact will the interview have on all persons involved, including the informant and others who may be present?

1. Three-year old Reagan arrives with both his mother and father at a university speech and hearing center. The interview and testing are planned to be conducted simultaneously, although Reagan indicates he does not want to leave his parents. How should the diagnostic team proceed?
2. Mrs. Lewis comes with her husband who is very depressed over his recent stroke and resulting physical and language problems. With whom does the diagnostician, Mrs. Sekeley, hold the interview? Will the interview and testing sessions be distinct or integrated? If integrated, what is Mrs. Lewis' role?

3. Fourteen-year-old Norris is brought by his very anxious mother, Mrs. Tempio, for help with his stuttering problem. Who is interviewed? What is Norris told about the interview? What is Mrs. Tempio told?

4. Four-year-old Kim is brought to a setting in which one diagnostician is to hold both the interview and testing sessions on the same day. No provisions are available for another person to care for Kim during the interview. Since Kim is a very active and at times an out-of-control child, the mother is not able to attend well to the questions she is asked. Indeed, Kim is quite disruptive and very little interviewing is possible. What should the diagnostician do to obtain the interview information he wants?

Launching the interview

After the diagnostician has dealt with the structure of the interview as part of the total diagnostic context, he must begin the actual interview. Earlier we stressed approaching the interview as a coalition between the informant and the diagnostician. We therefore suggest the diagnostician launch the interview by explaining the purpose of the interview and the importance of the informant in this process. For example, the diagnostician may want to begin in the following manner: "Mrs. Amaddio, we are glad that you were able to come with Pam today. Before we test her, I'd like to spend a little time talking with you so that I can better understand her problem as you see it. Since I will see Pam for such a relatively short time and cannot observe everything about her, I will have to rely on you to tell me the things that I cannot observe. This will be very important in helping me understand many aspects of Pamela's problem, why she is having the problem, and what we can do about it." Such an introduction explains the purpose of the diagnosis and also includes the informant as an integral part of the process.

Plan how you would introduce the purpose of the diagnosis and explain the informant's role to the following informants. How would the diagnostician explain the purpose of the interview to the following people? What language would he choose to do this?

1. Mrs. Reidel, a social worker with the department of child welfare, has brought 10-year-old Darren to the community hearing and speech agency. Darren lives at home with his mother and seven other siblings.

2. The diagnostician, Dr. Lipkowitz, is to begin an interview with Dr. Whitney, a well-known pediatrician in the community, whose 7-year-old son is hypothesized to have a minor articulation problem.

3. Miss Mayfield is to interview Mrs. Lund, a working-class white mother of 4-year-old Sandra.

4. Mr. Sugarman, a public school diagnostician, has scheduled an interview appointment with Mrs. Becker, the fifth grade teacher of Kathy who has a stuttering problem.

After introducing the purpose of the diagnosis, we suggest the diagnostician acknowledge the information he has received about the patient prior to the interview. For example, he might say, "I appreciate your taking the time to fill out the questionnaire we sent you. I was wondering if Bethany's speech has changed any since you returned the form?" Or in another instance, the diagnostician might say to the wife of the patient, "Dr. Kronenberg said your husband had a stroke 2 months ago. Tell me what changes you have seen in his speech? Mentioning the information he has received lets the informant know the scope of information that the diagnostician possesses and serves as a starting point to talk about the problem. If the informant has submitted information, it lets the informant know that the diagnostician has read what he has written and that its content need not be repeated. If reports have been sent from persons other than the informant, we also feel the diagnostician should mention these, unless explicitly asked not to by the one who sent the report. Letting the informant know what information has been received allows for more open, direct communication.

We want to point out, however, that acknowledging the receipt of information from other sources is quite a different matter from sharing the contents of that information. For example, while a diagnostician may say, "We have received reports from Dr. Nordell (the school psychologist) and Mrs. Elson (the child's teacher)," we do not feel the diagnostician should report another person's findings. Usually reports from other professionals will indicate what information has been given to the patient or parents. If not, and the informant asks about the other professionals' findings, the diagnostician may simply say, "I suggest that you ask Dr. Nordell these questions as he was the one who tested your child, and he will be better able to explain his results."

Acknowledge receipt of information in the following situations.

1. A parent, Mrs. Weiss, has returned a children's speech and language history form with most of the items left blank.
2. The diagnostician has received a report from the neurologist in charge of Mr. Zeitz during his recent hospitalization following his stroke. Mr. Zeitz claims he does not know what happened to his speech.
3. Mr. Kronenberg has completed a history form in exacting detail. He has also mentioned that he is seeing a psychiatrist, from whom he has requested a report be sent to the hearing and speech center. The psychiatrist's report has not been received at the time of the interview.
4. The diagnostician has received no information other than basic identifying information about Ray Harold, a 20-year-old man with a voice problem.
5. A parent, after learning that the psychologist who tested her 5-year-old son Bart has sent a report, asks what IQ her son received.

Collecting the interview data

Having explained the purpose of the diagnosis and acknowledged the available information, the diagnostician is ready to begin asking the questions he has planned in order to get the information he wants. It is generally a good idea to begin the question–answer process in a nonthreatening manner. The diagnostician will want to be sure the informant can feel successful in responding to the initial question. With some patients the diagnostician may begin by asking a general question first such as, "Have you seen any changes in John's speech since you filled out the history questionnaire?" Or if the informant has not provided any previous information, perhaps the diagnostician would begin by saying, "How would you describe Larry's speech and language problem?" or "What concerns you about Larry's speech and language problem?" Such a general circumscribed amplification question allows the diagnostician to assess the informant's level of understanding of the problem and also focuses the interview immediately on the patient's speech and language. Emerick (1969) has suggested that the diagnostician listen before he talks, thus allowing the informant to let you know where he is. From this the diagnostician can better determine how to employ his preplanning strategy. Such an approach also subjects the clinical hypothesis to test without first limiting the range of possible topics or biasing the focus of the interview.

If the diagnostician senses that the informant may not initially feel comfortable in providing a relatively lengthy and unstructured response, he may alternatively choose to begin the questioning by asking for some very specific, readily obtainable information such as identifying information or clarification of some item on the history form. For example, "Is your address still 2897 Berkshire?" or "You mentioned on the phone that you saw Dr. Warner at the psychology clinic. When did you see Dr. Warner?"

Having started with a general question, the diagnostician can continue by picking up a point in the informant's reponse and asking for further information about that point. For example, if Mrs. Ledowsky says that 4-year-old Amy stutters and has a hard time getting her words out, the diagnostician might then ask Mrs. Ledowsky to describe further what it is that Amy does when she stutters, what situations make her stuttering more or less severe, or if she has noticed any letters or words that Amy has particular difficulty with. If the diagnostician has framed specific questions about Amy's speech and language, he will then want to insert those questions here.

In proceeding through the interview, we find it helpful to approach the questioning by general topic areas. The topic headings of the speech and language history questionnaire can serve this purpose. These topics include identification; statement of the problem; speech, language, and hearing history; general development, including pregnancy and birth history as well as developmental history; medical history; behavior; educational history; and home and family information.

The extent to which each topic is explored will depend on the information available prior to the interview, the design of the interview, and the informant's ability to provide the requested information. If detailed information was available, the diagnostician may only need to address a few topic areas. If little information was available, the diagnostician may need to initiate each new topic area with a general, circumscribed amplification question, followed by more structured questions to gain the specific information needed. In this manner the diagnostician can balance open and closed questions, gaining the kind of information both have to offer. Approaching the interview by general topic areas helps the diagnostician remember what information he planned to obtain without being bound to notes, and thus leads to more thorough and smooth data collection in the interview. A topic approach to interviewing helps guard against simple rotelike presentation of a series of nonrelated, preplanned questions. Finally, approaching the interview from the topic areas also allows the informant to see the continuity of the interview and helps him understand why certain questions are being asked.

As mentioned previously, we suggest the interview begin or at least very early focus on the patient's speech and language. The patient's speech and language problem is what initiated the visit and therefore it is a logical point to begin from both the informant's and the diagnostician's perspectives. The informant undoubtedly expects to talk about the problem, and thus discussing the speech and language problem provides an initial common ground between the informant and the diagnostician. After the informant has been able to say what he wants to about the speech and language behavior, and the diagnostician has been able to ask the questions he has framed, the diagnostician will then want to move the interview to other topics.

Many of the remaining topics will help the diagnostician understand causal factors, although the purpose of some of these topic areas may not be obvious to the informant.

We suggest that in moving on to these other topics the diagnostician may want to introduce the new area by explaining why he is interested in such information. For example, in addressing medical history, the diagnostician may say, "I would now like to discuss your child's medical history as sometimes we can identify illnesses or accidents that may be related to his speech and language problem. How has Arick's health been?" Or if considerable information is available, the diagnostician may say, "You mentioned on the history questionnaire that Arick has had several earaches. For what period of time did he have these, and how were they treated?" Or when introducing questions about general behavior, the diagnostician might say, "I'm interested in getting a picture of Jimmy's other behavior so that I can put his speech and language into broader perspective. Let's start by telling me how he spends a typical day from the time he gets up in the morning until the time he goes to bed at night."

Along with gaining the information he wants, the diagnostician will have to execute the recording procedures he has decided on if these are to be done within the interview session. If he has planned to tape-record the interview, he will need to explain his purposes in recording the session and gain the informant's consent. If the diagnostician has decided to write information down only after the session, he will need to pay close attention to the specifics given. If identification data has not appeared in written form, most diagnosticians will want to make sure this information is recorded accurately at the time it is given. Whatever method of recording the diagnostician chooses, he will need to let the informant know what he is doing and keep check so that his recording does not interfere with the interpersonal interaction.

The real skill involved in interviewing is being able to adapt the questions and recording of information to the individual characteristics of the informant. The diagnostician may well approach the interview via topic areas and have settled on a recording method; however, the specifics that evolve are very much dependent on the interpersonal dynamics that take place between the diagnostician and the informant.

Closing the interview

After the diagnostician has gained the information he wants in the interview and the informant has been given ample opportunity to offer what he wants, the diagnostician will need to close the interview. Molyneaux and Lane (1982) consider this to be a "special" part of the interview and these last minutes should be used effectively. He can do this by thanking the informant for his cooperation and the information he has provided. He then will need to specify what is to happen next and when and how he will get back to the informant. For example, he might say, "You have been very helpful in giving me a lot of information about Perry. While we could probably continue to talk for some time, I would like to begin testing Perry before he gets too restless. You may remain in the waiting room while I am with Perry. After we are finished, I will again meet with you to discuss my findings and then plan our next steps."

This project is designed as a role play between one person designated as a student diagnostician and a second person who will serve as the informant. The diagnostician plans to gain the following information as a part of the interview.

1. The student diagnostician wants to tape-record the session. He must explain his purpose in wanting to record the session and ask for the informant's consent.

2. The diagnostician wants to get a more detailed description of a 5-year-old child's language comprehension. Information available prior to the interview simply stated, "He doesn't seem to understand everything said to him."
3. The diagnostician has no information pertaining to developmental milestones.
4. The child has been described by the referring pediatrician as "irritable," "difficult to manage," and "prefers to play alone."

The diagnostician is to gain the same information from the following three informants role played by the second person. How will he modify his approach and interactions to gain this information?

1. Mrs. Robbins is a middle-class housewife who is concerned about her adequacy as a mother. Her husband tends to blame her for Raymond's unmanageable behavior, claiming that if she knew how to manage him, Raymond would not have all of his current problems. She fears that Raymond may be retarded and is very concerned about the cause of his language and behavior problems; however, she attempts to present him in the most favorable light and to minimize his difficulties.
2. Mrs. Watkins is a lower-class mother who communicates her information and impressions about her son through a "restricted code." While she knows Arnold is not "stupid," she has little knowledge of other factors contributing to speech and language functioning. While her understanding of Arnold's problem is limited, she very much wants to do whatever is best for him.
3. Mrs. Roth is a social worker in the residential treatment program where Joshua has been living for the past 8 months. She is young and only recently out of school. She has been trained in process recording and tells the diagnostician that she feels use of the tape recorder for interview is inappropriate. Mrs. Roth has relatively little information about Joshua since she just recently was assigned his case. In addition, she has had little experience with children with speech and language problems. She is, however, very interested in learning about speech and language in general as well as learning specifically about Joshua's problem.

Following the role with each informant, the participants and observers may want to discuss the following points.

1. Interpersonal interactions: How did each participant behave toward the other one? What was each participant feeling during the interview?
2. Information flow: Did the informant give and get information he wanted? Did the diagnostician give and get the information he wanted? Was all the relevant information exchanged?

Clinical testing

Orienting procedures

At the outset of clinical testing, patients must be given information that orients them to the diagnostic session. Structure is provided that lets a patient know what is expected. A balance must be maintained between formality of testing and informality of interaction. Natural interests and spontaneous responses to the setting and the materials, including getting off the subject, must be allowed for if interest in the procedures is to be maintained throughout the session. Anxiety, boredom, restlessness, negativism, frustration, and anger must be combated. The initial contract should specify in some sense the roles each will play—this is what I do, and this is what you do. Within this framework, the patient may be given choices.

For the child it may be well to establish more rules at the onset of the testing session. First, we are going to sit down; then we are going to look at some pictures; then you can tell me the names of my pictures—various ways of putting structure into the session so the child knows what he is doing, why he is doing it, and what may be coming next. After the ground rules are laid, the child can then be given choices of things to do, which task to do first, which chair to sit in, what to do next, how long to do it, when to take a break, and so forth. The child can be made an assistant to the diagnostician. He can help get out the materials, put them away, turn pages, and arrange the tables and chairs; he can assist in any number of activities that turns him into an active participant in his session. Being a part of the decision-making process keeps a child interested, motivated, curious, and in some control over what happens to him.

The choices offered can be structured in such a way that each alternative is acceptable to the diagnostician. For example, if in the testing room two chairs are placed, one red and one blue, the child can be asked, "Which chair would you like, the red one or the blue one?" He is given a choice; but the choices are limited, and both chairs should be appropriate for the child. Giving assent to a child's wishes gives him a feeling that he has a part to play in decisions that will affect him in some way.

Carrying out the testing strategy

The diagnostician has a plan for testing the patient and the necessary materials ready for doing so, including backup procedures that may be necessary for testing alternative hypotheses. The plan is made up of a series of "puzzle pieces," some more detailed than others. Gathering all the pieces is now essential for filling in the plan. It was suggested in the last chapter that the diagnostician develop a flowchart representing how he might move from one procedure to the next, indicating alterations of procedures that would not affect the accumulation of data.

The general flowchart of most help is that which first proposes a tool to obtain base line data about the behaviors of interest, followed by tools that provide more specific detail. Establishing base line data about the cause–effect relationship gives immediate information, and in the case when the patient cannot or will not continue, the diagnostician has some information to use.

A common tool used to establish early base lines is conversational speech, a basic tool for any speech and language disorder and sometimes considered a routine procedure. For an adult patient this can be incorporated as part of the interview, providing the diagnostician specific data about speech and language while providing the patient with an opportunity to discuss his problem. For young children, however, converstaion is not easy and a conversational situation will generally have to be structured. Probably the least successful structure for young children is the question-asking approach. Children meeting strangers do not respond well to direct questions—even of the most innocuous types like "What is your name?" Children, on their first contact with an adult, must be drawn into verbal interaction. They must understand that they can respond in their own manner, and with all their adequacies and inadequacies.

The use of parallel talking with children is often effective. The diagnostician can select an activity that initially requires no speech; for example, while playing together with some toys of interest at a stand-up sandbox, the diagnostician can comment on what he is doing and what the child is doing, slowly adding to his comments instructions for the child to follow. "Let's take our cars to the garage." Does the child proceed to do so; be sure to wait and see.

Children are inquisitive; their curiosity often "gets the best of them," and it can be used to advantage by the diagnostician. Let children look into things, discover things, be surprised by things, laugh at things, and enjoy their surroundings. A technique for stimulating conversation that takes advantage of children's curiosity is the old hiding trick. The diagnostician can have a flannel board set up and a big bag of carefully selected pictures that is his secret. The child can be intrigued by the examiner's interest in the bag until he wants to get into the bag. Once the "stage is set," the child can be instructed to close his eyes, reach in, take one picture, and put it on the flannel board. The flannel board could have sections: the city, the farm, the house, the department store, and so forth. The pictures in the bag can relate to these sections. When the child pulls out a picture the examiner can say, "Oh, you found a cat; I think that goes in the house. Let's put it in the house." Natural spontaneity is required of the diagnostician. Verbal overreaction on his part can set off overreaction in the child.

Does the child follow the instructions? Further questions can be asked, "Where did you put the cat? In the house?" In this way the diagnostician can model various speech and language structures for the child to use when it is the diagnostician's turn to close his eyes, reach in the bag, take one picture, and put it on the flannel board. Depending on the child's disorder, the diagnostician can structure this technique to get at any aspect of speech and language: reception, comprehension, integration, formulation, repetition, and production. He should know at what age levels the tasks he designs can be performed by children; that is, he selects his activity and his verbal stimuli according to normative information. A carefully structured activity such as the preceding usually gets a child to interact verbally; and through it the diagnostician obtains baseline data, a spontaneous language sample, and, as well, sets up a comfortable interpersonal relationship. Since talking and listening are the mainstays of diagnosis, this procedure may provide enough data to understand the effect component of the cause–effect hypothesis.

There are many general suggestions that could be offered for working with children. Among them we list the following that the diagnostician may find helpful.

1.   Remember that most children are easy to test. They go through the paces in a remarkably matter-of-fact manner. Take a hint from this. Make your manner likewise. Assume that "here is something we are going to do." It may be enjoyable but that is really secondary. In most cases, time is saved and the actual creation of emotional reactions is avoided if the diagnostician does not approach the testing as a thrilling, exciting game that the child is going to "just love." Any extremes of emotion by the diagnostician may create problems in the child. There is no need or justification for building up an atmosphere of excitement in anticipation of a fascinating game. The older the child, the more apparent this statement becomes. You are securing a representative sample of the child's speech. The more simply and efficiently this can be done, the less wear on the diagnostician and child.

2.   Administer the tools quickly and efficiently. For most children the process must move along at a reasonably good rate in order to hold their attention and to prevent prolonging the testing beyond its maximum usefulness. But do not push the child too fast. You do not need rapid-fire responses. If he appears interested in looking at a test picture or talking about it, let him. Rapidity of administration varies greatly from child to child. Do not expect a response on every item—let some of them go and pick them up later. Struggling to get a response from the child on every item by asking again and again or saying, "You know that" can build up a condition of nonresponding.

3.   Allow children to have temporary diversions during the testing. They should be able to make comments, ask seemingly irrelevant questions, and get up and move around without

being made to feel guilty. On the other hand, too much freedom or too prolonged distractive activities may be disastrous. The diagnostician should maintain control of the testing situation. This control can be gentle though insistent. In most cases it is sufficient to direct attention to the testing materials after brief diversion. At other times it may be necessary to say or imply, "We have played a while, now let's go back to this."

4. Be careful of asking the child if he wants to do something. This often sets off negativism, and what if the child says "no" to a task you had every intention of doing. The diagnostician then runs the risk of the child discovering that his wishes may be ignored. So guard against requests that you suspect may be met with refusal. Negativism cannot usually be reduced by prodding to respond and certainly not by displaying disapproval of his "uncooperative" behavior. When a child is thrust into a potentially threatening (to his way of feeling) situation, he has a right to be negative until such time as he can evaluate the situation. Negativism is often acceptable behavior that does not need to call forth any particular emotional reaction on the part of the diagnostician.

5. The use of reinforcement must be considered carefully for maintaining continued participation. Verbal reinforcement usually works, but in some instances other primary and secondary reinforcers will be needed. But the reinforcing device should not impede the flow of testing. A device that helps to keep young children moving to completion is the use of a timing device. A nonworking clock can be set, and the examiner can point out where the big hand must go before the child can stop. "In 10 minutes we will be done with this." Children often have vague time concepts and 10 minutes will not be too meaningful. The diagnostician and child can move the hand on the clock to show the passing of time, making the hand arrive at the designated place at the time the testing is over.

6. There is also one rather specific suggestion we would like to offer. When doing speech mechanism examinations with children, never assume that you will get to look in their mouths as often as you would like. Make every observation count. If the child cooperates the first time, do as much as you can, look for everything you can, do one task immediately after another as there may be no second chance.

Once the interaction pattern has been established and some baseline of information obtained, the diagnostician can move into his more detailed and specific clinical testing. Each tool is introduced matter-of-factly. "Now we are going to look at some pictures, and I want you to tell me the name of each one. I'll help you if you don't know the name. You turn the pages." Or "Mrs. Valrille, I have a test to give you to help us understand your problem better."

Knowing when to discontinue using a tool is as important as knowing when to use a certain tool. It requires knowing when enough details about the behaviors under study have been obtained or when a patient no longer is performing adequately or with interest. There is no rule to follow other than knowing what information is being obtained and how useful it will be in discovering the essentials of the clinical problem. For example, one of our favorite observations was of a child who was asked to repeat sounds in sequences. The sequences were created by the child who threw a set of dice (wooden blocks) on which the sounds were printed. Dice were added or removed to change the length of the sound sequences to be repeated. This procedure continued, to our way of thinking, beyond its meaningfulness, and after a time the child confirmed this by saying: "When are we going to stop playing with these stupid blocks?" The student was spending too much time getting details at the risk of losing the child's interest and cooperation.

When using standardized tools, the intent is to complete the test if at all possible or else the normative data will not be usable. Some tools are designed to establish basal and ceiling levels of performance such as the Expressive One-Word Picture Vocabulary Test (Gardner, 1979). Others require completion in their entirety, for example, the Photo Articulation Test (Pendergast, Dickey, Selman, & Soder, 1969). Still others supply a screening portion to help make decisions about going on to the remainder of the test for added details such as the Illinois Test of Psycholinguistic Abilities (Kirk, McCarthy, & Kirk, 1968). However, even with such tools, testing should be discontinued if the patient is evidencing significant difficulties in performance or attention that could hinder any remaining testing. When tools are designed to present items graded for difficulty level, they are easier to use than those that are not.

Another situation that occurs is with the patient who manifests immediate behavior indicative of his clinical problem, for example, the adult stutterer who stutters significantly from the moment the diagnostic session begins. The diagnostician knows he has a prosody disorder. Can testing be discontinued? If the diagnostician's intent was only to discover this fact, then testing could be discontinued. However, diagnosis is designed to obtain more than an obvious sample of manifest behavior. He will go on to obtain as many details about the disordered prosody in as many situations as possible, exploring the full range of cause–effect relationships. He works toward gaining as much information as possible to answer any number of clinical questions for making management decisions.

At other times the patient does not readily manifest the behavior reported by the referring source. This is seen to occur quite frequently in young children reported to be stutterers. If anxiety-provoking situations create greater nonfluencies, we should expect that a child coming into the strange diagnostic setting, meeting strange people, and being separated from his parents would be anxious and would demonstrate the nonfluencies that concern his parents. However, we have seen many instances where the child performed with little or no hesitation in verbal interaction, nor did he reveal any disfluencies.

The diagnostician should question the situations under which the child was asked to perform. Was there enough immediate situational stress present to elicit disfluent speech? How could the diagnostician introduce communicative situations that might elicit the stuttering behavior for which the child was referred? Various techniques have been developed based on environmental stress as a causal factor in stuttering. We also have seen instances when the child seemed to be very happy, relaxed, and highly verbal but began to present disfluencies when "stress" was introduced into the interpersonal interaction. One technique found to elicit these nonfluencies has been to ask the child questions rather rapidly, without giving him the opportunity to answer or express himself fully. These instances seem to bring out the nonfluencies. But it does not appear to create any particular anxiety in the child or emotional stress. What we see is often in line with what parents report; he is excited and wants his turn to talk, but it is not an easy talking situation. We like to have the parents observe in these situations to confirm the behaviors we hear or do not hear as the case may be.

We will now proceed to a series of diagnostic situations reflecting different aspects of data collection. Only the schematics of the patient background and tools will be given. The student is encouraged to fill in the many missing details that may have led to these data collection circumstances.

Mr. Robert Chester saw the following three patients:

1. Edward James, a 4-year-old boy, diagnosed as severely hypernasal because of inadequate velopharyngeal closure;

2. Mr. Donald George, 47 years of age, diagnosed as having a severe articulation problem due to paresis of the speech musculature;

3. Carl Richard, 5 years old, medically diagnosed as having spastic cerebral palsy. For each of these patients, Mr. Chester performed a speech mechanism examination. For Edward James, he concentrated his procedures on evaluating the extent of velopharyngeal closure. For Mr. George, he concentrated on the articulatory musculature. For Carl Richards, he concentrated on the phonatory, articulatory, and resonatory mechanisms. Considering his procedural concentration, what speech and nonspeech activities would Mr. Chester use for each of these patients. As a general guide to speech mechanism examinations, Appendix IV presents a speech mechanism examination form. This form is designed primarily as an overview speech mechanism examination; it does not provide many of the details that may be necessary to proceed with the examinations of the preceding clients. To assist the student in designing their specific procedures and observing the responses, the following references are offered: Darley (1964), Darley et al. (1969a, 1969b, 1975a, 1975b), Hixon and Hardy (1964), Mason and Grandstaff (1970, 1971), McWilliams et al. (1968), Mysak (1971), Dworkin (1978), Dworkin and Culatta (1980), and Kuehn (1982). A quote from Darley can serve as a further procedural guide in planning your examination:

> . . .speech is no slow-motion summation of the movements of dissociated though adjacent structures; a static view in the course of somewhat artificial activities will not truly tell us about the dynamics of the speech mechanism *in speech*.
>
> We must discover malfunctioning of the speech apparatus during utterance. Observation of the deviation in speech may unveil the deviation in structure or function. Lifting of the tongue outside the mouth may not be duplicated within it; the tongue may rise in silence and during breath holding but not in speech or during exhalation. The smooth function of a single part may break down when built into a complex pattern of overlapping movements requiring efficient coordination. A compensatory movement used to overcome an anatomical or physiological deficiency may serve well in isolation, but it may create more problems than it solves when it is fitted awkwardly into a sequence. It is manifest, then, that we must supplement tests of function of individual parts with a thorough appraisal of the structures operating simultaneously *in speech*. (Darley, 1964, pp. 103–104)

Each of the following patients has been hypothesized as having a voice disorder. No causal factor has been hypothesized:

1. John Herbert, 7 years of age, in the second grade,
2. Fred Josephs, a high school athletic instructor, aged 29 years,
3. Margaret Josephina, aged 16 years, and lead cheerleader of her high school,
4. John Pardio, aged 72 years, a retired farmer.

Mr. Julius Weiss, the diagnostician, has planned the following general procedures, not necessarily in this order, for these four patients:

1. General conversational speech,
2. Procedures for habitual and optimal use of the voice,
3. Controlled measures of voice use: words, isolated vowels, phrases, sentences, situational roles.

From these general procedures, develop a specifically outlined plan adapting these procedures for each of the preceding patients. Consider how the following "rules" may apply to your procedures.

1. Listen to one component of the voice at a time.

2. Listen only for disordered characteristics.
3. Describe the voice characteristics in perceptual (product) terminology.
4. Do not use causal terminology for a description of the voice characteristics.
The following references will be helpful for determining the procedures you might use: Boone (1977), Moore (1971a, 1971b), Perkins (1971a, 1971b), and Wilson (1979).

Mr. William Cross will be seeing the following two aphasic patients.
1. Mr. Jack Metz was referred by Dr. Tom Harris for diagnosis and therapy. Dr. Harris diagnosed him as aphasic with accompanying visual problems. What procedure might Mr. Cross introduce into his testing to determine the type of visual problem and if the problem interferes with Mr. Metz's language functions?
2. Mr. James Grogan, aged 41 years, was referred to determine the appropriateness of language therapy. Mr. Grogan's family doctor, Dr. Ken Maras (general practitioner) felt he might not benefit from therapy because of his "emotional lability, extreme depression, disorientation, and loss of intellectual function." Mr. Grogan has been diagnosed by Dr. Bill Burcham (neurosurgeon) as aphasic after removal of a tumor of the left temporal lobe.

There are many factors about these two patients affecting the selection of tools and data collection. Assume that Mr. Grogan is aphasic; concentrate on how you would make your observations of the factors mentioned by Dr. Maras. What tests for aphasia and other tools might you select? How would you interpret Dr. Maras' remarks about Mr. Grogan's emotional and mental status in light of associated factors often seen in aphasic patients? How do neurologists examine the functions presented in Mr. Metz's and Mr. Grogan's referral? Look into general neurologic examinations, visual field testing, mental status, orientation and so forth. The following references will assist you: Brookshire (1973), Chusid (1970), and Mayo Clinic (1971).

The following patients were found to have speech sound errors with no disruptions of the speech-producing mechanism. Adapt the stimulability (integral stimulation) procedures suggested by Milisen (1954) to each of these patients. Consider how you would stimulate for each of the sound errors.
1. Brian, 3 years of age, made errors of omission and substitution on all fricatives and affricates.
2. Sheila, 7 years of age, made distortion errors on the /θ, s, z, tʃ, and dʒ/.
3. Mr. Danny Nichols, 23 years of age, made distortions on all productions of the /r and ɝ/ phonemes.
Consider the following in planning your stimulability procedures.
1. Gaining and maintaining attention
2. Examiner–patient physical proximity
3. Teaching the stimulability technique
4. Number of stimulations to apply
5. Signaling the patient to respond without intervening verbalization
6. Amount of auditory, visual, and phonetic placement information to provide
7. Use of phonemes the patient can produce
8. Use of stimulation in isolation, nonsense syllables, and words

Mr. Jack Russo will be screening four groups of individuals suspected of having errors of sound production. He is given 10 minutes with each person. He plans on using word productions for obtaining his information. When he is finished, he wants to know:
1. Are errors present that are outside expected norms?
2. How many errors are present?
3. What is the type of error?
4. What position in the word does it occur?
5. Are there any patterns of consistency?
For his test words, Mr. Russo will go to the objective standardized articulation tests, and select 20 words for each population. He will develop a recording–scoring form for each screening. How will he do this for the following groups?
1. Four-year-old children in a large nursery school,
2. Nine-year-old children in a Catholic elementary school,
3. Fifteen- to seventeen-year-old mentally retarded adolescents in a vocational workshop for the retarded,
4. Adult male prisoners in the state penal institution.

You are to be seeing 5½-year-old Aiko Morimoto who is suspected of a language-learning problem. Aiko arrived in this country from Japan when she was 4 years old. Japanese is the primary language spoken at home, although Aiko has been exposed to the English language, including one year of nursery school. A question has been posed to you regarding her language-learning abilities and whether she will be able to function in a regular first-grade class. What information would you collect on this child and what tools would you use? Consider the approach suggested by Dulay, Hernández-Chávez, and Burt (1978), and Burt, Dulay, and Hernández-Chávez (1978).

You have been asked to see two adult patients, each with a type of cerebral palsy that was identified soon after birth. The first patient, Mr. Stanley Acree, is 28 years old and has been medically diagnosed as an athetoid type of cerebral palsy. The second patient, Mrs. William Garfinkel, is 32 years old and has the spastic type of cerebral palsy. In collecting data on these two patients, how will you determine the relative importance of historical and contemporary causation? The assumption is that both patients' speech mechanisms are affected by the neurologic condition. What data will you collect and what are your expected findings? Use Platt, Andrews, Young, and Quinn (1980) and Platt, Andrews, and Howie (1980) as resources.

Tool administration

To administer the tools he has selected, the diagnostician must have general knowledge about tool presentation as well as the specific knowledge about each tool he is planning to use. As a part of tool administration, the diagnostician also concerns himself with accurate recording procedures.

• *Tool presentation.* The diagnostician must know each tool and its specific administrative procedures. He must understand all the stimulus–response variables that exist in any given tool. Many tools specify the basic stimulus–response modalities being tested but make little or no mention of other modalities necessary to complete the task. For example, the Northwestern Syntax Screening Test (Lee, 1969) aims to test auditorily presented syntactic "reception and expression"; however, successful completion of this tool also requires rather astute visual perception. Many tools for measuring comprehension of language are of this type, requiring both auditory and visual processing of information. Some tools provide an auditory stimulus for presentation that is only incidental for facilitating a response. The Templin–Darley Tests of Articulation (Templin & Darley, 1969) provide a stimulus frame to elicit the name of the item pictures: "We fasten the ____ ," where the expected response is *zipper*. However, if the patient can understand that he is to name the picture, the auditory stiumlus can be abandoned in testing. Many tests require visual interpretation of a picture in order for the patient to respond, which has always created a certain amount of consternation among diagnosticians. Tests are frequently criticized for lack of adequate pictorial representation— "No wonder he can't name cat, the picture looks more like a dog."

There are some tools that provide for alternate modes of stimulation and response. Examining for Aphasia by Eisenson (1954) exemplifies this. In many of the subtests, if the aphasic does not or cannot respond to one mode of stimulation, an alternate will be provided. Presumably the data obtained with the alternate methods is equally adequate, although this is not stated in the test manual. Research evidence provides some information that, at least for naming tasks from visual stimulation, the examiner could use pictures, objects, photographs, or line drawings to elicit equally appropriate naming responses from aphasics (Corlew & Nation, 1975).

As well as stimulus–response modality variables, the diagnostician should be completely aware of all the speech and language levels represented in the stimulus items. Again, many tools specify their primary purpose as testing for a certain linguistic level, whereas the test items require processing of more than one level. For example, the Denver Auditory Phoneme Sequencing Test (Aten, 1979) requires auditory presentation of pairs of words that are either the same or different. The question that arises is how the completion of the task is to be interpreted—on the basis of discrimination of speech sounds or on the basis of semantic comprehension since the stimuli are words. The same is true of any "discrimination" test based on word pairs. Any tool designed for syntactic comprehension would probably also require semantic comprehension. Because of this, the Assessment of Children's Language Comprehension (Foster et al., 1973) first determines if the child comprehends all the test words (semantic level) before putting them into combinations called critical elements, interpreted as syntactic word orders.

There are few tools that are relatively "pure" in terms of stimulus–response modalities and levels of language being tested. The diagnostician must rely on his analysis of the test items, remaining alert to the fact that there will be variables incidental to the test designer's basic concern.

Tools are essential to the diagnostician. They provide detailed ordering of the stimuli to be presented and ways for observing specified response levels. Required in all these tools are administration procedures that the diagnostician uses if at all possible or if they are applicable to his patient. Most tools come with manuals or instructions for administration— how to present the items, what order they come in, establishing basal levels and ceiling levels of performance, alternate stimulations, number of stimulations, score forms for recording purposes, response scoring systems, and so forth.

It should go without saying that before using a test instrument for its explicit purposes, the diagnostician should be well grounded in its administrative procedures, particularly with methods of recording and scoring the responses. Without question, students in training should obtain good groundwork in tests and measurements that will give them the background and respect for the careful use of instruments of measurement—background that can be utilized for learning each new tool that is developed in their profession.

Some additional remarks are necessary about changing the standard instructions that accompany testing tools. If possible, the diagnostician using structured objective tests should present them according to their standard instructions. However, varying the stimulus presentation sometimes allows a patient to respond better. For example, young children at times have difficulty responding to the phrase "Show me" or "Point to ____ " — the recommended stimulus presentation for the Peabody Picture Vocabulary Test (Dunn & Dunn, 1981). By making a slight alteration in directions and saying "Touch ____ ," "Put your finger on ____ ," or "Put the penny on ____ ," the child will respond. Stimulus phrases such as "Make ducky sit on ____ " also motivates a child, who has long since become disinterested in "showing me" or "pointing to" the said picture.

When presented initially with standardized items from a test, some patients may not grasp what they are to do. At this point it may be very appropriate to alter the task considerably. When altering the standard presentation, the diagnostician must be aware of the possible invalidation of the tool and be cautious of using the normative data that has been gathered under the standard presentation. While it is unlikely that "Touch *boat*" or "Put you finger on *boat*" substantially changes a child's level of vocabulary comprehension, other presentation modification may. For example, if the child is asked to "point to what grandma and grandpa have on their lake," the child is responding to the visual representation of boat rather than the spoken word, *boat*. These two tasks are not equivalent. However, when a patient cannot or will not respond to the stimulus, the diagnostician may resort to repetition as an alteration of the stimulus–response mode. Repetition of stimuli has often been used as a major testing method even though its use has been heavily criticized. To us, imitated or repeated responses tell the diagnostician something about underlying language processes. Repetition may be different from spontaneous responses, but repetition cannot be accomplished without certain internal processes being intact. If repetition is the only way a test can be used with a patient, alter the test format; repeated responses are far better than no responses. On the positive side, if the patient matches the model, it is demonstrable evidence that he can produce the response, which may be evidence that his speech and language disorder can be changed. Given certain cautions about using repetition as a mode of eliciting responses, it can be used efficiently as a method of data collection.

Every other source of speech and language stimulation that occurs in the diagnostic session (the immediate speech and language environment) must be structured just as carefully as the items from selected tools. Frequently, diagnosticians forget that their spontaneous remarks may be too complex to be comprehended by the patient. If the diagnostician expects the patient to respond, he must monitor all the verbal stimulation he provides. For example, a 3-year-old child with a language disorder may respond marginally to yes–no questions, but not to "wh" questions other than *who* or *what*. Using graded verbal stimuli, the diagnostician can discover, through conversation, the general level at which a child with a language disorder may be able to comprehend and formulate responses and the point at which he no longer can respond.

As well as controlling the complexity of language stimulation, the diagnostician must take care not to overstimulate. Overstimulation sometimes occurs with young children who are not talking or giving any indication of comprehension. It is also seen with aphasics who have comparable language difficulties. The diagnostician may resort to an overinflected, loud, singsong speech pattern—a truly dreadful type of overstimulation. When observing this behavior, we sometimes think that the diagnostician hopes the patient will talk because he talks this way. Overstimulation is also seen by the use of extensive questioning: "What is this? What is your name? What is that? Did you come with mommy?"—endless questions that the patient may not be able to answer, does not want to answer, or is not given time to answer.

• *Observation and recording.* How to observe and record the patient's responses is fundamental to data collection. Everything the diagnostician needs to learn about the patient may well be right before his eyes and ears; however, if he is not able to see, hear, and keep track of what is there, he may lose the very information he needs.

The diagnostician should maintain close scrutiny of all the behaviors exhibited. No behavior should be thought of as simply incidental; it should be observed, recorded, and considered in terms of its relationship to the clinical hypothesis. Frequently, significant responses emerge from unplanned or unorthodox stimulus presentation. For example, a diagnostician was testing Joe whose causal hypothesis was a significant hearing loss. In the test room, Joe was not responding to any auditory stimulations. He did not turn his head toward any sound source, differentiate between sound toys—nothing. An observer was behind the two-way observation mirror and tapped lightly on the glass. Joe turned toward this sound source. To check this response, the examiner in the room engrossed the child in play, the observer repeatedly tapped and the child repeatedly turned. The diagnostician had observed a response to sound. Information was obtained for their clinical hypothesis from an unplanned stimulus.

Planned or unplanned, every behavior may offer a source of information to the observant diagnostician. Even crying behavior, while it might impede other data collection, is useful. For example, 2-year-old Bonnie, whose causal hypothesis was inadequate velopharyngeal closure secondary to a repaired cleft palate, was being seen. She seemed terrified of any procedures that might mean discomfort for her and cried excessively at the onset of the session. The diagnostician here could be both comforting and observing. Is the crying behavior nasal? How nasal? Does it vary with the intensity of the crying?

The diagnostician's planned use of the SLPM as a framework for observation makes it possible for him to organize the many variables under study. He can plug in the various behaviors as they occur. Each relevant behavior can be recorded as a product, a behavioral correlate, or as associated behavior. The diagnostician can record the details he obtains from his observations until he builds up enough information to signal that the diagnosis can be concluded. Observing all behaviors from this framework prevents the diagnostician from unwarranted interpretations of isolated responses.

While the diagnostician has the SLPM framework for observing his patient's responses, he must know how to record the details he observes. He needs some means of capturing what the patient is doing so he may analyze, refer to, and report that data at a later time. He must know how to use notational systems for recording his data. He can use test forms, behavioral observation forms, and systems of his own making as long as the recording of the data reflects the reality of the data collection session. It is the rare circumstance when the diagnostician does not have to make constant, on-the-spot records of his patient's responses. When recording his measurements, he immediately interposes himself between the actual response and his recording of that response. At the moment of response the diagnostician usually records his impression of the correctness of the response and the quality of the response, particularly if he has judged the response as incorrect. He does this by comparing the response to some internal criteria for adequacy.

Recording in its limited sense would be description or getting down what the patient said. Any other type of recording requiring judgment of the correctness and quality of the response is scoring. Thus, recording and scoring of responses are intimately bound together; seldom is all scoring done after all responses are made. The diagnostician generally must record and score each item as it occurs for later use.

In some instances, especially in student and research-oriented diagnostic settings, the diagnostician may want to record all or part of the clinical testing in its entirety. He may choose to employ a video or audio tape recorder which will allow him to capture on tape the patient's speech and language product. To be useful, however, the diagnostician will have to use several precautions in taping. With either an audio or video tape recorder, he must be sure the recorder is working correctly. How often have diagnosticians thought they were recording, and the tape was never turned on. The tape and recorder must be of sufficient quality for the diagnostician to capture the information of interest. Thus, for example, for judgments of voice quality or close phonetic transcriptions, good tapes and recorders must be used. The patient must be positioned optimally for the camera or microphone; sound level meters must be monitored. Finally, especially for audio recordings, a gloss of what is said must be provided so that the diagnostician can interpret the sample when the contextual clues have been removed. In providing the gloss, the diagnostician must be careful not to speak over the patient. Finally, extraneous noise and voices must be kept to a minimum, including preventing the patient from handling the microphone.

Even if the diagnostician chooses to audio- or videotape-record his patient's responses, he still will need to transcribe the tape in some form. Regardless of whether or not the diagnostician is making the judgments "live" or from recordings, he has basically three procedures available to him for scoring the response, and most scoring protocols accompanying tests use one or more of these.

1. He can determine if the response is correct or incorrect.
2. He can judge the quality of the response along some scale.
3. He can describe the response.

For example, when the diagnostician records that Bertheva made a /b/v/ substitution error, he has used both the descriptive and correctness procedures—noting the type of error is automatically making a statement of correctness. The recording procedures of most tools greatly depends on the complexity inherent in the response required or the information the diagnostician wants to obtain from the response. Where categorical responses of the yes/no type are required, the diagnostician can score them as right or wrong at the time the response is elicited. Where more complex responses are elicited, the choice is often to describe: to record what the patient did for later use in multidimensional scoring.

At first glance it would seem easy to at least differentiate a correct response from an incorrect one. However, we know this is hardly true. Our experience indicates that the range of variability for judging correctness of certain types of responses may be broad, particularly considering responses in context; that is, a sound produced in isolation is usually easier to judge than a sound produced in conversational speech.

There are no absolute criteria for perceptual measurements; experimenters obtaining intra- and interjudge reliability will attest to this. Shriberg (1972) confirms this impression in his study conducted to determine the perceptual judgments made on the /s/ and /r/ phonemes. And yet, the diagnostician must develop internal criteria for making accurate perceptual measurements on the response made by the individual patient. Unlike the experimenter, he usually cannot obtain interjudge reliability of his response recording. Instead, he relies on his own established reliability for each tool he uses. Tools such as Wepman's Auditory Discrimination Test (1958) and the Full-Range Picture Vocabulary Test (Ammons & Ammons, 1948) rely basically on categorical scoring; the primary interest of these tools is the correctness of the response, not the type of error made. A major test for aphasia, the Minnesota Test for Differential Diagnosis of Aphasia (Schuell, 1965), uses a correctness scoring procedure and because of this draws some criticism.

Many of the measures taken of speech and language responses cannot be scored as right or wrong. Instead, responses are qualitatively recorded. Rating scales are frequently used as qualitative recording devices, particularly for disorders such as voice and stuttering. As well, rating scales are used to provide estimates of severity and intelligibility. As he listens to the response, the diagnostician judges the kind, amount, and degree of variation that occurs. Thus, the ability to plot responses on these psychological scaling procedures is dependent on the diagnostician's knowledge of the range of variation that can occur.

The most common scales are those that ask for three judgments, for example, *mild–moderate–severe, low–average–high,* or *poor–average–good.* Others, however, may require the listener to rate behavior on a scale from 1 to 5 or 1 to 7. The presumption made is that the intervals on these scales are equal and can be converted to numerical quantities. The diagnostician must be trained to judgmental criteria if he is to use these scales appropriately. If not, he will not know if the pitch is *high–appropriate–low*; if the distortion is *mild–moderate–severe*; or if the amount of nasality is *absent–mild–moderately severe–severe–extreme.*

We have often asked classes of students in training to rate speech responses on various scales. The variability of ratings is always amazing. It becomes readily apparent that interjudge and intrajudge reliability is crucial to accurate recording of responses. Our profession is in great need of training tools to assist students in developing perceptual criteria for various speech and language behaviors they will be asked to rate. In educational programs and research settings the use of audio- and videotape recorders is advocated. Recording all or part of the diagnostic session has unquestionable advantages and allows for later interobserver reliability and more studied analysis.

Many tools use some form of rating scale for recording responses, either for the entire test or for selected subtests. For example, in the Boston Diagnostic Aphasia Examination (Goodglass & Kaplan, 1972) *articulation* is rated throughout a number of subtests. Their scale rates articulation on a *normal–stiff–distorted–fail* continuum.

Because the diagnostician is generally interested in the type of error made by the patient, he also employs descriptive recording procedures. In this procedure the diagnostician puts down on paper the "exact" response made by the patient. He will then categorize the response into a "type of error" category and may at the same time record a correctness judgment. If Fred was asked to name pictures and was shown a fish and he said *"bird,"* the diagnostician would record the word *bird,* score it as incorrect, and categorize it as a type of error; perhaps in this case an in-class semantic error. Or in another example, when Diane points to the incorrect picture on the Peabody Picture Vocabulary Test (Dunn & Dunn, 1981) and the diagnostician records the number of the picture to which she pointed, he then has obtained some information about the types of vocabulary comprehension errors Diane is making. Or yet another example: Listening to Jill's voice the diagnostician records that it is breathy and hoarse. In this instance the diagnostician bypasses recording what Jill says and instead describes categorically the dimensions of voice quality he has heard.

Testing tools available abound with various examples of the use of the descriptive recording–scoring procedure.

Many tools utilize all three recording–scoring procedures. Since speech and language behavior is not unidimensional, tools are designed to obtain several dimensions of behavior from a single response or from a series of responses. Tools like this require multidimensional scoring, isolating as many dimensions as can be observed and recorded simultaneously. Experimental and clinical studies have been instrumental in isolating important dimensions of speech and language disorders. For example, Prins and Lohr (1972) studied 46 visible–audible variables of stuttering behavior. From their analysis of the data they identified 10 factors that, to them, identified the dimensions of stuttering behavior. For the diagnostician, studies such as these assist in determining which behaviors to observe and which provide the most differential information, rather than observing a set of variables that all give similar types of information.

When using standardized and objective tools, the diagnostician is obliged to record and score the response accordingly if he wants to use the standardization data available. However, at times he may find that using only the recommended procedures limits the information he might obtain. Therefore, he may choose to amplify on the recording–scoring procedures to gain additional information. This is particularly true in tools like the Minnesota Test for Differential Diagnosis of Aphasia (Schuell, 1965), which uses primarily correctness scoring procedures. The diagnostician would probably amplify his recording, adding descriptive procedures to gain data about the type and quality of the responses made to the test items. The diagnostician must always remember that he learns more from knowing what the error is than from knowing an error occurs.

CLOSES THE SESSION

As well as knowing how to open his clinical testing session, the diagnostician must do some planning for closing the session. Children who have been separated from their parents now must be separated from the diagnostician. We have seen instances of children who have screamed because it was time to go home. No matter how the session started, the patient usually comes to realize that the diagnostician is working with them to solve a problem. Even very young children have an awareness that this event is meaningful. Abrupt separations can lead to negativism when the next appointment comes. Patients who leave with good feelings return for therapy with good feelings.

Closing the session is actually initiated at the beginning of testing. Patients can be informed how long the session may be and periodically informed that there is only so much time left. Closing the session, then, is task oriented; each tool completion leads to final completion.

For children, it is especially important that the last task be one designed to give them as much praise for success as possible and one that places little demand on them. As an aside, we want to emphasize that throughout testing, where possible, a tool should be ended with successful performance by the patient. For example, using the Woodcock–Johnson Psycho-Educational Battery (1977), we will continue "testing" after the ceiling has been reached, making up names for two or three successive plates that we know the child can point to successfully. Praise at this time for his success also assists in gaining cooperation to move on to the next task.

At times when the patient knows he is doing the final task, his performance is affected. Generally, being glad the session is coming to an end, his responses may become perfunctory and careless. Nontypical responses may occur. Thus, it is wise to use final procedures that are either very different from others used or those that may be less essential to the diagnostician's findings. Some diagnosticians use a period of free play with children to close the session. With adults, general conversation is appropriate. When the end of the session has come, it should be stated as such, and the patient given the opportunity to respond about his feelings of what took place and what is going to happen next.

SUMMARY

In this fourth step of the diagnostic process, the diagnostician implements his clinical design; he collects his clinical data. Here he applies the information studied and organized in the previous steps. He also calls on his knowledge and professional skill in tool presentation, response observation and recording, and interpersonal interactions. These sources of information allow him to adapt his design to new data and to the individual needs of the patient he sees.

Three tasks are involved in collection of the clinical data.

1. The diagnostician first *prepares for the diagnostic session.* He must ready the room and his materials, ensuring that his physical props are in order. He also will establish his initial contact with the patient. In doing this he prepares the patient for what they may expect to take place, and he himself samples what he may expect from them.
2. The diagnostician then proceeds with *collecting his data.* Usually this includes both an interview and the actual clinical testing. These may or may not occur on the same day. Both the interview and testing will include tool presentation, adaptation to new information and the interpersonal context, and recording systematic observations.
3. Finally, the diagnostician will need to *close the testing session.* Here he will want to let the patient know how things stand and what next steps will be taken.

KATHERINE COMPARDO: CLINICAL TESTING: COLLECTION OF THE DATA

Conduct an interview with Mrs. Compardo. The interview has been structured so that Katherine is playing quietly in a sandbox in another corner of a large room. Mrs. Compardo and the diagnostician can thus interact without distraction as Katherine is actively involved in her play. Table 7-1 sketches part of this interview. The student is encouraged to complete the interview through role play. Refer back to Chapter 6 where further information needed about Katherine has been delineated and where questions have been framed and to the children's speech, language, and hearing history questionnaire that Mrs. Compardo has completed.

Table 7-2 outlines the initial contact and clinical testing done with Katherine based on the tools that were selected in the previous chapter. Not all tools and observations are discussed but enough to provide an example of how the diagnostician proceeded with his testing strategy and recorded his observations of the responses that were made.

PATIENT PROJECTS

The student is now directed to go back to the patients presented in chapter 4 and carry out a role play with other students, assuming the role of the informant and the patient. Conduct the interview and execute the clinical testing using the tools selected for that patient.

STUDY QUESTIONS

1. The student should become familiar with the various orientations to interviewing. Each has something to offer the diagnostician of speech and language disorders. As a project, develop an outline of the common principles of interviewing revealed in the following: Bingham and Moore (1941), Emerick and Hatten (1979), Garrett (1972), Rogers (1942), Stevenson (1971), Sullivan (1954), and Molyneaux and Lane (1982).

2. As well as the questions he designs, the diagnostician should consider the use of tools that have been specially designed as interview techniques. These are available as commercial tools and are also present in the research literature. What specific information would the following provide: Verbal Language Development Scale by Mecham (1959), the Vineland Social Maturity Scale by Doll (1965), the Receptive–Expressive Emergent Language Scale (REEL) by Bzoch and League (1971), the Denver Developmental Screening Test by Frankenburg and Dodd (1967), and The Child Behavior Checklist by Achenbach (1981).

3. Hannah and Sheeley (1975) have presented a seven-stage sequence flowchart for audiologic evaluation. Their overall concern is how audiologists might select testing procedures to arrive at a diagnostic profile. Compare their model of test selection to the framework being developed in this book for the diagnostic process, particularly as it relates to the selection of tools and collection of data steps of the process.

4. The student should explore the tools in Appendix III for uses of scaling (rating) procedures. Are the criteria for rating clearly established by the test designer?

5. "Auditory discrimination" has always been difficult to conceptualize and measure. How have the following test designers gone about this task: Templin Picture Sound Discrimination Test (Templin, 1957), Goldman–Fristoe–Woodcock Test of Auditory Discrimination (Goldman et al., 1970), the Test of Listening Accuracy in Children (Mecham et al., 1969), and Wepman's Auditory Discrimination Test (1958)? How have they provided for administering the auditory stimuli, what type of stimuli have they chosen, and how do they record and score the responses? Would all of these tools give you the same information about "auditory discrimination?" Review Locke's (1980a, 1980b) criticism of such tests and consider adaptation of his approach to the diagnostic setting.

6. Different tools have been designed to measure similar behaviors. What do the following tools offer for measuring formulation of various aspects of syntax (grammar): the expressive portion of the Northwestern Syntax Screening Test (Lee, 1969), the Berry–Talbott Test of Language (Berry, 1966), Lee's Developmental Sentence Scoring and her Developmental Sentence Type analysis (1974), the expressive portion of the Michigan Picture Language Inventory (Wolski, 1962), the Carrow Elicited Language Inventory (Carrow, 1974), Oral Language Sentence Imitation Test (Zachman, Hulsingh, Jorgensen, & Barrett, 1976), and Patterned Elicitation Syntax Screening Test (Young & Perachio, 1982). How many different types of stimuli are used for these tasks? Do they represent what might be considered as stimulus alterations?

7. Review the administration procedures for several tests of phonology and phonetic structure. What differences are evident in administrative procedures? Could the procedures from one test be used with a second test without affecting the reliability or validity of the results? Start your review with a comparison of the Natural Process Analysis (Shriberg & Kwiatkowski, 1980), the Assessment of Phonological Processes (Hodson, 1980), and the Photo Articulation Test (Pendergast, Dickey, Selman, & Soder, 1969).

8. Tests for young children are generally developmental in nature, although the orientation behind the tests may differ. For example, the Sequenced Inventory of Communication Development (Hedrick, Prather, & Tobin, 1975) generally follows child development models by testing performance by ages and stages. On the other hand, the Preschool Language Assessment Instrument (Blank, Rose, & Berlin, 1978) is considered to be a test based on discourse analysis. How do these two tools differ in the manner in which they collect data?

Table 7-1. Interview with Mrs. Compardo

Diagnostician's aim	Diagnostician's and Mrs. Compardo's statements (D = Diagnostician, C = Compardo)	
Explain the purpose of the interview.	D:	Mrs. Compardo, before working with Katherine I'd like to spend some time talking with you about her speech and language. Your information will be most useful in helping understand her problem and in giving us a broader picture of her. We'll be working together in determining Katherine's problem and in doing something about it.
	C:	I'm glad to finally be here today. I really don't know why Katherine is having trouble talking, and I hope that we'll be able to do something about it.
Acknowledge the information received prior to the interview.	D:	I appreciate your taking the time and thought to have filled out the history questionnaire so completely. I have gone over it carefully and it has helped me plan what I will be doing with Katherine today. It also has helped me think of a few other things I'd like to ask you.
	C:	On some of the questions, I just wasn't sure what to say.
	D:	I know that sometimes it's hard to know just what is intended by some of the questions. We'll be discussing some of those here.
Inform parent of recording method chosen.	D:	From time to time, you may see me jotting notes down. Some of the things you say I will want to write down exactly as you have said them so that I will be sure to have the correct information.
Begin interview proper with a general, circumscribed amplification question that addresses the speech and language problem.	D:	Since you completed the history form, have you noticed anything else that you might like to add about Katherine's speech and language?
	C:	Not too much has changed, although I think she is starting to call the cat "nana"—our cat's name is Nerja. She also has really been involved in picture books. She's always trying to get me to read to her. One other thing I've been noticing lately is that compared to my other children, she is really a messy eater. She uses both hands and really makes a mess.
Follow up open question with a more structured question based on earlier response.	D:	By messy eater, what do you mean? Does she play with her food, or does she seem to be having trouble keeping food in her mouth?
	C:	She's a good eater; that is, she likes to eat and doesn't really play with her food. Rather, she's just sloppy in the way she eats. Her milk is always running out of the corners of her mouth or bits of food fall out of her mouth. She also doesn't chew her food very well, swallows huge bites, and sometimes gags. As a baby she accepted solid foods much later than my other children did and had problems moving the food around in her mouth to chew it and swallow it. I didn't think we'd ever get her off baby food. I wish we would have owned stock in Gerber's.
Follow up point made by parent to get further information having to do with Katherine's understanding.	D:	One thing you said a little earlier I'd like to discuss a little more. You said Katherine is always trying to get you to read to her. What kinds of books does she like? Does she seem to like the stories, or is she mostly involved in looking at the pictures?
	C:	Katherine used to favor books like the ABC's and simple picture books, but now she seems to be bored by those. She likes books that have more of a story to them. She loves the *Three Little Pigs* and some of the Dr. Seuss books.

continued.

Table 7-1. Interview with Mrs. Compardo—cont'd

Diagnostician's aim	Diagnostician's and Mrs. Compardo's statements (D = Diagnostician, C = Compardo)	
Insert planned question relevant to topic area under discussion.	D:	Can you give me other examples of situations in which Katherine understands the language used?
	C:	Well, since she loved the *Three Little Pigs* so much, I bought her the record at the grocery store—you know one of those 49¢ records that she later can play herself. Now she wants me to play that over, and over, and over. She laughs when the pigs say "not by the hair of my chinny, chin chin," and sometimes blows when the wolf says "then I'll huff and I'll puff and I'll blow your house down."
	D:	Can you think of any other situations. Sometimes it's tricky to know if a child understands the words we say to them or gets the message through our gestures or other clues. Can you think of any situations in which it was quite clear that Katherine understood what you said rather than what she saw?
	C:	Let's see . . . oh, the other day I was busy cooking in the kitchen and I wanted a magazine that I had left on the nightstand next to our bed. I asked Katherine to go upstairs and get it, and she did. Sometimes she won't do what I want her to, but I think that's more a matter of stubbornness than not understanding.
Continue role playing the remainder of the interview		

Table 7-2. Initial patient contact and clinical testing with Katherine Compardo

Diagnostician's tasks	Information obtained
Room	
The room selected was a large nursery with a stand-up sandbox and several well-demarcated areas. In one corner was a kitchen setting with children's furniture; the sandbox was in another area; a chalk board and cabinets with toys behind closed doors were in the room. In a separate area was a child's table and chairs. Each area was set up with materials for use with Katherine.	
Initial client contact	
Katherine and her mother were met in the lobby of the agency. The diagnostician sat and talked with both of them. Katherine was seated next to her mother, and the examiner pulled up a chair to face them.	Katherine responded to "Hi Katherine" by smiling. The examiner reached out to hold her hand and she took it. They held hands while the conversation took place. Katherine made no verbalizations.
Separation	
Initially, all three went to the nursery. But it seemed to the examiner, and the mother confirmed it, that Katherine would have gone with him.	Katherine became engrossed in the sandbox while an interview with the mother proceeded. The interview lasted a short time, since so much information

continued.

Table 7-2. Initial patient contact and clinical testing with Katherine Compardo—cont'd

Diagnostician's tasks	Information obtained
Separation—cont'd	had already been obtained. After the interview, Katherine was asked if it was all right for her mother to leave the room; she shook her head "yes" and only momentarily followed her mother with her eyes. Still no verbalization had occurred.
Orienting procedures	
The diagnostician went to the sandbox with Katherine, commented on what she was doing, and joined in the activity.	She responded appropriately to the following instructions as well as to others of a similar type: "Put some sand in the bucket," "Put the dog in the house," "Where's the cat?" "Put the cat by the dog," and "Put some sand under the house."
	During this task she made several unintelligible "screeching" sounds. When asked to name the dog and cat, her responses were /ɔʔɪ/ and /æʔ/.
Tools	
Katherine was asked to come to the table to do some looking at pictures, listening, and talking.	She moved immediately to the table and sat in a chair.
Peabody Picture Vocabulary Test and Vocabulary Usage Test were used for a combined comprehension, formulation, and repetition task.	
The Peabody Picture Vocabulary Test was used for comprehension as it is used in the Vocabulary Usage Test; after the Vocabulary Usage Test item was given, Katherine was asked to repeat it.	Example plates: she pointed correctly but did not respond to the vocabulary usage items, nor would she attempt imitation of the words.
	Comprehension was tested through plate 15, at which time Katherine got up from her chair, shook her head "no," and ran back to the sandbox.
Took her to the kitchen area to explore the area.	Again, she demonstrated ability to follow directions and seemed to know the relationship among the various pieces of furniture in the area.
Asked her if she would do some talking for me, since I need to know how well she can do.	She shook her head "yes," reached out for my hand, and started toward the table.
Asked her to imitate a new way of getting to the table. We jumped in place, hopped, stood on one leg, ran several steps, and several other motor tasks.	She attempted all tasks and performed them with some awkwardness.
Direct repetitions of sounds and words were attempted. The diagnostician held Katherine on his lap so they were face-to-face, emphasizing to her how much he wanted to hear how well she talked.	

	ITEMS SIMULATED		RESPONSE
Vowels	/a,i,æ,o,u/		All repeated
Consonants			/b/
	/p/	voicing	/b/
	/d/		/di/
	/t/	voicing	/d/
	/k/	fronting	/d/
	/g/	fronting	/d/
	/m/		/b/
Words	Shoe		/d/
	Button		/bʌfə/

She would attempt no more imitation of speech.

continued.

Table 7-2. Initial patient contact and clinical testing with
Katherine Compardo—cont'd

Diagnostician's tasks	Information obtained
Tools—cont'd	
Imitation of speech musculature movements.	Tongue protrusion: seemed to be trying but could not protrude it
	Tongue lateralization: moved it to the left but not to the right
	Lip protrusion: again, seemed to try but did not accomplish.
	Other observations: tongue appeared to be held flat in the mouth; saw little tongue tip activity; rather constant drooling with little effort to swallow the saliva; she tended to wipe if off with her hand.
	Gave cereal to eat, she chewed and swallowed; she drank water from a cup.
One last chance to elicit names. Had her open the toy chest and explore the toys, but she was not given any until she said the name. Stimulus: "What is it?"	She understood, produced. /i/ for doll, dog, cup, and /hɪʔʌ/ for shoe, cat, and spoon.
Guided observations throughout the session.	See previous comments.
	She appeared to have an awkward gait with some toeing in, no facial asymmetry, licked a lollipop that was given at the end of the session.
Interpersonal interaction.	She responded well to the tasks, although she made it clear when she was finished. She seemed to enjoy doing things with the diagnostician and did go along with some tasks, that she might not have enjoyed.

Chapter 8

Clinical data analysis

Analysis of the clinical data is the fifth step of the diagnostic process. All of the data obtained during the interview and clinical testing is now ready for analysis—determining what significance the data may have for solving the clinical problem. Analysis of the clinical data is only an epilogue to collecting the clinical data and a prologue to interpretation of the data.

At the outset it is important to realize that this step of the diagnostic process is somewhat artificial, since data analysis is seldom separate from either its collection or interpretation. The diagnostician cannot wait until all testing is completed before beginning some analysis and interpretation. For example, he may alter his test procedures during the testing session because of preliminary analysis of the data being obtained. Similarly, when the diagnostician scores and analyzes the data for significance, he cannot always keep separate interpretive evaluations.

However, we consider analysis of the data to be an important step to consider separately, particularly for the diagnostician in training. It is designated as a separate step primarily to illustrate the mental processes that occur during clinical data analysis. Unlike the researcher who may lay out all his data and determine its significance through a series of statistical analyses, the diagnostician must do an ongoing analysis—he cannot wait until all his data is in before he determines if it is significant. But the diagnostician must develop the mental operations of this step, thought of as the nonjudgmental organization of the "facts" that have been obtained during clinical testing. The diagnostician needs to develop the skill of scoring the data, objectifying the data, comparing the data to normative data, and organizing the data in relationship to the hypotheses—all without interpreting its meaning. It is a phase of data analysis, not data interpretation.

Developing this step assists the diagnostician in keeping bias out of the diagnosis; it forces him to stay with the "facts" before entering the interpretive stage. This step is therefore analogous to the stage in research where the results are reported prior to any discussion and interpretation of their meaning.

To accomplish the clinical analysis the diagnostician engages in three tasks. First, he objectifies the information. Second, he categorizes and orders the new data in reference to the clinical hypothesis. Third, he determines the strength or significance of the data for supporting or refuting the clinical hypothesis.

OBJECTIFIES CLINICAL DATA

As the first task in data analysis, the diagnostician objectifies that data obtained. Included in this task are scoring and comparing the data to normative information.

Scores clinical data

The diagnostician sits down with all his tools, scoring protocols, manuals, notes, tape recordings, and his memory and scores all his new information. He wants to find out what he has and how good it is. Actually much of the objectification and comparative analyses of the data occurred while they were being collected. Responses and descriptive statements were recorded, how the client performed, and what he did. The conditions under which the data were obtained were noted, particularly those that would be reflected in the reliability and validity of the information. Thus, in this first clinical analysis task all the data that have not yet been scored are now objectified, and the data recorded and scored during the collection step are reviewed for accuracy and completeness. Greater detail and specification are added.

The diagnostician objectifies the interview information and the patient's performance on the tools by whatever method of scoring he has available—numbers, descriptions, and qualitative judgments as discussed in the previous chapter. He describes what the patient said and did, rates the performance according to perceptual criteria, determines pass-fail responses, judges the correctness of the response, describes the type of errors made, counts the number of errors made, and records the consistency of the errors. He notes the situations that resulted in error responses, in better or normal responses, and in response variability, and he judges the extent of the errors—how many errors were made out of how many responses. The diagnostician goes through many general and specific procedures to objectify the patient's response to the tools that were presented.

All these analysis procedures are attempts to specify the degree and extent of the variation and not, at this time, to judge the presence or absence of a speech and language disorder. For example, if the diagnostician used a phonetic structure test to determine the errors 4-year-old Donald made and discovered that he made 43 errors out of 50 possible responses, he would know how many errors Donald made. He might then ask, What are the characteristics of the errors? Were the errors primarily omissions, substitutions, or distortions? What sounds were used in place of other sounds? What sound features were characteristically in error? Were early developing sounds used in place of later developing sounds? What processes account for these error patterns? Was manner of articulation affected more than place of articulation? Were voiced sounds used for voiceless sounds? These and other details of Donald's errors could be "scored" and analyzed by the diagnostician. All these provide much greater information for interpretation than just knowing he made 43 errors out of 50. Edwards and Shriberg (1983) discuss multiple ways a deviant speech sound system might be analyzed and Hodson and Paden (1983) discuss their specific phonological approach.

From his objective analysis the diagnostician also provides summary descriptions that characterize the details of the variation, noting any variables that may interfere with the reliability and validity of the data—the reliance he places on the data as being "good" data. Objectification, then, is the analytic procedure by which the details of the patient's disorder are specified. This results in data of basically two types, quantitative (numerical) and descriptive.

Most objective standardized tools provide for some quantification of the results obtained, usually for comparative purposes. For example, the test form that accompanies the Photo Articulation Test (Pendergast et al., 1969) derives a series of numerical scores concerned with the number of errors the patient makes in relation to the total number of responses, sound categories, and positions of the sound. The Expressive One-Word Picture Vocabulary Test (Gardner, 1979) provides a basal score and a ceiling score from which a raw score is derived. The Assessment of Children's Language Comprehension (Foster et al., 1973) for Part A of the test scores number correct and for Parts B, C, and D scores percentage correct. Students are encouraged to review chapters 6 and 7 and Appendix III for discussion of tools, and to study the scoring protocols for each tool they consider using.

Diagnosticians often use a spontaneous speech and language sample to gain information about the level and structure of speech and language development. Because of its importance in obtaining information about the typical use of speech and language, its validity, reliability, and form of analysis is crucial. The spontaneous speech sample seems to be one of the most frequently studied tools. Beyond the methods used to elicit the sample and considerations given to its reliability and validity (Minifie et al., 1963), the diagnostician must also be able to record, transcribe, and analyze (score) the responses accurately. There are a number of quantitative and descriptive forms of analyses derived from a spontaneous speech and language sample (Crystal, Fletcher, & Garman, 1976; Miller, 1981)—mean length of utterance (Brown, 1973b), mean length of response (Johnson et al., 1963; Shriner, 1969), number of different words and structural complexity score (Johnson et al., 1963), length complexity index (Miner, 1969; Shriner, 1967), developmental sentence types (Lee, 1966; 1974), and developmental sentence scoring (Lee, 1974).

While the spontaneous language sample is probably most often used for a syntactic analysis, it also provides a connected speech sample for phonological analyses, and may be used for various semantic and pragmatic analyses. When the latter two analyses are attempted some means of recording the context is essential. This may range from glosses on the audiotape, to notes written simultaneous with the recording, or ideally a videotape recording.

Many tools and procedures used for diagnosis are not amenable to numerical reduction, nor is it desirable to do so. For example, there is still no number that describes a hoarse voice or the results of an interview even though Molyneaux and Lane (1982) have developed a systematic analysis system for interview information. Metric analysis is only one way of scoring data. Data is also objectified through the use of clear descriptions of the behaviors observed. Generally it is not enough simply to get a score that reflects performance; the diagnostician will want to provide more descriptive information, describing the patterns of behavior of his patient. Some of the objective and standardized tools provide for analysis of behavioral patterns. For example, using the test form that accompanies the Templin–Darley Tests of Articulation (Templin & Darley, 1969), we see that it provides for an analysis of the patterns of misarticulations with some emphasis on the differences in production between phonemes as singles and phonemes in blends.

Since so many tools used in diagnosis do not provide detailed pattern analysis, the diagnostician must develop his own system for scoring and analyzing the information he has obtained. The diagnostician does not have to be bound to the test designer's analysis recommendations or limitations. He can expand his analysis in any way suggested by his funds of knowledge about speech and language and its measurement. As an example, many phonetic structure tests score the response only by type of error—substitution, omission, distortion, or addition. The diagnostician can analyze the results beyond this. He could do a distinctive feature analysis (McReynolds & Huston, 1971), a kinetic or acoustic analysis (Van Riper & Irwin, 1958), or a phonological process analysis (Weiner, 1979; Shriberg & Kwiatkowski, 1980; Ingram, 1981). Rather than just analyzing the type of error that was made, he can analyze how the error was made in relationship to how the sound should have been made, describing this comparison from a number of perspectives. However, there are a number of viewpoints regarding what constitutes a set of phonologic processes. Khan (1982) reviews 16 major phonological processes.

Information from these analyses is important for management decisions. If a diagnostician analyzed the results of testing with Mrs. Wicker, an aphasic, only in terms of correct or incorrect response, he would miss data of importance for interpretation of the results. If Mrs. Wicker misnamed 90% of the pictures requested, the diagnostician would be fairly certain that she has a "naming" problem. However, if he knows what type of responses she made, he has more information about her problem. Are low-frequency nouns (hammock) replaced by high-frequency nouns (bed), or by a statement of use (you lay on it), or by a descriptive qualification (it's canvas—you know, for outside, for the breeze)? From this analysis the diagnostician can say much more about the type of naming problem as opposed to saying only that a naming problem exists.

A wide range of descriptive analysis methods have been developed. The influence of linguistic science on clinical analysis of language behavior has been significant. Often, however, some of the analysis systems offered are too complex or time consuming for diagnostic use. In the future we hope to see more clinical adaptations of these analysis systems.

Descriptive objectification focuses on behavior in context, on describing patterns of behavior. From this pattern analysis the diagnostician attempts to discover the principle by which a specific patient may be generating his speech and language behavior—a principle that puts the diagnostician in a better position for interpretation and management.

Scoring the data sets it up for the comparative analysis. Careful scoring objectified the data to provide greater reliability and validity to the diagnostician's observations. He has viewed the data from more than one perspective, objectifying it in order to gain greater security for his comparative analysis—to prevent impressionistic comparisons.

In the last chapter we suggested a project for gathering data on several patients using the speech mechanism examination. Now that you have examined this tool (Appendix IV) and considered what data you might collect with it, determine how you would score your findings. Consider both quantitative and descriptive procedures.

We now proceed to a series of patient examples for the reader to objectify. For each, score the data presented through use of numerical and descriptive analyses.

Chloe Paxton, aged 5 years, 5 months, was given the Templin–Darley Screening Test of Articulation. She correctly produced 22 out of the 50 responses required. The substitution errors made on this test were as follows:

Initial	Medial	Final
s/ θ	f/ θ	f/ θ
d/ ð	s/ ʃ	v/ ð
s/ ʃ	s/ ʒ	s/ ʃ
l/j	s/tʃ	s/tʃ

Distortion errors: The /r/, /r/ blends, and the /ɝ/ were consistently distorted.

Score these findings according to the test analysis procedures. Also do a kinetic and acoustic analysis as recommended by Van Riper and Irwin (1958). What additional information would a distinctive feature analysis provide (McReynolds & Engmann, 1975; McReynolds & Huston, 1971)?

The following are a series of observations made on Stanley Butts, aged 3 years, 8 months.

Stanley was first observed in the reception room by the diagnostician. He was building a block tower with his father. He verbalized /m: ba:/ and /ba ba/ repeatedly during this task. He built a six-block tower, and when it fell he said, "aw aw." The diagnostician pounded on the filing cabinet; Stanley did not turn to the sound the first time but did the second time. The diagnostician said "Hi" and Stanley repeated "Hi." Stanley entered the testing room quietly, and at the request of the examiner took his seat. When given a graduated color cone, he worked by trial and error for some time before working out the size relationships—finally he did, and he placed the pieces on the cone in order. He followed commands such as "turn on the radio, throw the ball, and put the ball in the basket." When he dropped objects, he would stand, screech, and quiver while he pointed to the object on the floor. He responded to a toy that made a noise when he picked it up by jumping up from his chair and running to the waiting room. He returned with the examiner, and after explanation and demonstration of the toy he played with it, repeatedly getting the toy to make the noise. While playing with colored plastic eggs he said /mo heg/—more eggs. He became engrossed in this activity, taking the eggs apart and putting them together. While doing this, he usually matched the colored halves correctly. When he made an error he said, "oh oh" and corrected the color match. During this activity he made no direct communicative interactions with the examiner. When the examiner again obtained his attention with a new task, Stanley immediately became interested. Throughout the observation period he could be easily distracted, changing from one activity to the next even when quite engrossed in his current activity. He frequently left his chair and went to the door but each time could be brought back to the table by being shown a new item.

Analyze these observations into a set of "scores." Where will your information come from for this analysis? How would you use the SLPM? What information do you have that might be causal, that might be effect?

The following are examples of the language formulation abilities of Gretchen Warner, aged 3 years, 7 months. A total of 40 responses were recorded during the course of the diagnostic session.

Gretchen used primarily three-word phrases; however, in the language sample the range was from one- to four-word responses. Phrases used were typically verb phrases; for example, "hear mommie," "ride car," and "eat cookie" and simple subject–verb combinations—"baby broke," "car gone," and "Gretchen jump." For questions and negatives the following types of responses were heard: "you pen, huh?" "mommie no sit," and "me no cookie." Other examples of her language responses were "me bite snake," "there barber," "no you turn," and "ride on a car."

How would you score these responses? What systems of analysis would you use? What would Leonard et al. (1982) tell you about communicative functions? Diagnosticians often rely heavily on an objective analysis of spontaneous speech and language responses obtained during a single diagnostic session. Many questions have arisen about the reliability and validity of such language sampling. Recommendations have been made that speech and language behavior should be sampled over two or more sessions and at different times during the day. This, of course, is not a likely practice in diagnosis unless diagnosticians extend their sessions over days or weeks. Can diagnosticians, then, ever obtain a reliable, valid, typical sample of a child's speech and language behavior? Are samples of behavior of language disordered children the same as language samples of normal children? If diagnosticians are to compare their disordered patients to the various systems of language analysis, which index of development will be best to use? How can these indices be used along with other data collected to assure the diagnostician that he is making appropriate analyses? See the previous discussions and references to the use of a spontaneous speech and language sample.

Compares clinical data to standards

All of the scored data are compared in some way to standard information (normative data from standardized tests and from the diagnostician's fund of knowledge), or the data are compared to intradisorder information (to other patients who have similar speech and language disorders).

The purpose of this comparative analysis is to plot the patient's performance and behavior against the standard behavior of the comparison group. Is he ahead of, behind, or comparable to others his age? Is he at the 25th, 50th or 75th percentile? Is his variation mild, moderate, or severe? Does he fall into Group I, II, or III? Ultimately these comparative analyses lead to clinical interpretations that conclude whether a speech and language disorder exists.

In order to perform his comparative analyses the diagnostician must have standard information to use for comparison. The standardized tests have such normative information for ready use. The diagnostician quantifies his patient's responses and compares them to the scores of the standardization group, but as discussed in chapter 6, standardized tools are not always applicable to a clinical population. At times the standardization group is not comparable to the patients seen in a particular setting, as in the case of a setting that sees a large population of black children (e.g., Terrell, 1983), or the procedures by which the standardization data were gathered cannot be duplicated with a patient with a speech and language disorder or within the time constraints imposed by the diagnostic session. Seldom in diagnosis can we duplicate the sampling procedures recommended by the experimental literature. At other times the standardization data may not extend to the age levels of the patients being seen. This is often the case for diagnosticians seeing many young children between the ages of 2 and 4 years. Few tools have been developed for measuring speech and language skills at this age level, and the reliability of the measures is frequently not stable. Finally, the standardization data may not reflect the theoretical orientation of the diagnostician and thus may not be suitable to him. Some of these difficulties are illustrated in the following two paragraphs.

Hollien and Shipp (1972) have presented normative data on the fundamental frequency of the male voice between the ages of 20 and 89 at decade intervals. This data was obtained through a sophisticated instrumental analysis in their laboratory, using the "fundamental frequency indicator" described by them as a "digital readout f_o tracking device." The information made available by them can be important for the diagnostician, but how can he use the same measuring device to arrive at his patient's fundamental frequency for comparative purposes? Most likely, he cannot. Instead, the diagnostician will have to rely on his clinical perceptual measures to determine his patient's fundamental frequency. He will have to use measures different from those by which the normative information was gathered and yet make a comparison to that normative information.

Many patients seen for diagnosis have disorders of phonetic structure or phonology. The normative data available regarding the development of "articulation" came from studies done some time ago and from a different theoretical orientation than is currently used (Poole, 1934; Templin, 1957; Wellman et al., 1931). There is a question about the current applicability of this information, a question addressed somewhat by Sander (1972). Using the data from Wellman et al. (1931) and Templin (1957), Sander demonstrated that the acquisition of phonemes is best viewed from an age range rather than as age norms. Further work along similar lines has been completed by Prather et al. (1975) in studying the development of articulation in children between the ages of 2 and 4 years. The work by Sander (1972) and Prather et al. (1975) indicates that the data that were heavily used may no longer be appropriate, and it assists in drawing more contemporary comparative analyses.

The primary basis for comparative analysis resides in the diagnostician's funds of knowledge about normal and disordered speech and language. The diagnostician throughout his training and professional life builds in standards for comparison. By way of illustration, many patients do not respond to direct, objective procedures for testing a specific speech and language behavior. Attempts to get young children to name specific words on a phonetic structure test are limited by the child's vocabulary ability, willingness to participate in a naming task, attention span, motivation, and other factors. Instead, the diagnostician may have to rely on spontaneous speech, repetition, and a little naming to obtain a sample of the child's use of phonemes. He must, however, compare this nonstandard sample to the normative data available if he is to make decisions regarding the child's abilities.

Of particular relevance to diagnosticians for comparative analyses are the data that characterize a disordered population (intradisorder comparison). Much information is available about groups of people with speech and language disorders, grouped behaviorally or causally, for example, stutterers, aphasics, voice disorders, or mentally retarded. In other areas little is known, or is just beginning to be studied; for example, language of the blind and visually impaired (Mills, 1983). This intradisorder information is crucial to the diagnostician. For example, if the diagnostician is to see 7-year-old Danny who is classified as educable mentally retarded, he will want to know how Danny compares to normal children his age and younger as well as to other educable retarded children (Chapman & Nation, 1981). In a sense standards for disordered behavior are established, and a new patient is compared with these standards to determine if he fits, that is, if he is typical of the general description of the disordered population.

It is easy to see why the diagnostician must be careful when drawing comparisons such as these. Just as normative data can be faulty and misused so can the data gathered on disordered populations. There have been many studies done with the intent of describing the typical speech and language behavior of a special group of individuals; however, the findings are dependent on how the group has been defined and the manner in which the data have been gathered and described.

Because of new information and changes in theories about speech and language behavior, the diagnostician must continue to renew his theoretical perspectives on the analysis of the behaviors that signal a speech and language disorder. The experimental and clinical literature provide much of the current information needed for data analysis. The student in training must develop and maintain an appreciation for the insights the literature provides for data analysis and interpretation.

You have just completed the diagnosis of Sheila, a 15-year-old girl with Down's syndrome. You have taken a spontaneous language sample. How helpful would the information provided by Stoel-Gammon (1980) be to you in a phonological analysis of the language sample? What would you expect of Sheila's language performance (Naremore & Dever, 1975)?

CATEGORIZES CLINICAL DATA IN RELATIONSHIP TO THE CLINICAL HYPOTHESIS

In this second clinical analysis task the new data the diagnostician has objectified are now listed and categorized in relationship to the clinical hypothesis within the SLPM framework. He now has many bits of new data that need to be inventoried; just as in the constituent analysis he inventoried the bits of information for deriving a hypothesis, he now inventories the new data for deriving his clinical diagnosis. The student is referred back to chapter 4 for the details and concepts presented about listing and categorizing. These same tasks are used in the clinical analysis and thus will not be reiterated here.

However, we want to point out once again the importance of the SLPM as an organizing principle for the diagnostician in clinical analysis. Gearing his analysis to the SLPM, the diagnostician would order his data within the components of the model, not just the hypotheses that were formulated. He should order the new data that falls into all the components of the model, even if his hypothesis did not include all the components. For example, the diagnostician might not have been focusing on input stimulation factors; however, if data were accumulated that fits into this component, he should consider it in his clinical analysis.

Using the SLPM in his clinical analysis, the diagnostician can go beyond the data that were obtained. Just as he did when formulating his clinical hypothesis, the diagnostician can list and categorize (order) the data in terms of both the factual data and the inferences he makes. For example, measures of structure and function of the speech mechanism may be objectified and provide direct evidence for associated causal factors. On the other hand, information about causal factors within the speech mechanism may come inferentially from behavioral (product) data. If the diagnostician heard excessive nasality (product), he might infer inadequate velopharyngeal closure as a potential causal factor within the speech mechanism. The SLPM demonstrates how these relationships can be drawn, giving the diagnostician support for some of the later interpretations he may derive from the data. If the diagnostician derives his hypotheses from the SLPM, it follows that his clinical analysis can rely on the same model. This listing and categorizing task provides the diagnostician with a pattern analysis—what data fit each part of the hypothesis—the distribution of details that specify causal factors and effects.

In chapter 4 we provided a constituent analysis form in some detail (Form 4-1), specifying the components of the SLPM, cause–effect categorization, statements of the problem, purposes of the referral, management considerations, behavioral considerations, and incidental information. This form is again useful at this step; however, the diagnostician can adapt its format for clinical analysis adapted more to each specific clinical hypothesis. This adapted format serves as a specific summary form to list and categorize the data obtained about each patient.

DETERMINES SIGNIFICANCE OF CLINICAL DATA

In this third task of clinical analysis all of the data now listed and categorized must be examined for significance, for its relevance to the clinical hypothesis, alternative hypotheses, or new hypotheses. The questions the diagnostician asks himself in this task are how can the data be used, how can it assist me in making my clinical interpretations, and is it relevant for deriving my clinical diagnosis? Again, the student should return to chapter 4 for a full discussion of the diagnostician's task, determining the significance of his constituents. The same process applies to determining the significance of his data in the clinical analysis. He is basically ruling in and ruling out data that provide him with support for interpretation.

The diagnostician continues to compare the data obtained with his funds of knowledge, with some emphasis on intradisorder comparisons. He uses his funds of knowledge to determine what data are supportive of causal factors, what data specify effects, and what data support a cause–effect relationship. He wants to know how confident he can be using the data to draw his interpretations. Does the data offer him a potential solution to the clinical problem, or does he start again?

As was done in chapter 4, the diagnostician can develop a significance table to systematically view the data that are now listed and categorized. The diagnostician is now engaged in "differential diagnosis"—a process applicable to all clients.

SUMMARY

In this fifth step in the diagnostic process the diagnostician scores, compares to norms, categorizes, and determines the significance of all new data collected during the interview and clinical testing sessions. While typically this step runs imperceptibly from the previous step (collection of the clinical data) and into the following step (clinical interpretation), we feel it is important for teaching purposes to discuss analysis as a separate step, thereby underscoring the objectivity that is its essential characteristic. To guard against bias, it is advantageous to develop this practice of nonjudgmental consideration of the data before it is interpreted.

The diagnostician is encouraged here to objectify his data both quantitatively and descriptively, using standard criteria from information available in his fund of knowledge, from his internalized perceptual norms, from intradisorder comparisons with clinical populations, and from standardized test norms. Descriptive analyses provide broader specification of the data and are particularly useful in planning patient management.

Three tasks comprise the clinical analysis step.

1. The diagnostician first objectifies his new data. He does this through scoring the data and comparing it to standards.
2. He categorizes the new data in relationship to the clinical hypothesis. This task is similar to the comparable task in the constituent analysis. He plots his data in accordance with his clinical hypothesis within the SLPM perspective. He inventories his data to determine what he has available to use for interpretation of the clinical problem.
3. The diagnostician determines the significance of all the data. Again, this task is similar to that performed in the constituent analysis. Here the diagnostician is attempting to discover the strength and relevance of his data for supporting or refuting the clinical hypothesis.

Table 8-1. Clinical analysis form for listing and categorizing data obtained on Katherine Compardo in relationship to her cause–effect hypothesis

CNS disruption	Physical process	Behavioral correlates	Products	Other information
Central language segment	Language representation Speech programming	Formulation Sequencing	All language levels "Aphasia" "Apraxia"	This would be specified as in Form 4-1 or specifically re: Katherine Compardo's hypothesis
See overall motor abilities See overall use of speech mechanism			See all information about the speech and language produced under all conditions (stimulability testing seems important here)	*Referral* Overall motor abilities Limited speech and language leads to several causal questions
See overall abilities on tasks of language, interpersonal reactions, and cognitive performance	Same	Same	Naming are the only responses from which to work	
	Use of speech musculature	See items related to speech and language product Stimulability testing		*Comprehension* See all responses to directions and Peabody Picture Vocabulary Test responses

KATHERINE COMPARDO: CLINICAL DATA ANALYSIS

Table 7-2 detailing the information obtained on Katherine Compardo, demonstrates the initial step in objectifying the new data that were obtained. Because of Katherine's level of performance, the data are primarily descriptive objectification—what Katherine did under what circumstances. Return to Table 7-2 and continue to score and do comparative analyses of the information presented. On what basis will you make comparisons of her data: norms from standardized tests, norms from your funds of knowledge about normal and disordered speech and language, and/or your knowledge about children with similar types of speech and language disorders—intradisorder comparisons? Katherine completed the Peabody Picture Vocabulary Test up to Plate 15; what information does this provide regarding comprehension of single words? What comparative analysis would you draw from her responses to comprehension stimuli throughout the testing session? Since Katherine gestures frequently review Wilcox and Howse (1982) to consider the relationship of gesture to comprehension. She responded appropriately to directions that had the following prepositions embedded in them: in, by, and under. What normative data would you apply for comparison to her formulated language? Are specific normative data needed? Continue asking yourself comparative questions for application to Katherine's clinical data.

In Table 7-2 the diagnostician recorded a number of the circumstances under which Katherine Compardo's data were obtained. Reading his remarks, do you get a clear feeling of how well Katherine performed on the tasks required? Would you be able to make a general statement about the reliability and validity of her performance? Do you think the diagnostician obtained typical performance, or are there indications that Katherine was withholding speech and language? One way of checking on validity is to compare the behavior obtained with behavior reported by others—in Katherine's case, the mother.

A clinical analysis form adapted from Katherine Compardo's clinical hypotheses might look like Table 8-1. On this form we have not categorized the specific response items from Table 7-2. Instead, we only point out generally some of the information that applies to the listing and categorization—emphasis is on the inferences that might be drawn from the data. The student is encouraged to specify the items for analysis and to add those we have not included. Table 8-2 should also be completed to determine the significance of the information obtained in relation to Katherine's clinical hypotheses.

PATIENT PROJECTS

For each of the patient projects on which you collected data through role play complete the analysis tasks discussed in this chapter. First analyze the tests you used following the analysis protocols provided with the tests. Then, relook at all of the data from other analysis perspectives, most importantly within the SLPM framework.

Table 8-2. Determination of significance of all the data on our example patient, Katherine Compardo

Data	Significance
Summary statement of information collected about language product, for example: The mother's reports are accurate; Katherine responds only occasionally in single-word responses that are often unintelligible.	What does this tell about language formulation? Can she formulate language, but does not produce it? Is the speech programming process affecting the output; that is, could she formulate the message but not program it for production?

STUDY QUESTIONS

1. What does the following literature offer to the diagnostician for data analysis and interpretation: Silverman (1973), differentiation between normal disfluencies and stuttering in young children; Ramer and Rees (1973), comparisons between standard American English and black English; Wiig and Semel (1973), comprehension differences between children with learning disabilities and normally achieving children; Morehead and Ingram (1973), early language acquisition of normal and linguistically deviant children; Yoss and Darley (1974), differentiating developmental apraxia from other articulation disorders; De Hirsch (1967), differentiating the speech and language behavior of the aphasic and schizophrenic child; Menyuk and Looney (1972), language performance differences between normal and language disordered children?

2. Sharf (1972) presented information that compares some of the measures taken and used for analysis of children's speech and language development. What suggestions does he offer that might assist the diagnostician? How would you reconcile his concerns about the use of age comparisons and the need to sample over time? What further information do the following offer for use of the spontaneous speech and language sample (Crystal, Fletcher, & Garman, 1976; Johnson & Tomblin, 1975; Miller, 1981; Shriner & Sherman, 1967; Shriner et al., 1969; Wilson, 1969)?

3. Seldom do diagnosticians use a physical analysis for specifying the details of speech and language variations. Physical analysis is most often used in basic research. How have Faircloth and Faircloth (1970) used graphic level recordings and spectographic information to support their findings that making diagnostic judgments about speech sound errors in isolated word production is not as valid as making them from connected speech testing?

Chapter 9

Clinical interpretation

After the clinical data have been scored, categorized, and their significance determined in relationship to the hypothesis, the diagnostician is then ready to interpret the data, the sixth step of the diagnostic process. This step is a synthesis and integration of all the preceding steps. It is the culmination of the diagnostic process, where the aim is to come to decisions about the nature and extent of the speech and language disorder and its causes. This phase of the diagnostic process in particular tests the diagnostician's problem-solving skills. He must now put all the pieces together into their most logical order.

Interpretation, clinical evaluation, has at its core patient concern, including the ethics of assessment (Messick, 1980). Interpretation lays the groundwork for management proposals. How he interprets the clinical data underlies the conclusions the diagnostician will draw, how he will communicate his understanding to others, and what management proposals he will choose. The clinical interpretation is, in a sense, the answer to the clinical questions that have been posed.

As the clinical analysis parallels the constituent analysis, the clinical interpretation parallels the clinical hypothesis. The constituent analysis sets up the information for the derivation of the clinical hypothesis and the clinical analysis sets up the data for the clinical interpretation. In many ways this step represents a continuation of hypothesis formulation. Only now the diagnostician has firsthand data and is better able to judge the strengths and weaknesses of the interpretation he offers. Probably many clinical evaluations are more accurately called clinical hypotheses with greater degrees of probability. The diagnostician hopes his interpretation has a high level of certainty.

DIAGNOSTICIAN'S TASKS

The diagnostician now engages in the tasks that will fulfill two of his primary job functions: to determine the nature and extent of the speech and language disorder and to understand the causal factors associated with it. To do this, we have proposed three tasks to be performed at this sixth step of the diagnostic process.

1. He interprets all the data, examining cause–effect relationships and formulating the basis for his diagnostic statement.
2. He formalizes his interpretation by stating his diagnosis, specifying his cause–effect relationship.

3. He supports his diagnostic statement through a formal support paper, a clinical evaluation, that considers his position on the clinical problem, offering his reasons why his diagnosis is more appropriate than other conclusions might be.

INTERPRETS ALL THE INFORMATION

The diagnostician's major function in this task is to draw reasonable relationships among all the cause–effect data. He asks himself if his interpretation bears a reasonable relationship to what is known in the field of speech and language disorders, if the causal factors used to explain the speech and language disorder bear a reasonable relationship to known facts, if he has enough facts and parsimonious inferences to support his interpretation, if his interpretation verifies the interpretations of other workers in the profession, if his interpretations provide new insights into speech and language disorders, and if his interpretations provide for appropriate management decisions to be made.

This first task draws heavily on the diagnostician's problem-solving abilities. Here the diagnostician figures out how the data best fit together to explain the problem, to explain the most likely cause–effect relationship. In essence, this task is the thinking process that allows the diagnostician to formulate his diagnosis.

As the culmination of the diagnostician's problem-solving skills, the interpretation task is based on information from all the previous steps and on all information used by the diagnostician as a "solver" of speech and language problems. All the information gained and examined in the earlier steps is brought together to contribute to the final diagnosis. If there were any uncorrected "errors" in the previous steps, they will probably be reflected in the interpretation. As mentioned previously, this step closely parallels Step 2 of the diagnostic process, the derivation of the clinical hypothesis. The reader is directed to chapter 5 for review of the information presented there, which is entirely applicable to this task.

From the clinical analysis step the diagnostician developed a clear perspective on the significant results of the assessment process. In the interpretation task he first brings together the constituent analysis data inventory with the new clinical analysis data. He can then see how much data have accumulated around the clinical hypothesis and the value of the data—their validity, reliability, and objectivity. He will also be able to determine what data might still be missing.

From these two data inventories the diagnostician can now focus on professional interpretation. What do these data mean? Does the patient have a problem? If so, what is the disorder and what may have caused it? His clinical hypothesis pointed the direction; now the diagnostician determines if he is on course. In the same way the clinical hypothesis offered the diagnostician a potential solution to the problem, the interpretation has a forward reference; it becomes the diagnostician's "solution" to the problem from which the proposed course of management comes.

Since the decisions made about the management of the patient's speech and language problem rest on the diagnostician's clinical interpretation, this step of the diagnostic process is crucial. If the diagnostician does not exercise extreme care in this final problem-solving state of diagnosis, inappropriate management decisions may easily result.

Overreliance on test scores

Some diagnosticians often resort to overuse of test results for interpretation, particularly in those settings that routinely use or require the use of certain test batteries. Instead of integrating all the data accumulated on the patient, they make interpretations based entirely on test scores. Some tests gain greater use this way than others. Each diagnostician must guard against replacing clinical evaluation with reporting test results. The use of test results (the clinical analysis) is only a part of the overall clinical interpretation. The diagnostician must differentiate between reporting test scores and interpreting clinical data. Overreliance on test scores can lead to faulty management decisions to say nothing of faulty diagnoses. If the diagnostician only uses a given tool, the only inferences and conclusions that can be drawn are dependent on the findings from that tool.

Drawing cause–effect interpretations

In his constituent and clinical analysis the diagnostician systematically viewed all information that specified what the disorder might be and any information that reflected potential causes of the disorder. His emphasis in interpretation is drawing the probable relationships among these sets of data. At times the relationship is easy to see: "Mr. Grogan has aphasia due to a stroke," "Mr. Catlow has no vocal tone due to a recent laryngectomy," and "Ms. Wicker's hoarse voice quality is currently due to the presence of large vocal nodules." At other times, relationships are difficult to impossible to draw. Cause–effect relationships are complex interactions; diagnosticians often do not see a direct cause of the speech and language disorder, particularly in young children with developmental disorders. Thus, the diagnostician's use of his inferential measurement strategy is vitally essential if he is to support his cause–effect relationship.

Interpreting the nature of the speech and language disorder requires knowing the characteristic patterns seen in the various disorders. The interpretation is two pronged. First, the diagnostician must differentiate the patient's disorder from other types of disorders, for example, a prosody disorder from a semantic disorder or a language disorder from a phonetic structure disorder. Second, he must go on to differentiate the patient's individual disorder pattern from characteristics of patients with similar problem types, that is, $stuttering_1$ from $stuttering_2$ from $stuttering_3$. The individual patterns of behavior presented by patients with similar disorders vary significantly. The clinical analysis should provide the diagnostician with needed information for making these differentiations, that is, if he has been able to observe enough speech and language behavior.

Interpreting the nature of the speech and language disorder is often easier than determining the causal background for the disorders or for the individual behavioral patterns seen. This is generally true because the speech and language behavior is more accessible to direct observation, while causal factors are often understood only through inferences from secondary behavior. The diagnostician's fund of knowledge about speech and language disorders and their causes is as crucial to clinical evaluation as it was in deriving the clinical hypothesis.

If the diagnostician has gathered his causal data carefully, he will arrive at a more likely probable causal basis for the disorder than arriving at a least likely probability. As we discussed, the diagnostician has three ways of relating causal factors. First, he can view the causal basis for a speech and language disorder from a purely historical perspective: What happened in the past that might account for the disorder. Second, he can view the contemporary basis for the disorder: What is currently operating that may account for the behaviors manifested—a processing viewpoint. Of course, the diagnostician has a third option—interrelating these two viewpoints about causal factors. In most instances he should attempt the latter.

234 Diagnosis of Speech and Language Disorders

The following are a set of findings on 4-year-old Adeline Eichelberger.
1. Language comprehension, integration, and formulation are delayed 1 year.
2. Intelligibility is severely limited.
3. Medically diagnosed at 1 year of age as having mild cerebral palsy.
4. Discovered moderate sensorineural hearing loss at 3 years of age. Bilaterial hearing aids recommended and used since that time.
5. Intelligence tested within normal limits within the past month.
   Interpret the causal factors operative in Adeline's problem from the three options for viewing causation: historical, contemporary, and combined.

How does the diagnostician go about drawing and interpreting the most likely cause–effect relationship? For example, how does he know that Craig's history of significant ear infections and hearing problems are related to his current errors of phonology? This assumed relationship would mean that at some point Craig was unable to hear the sounds of speech or to discriminate the phonologic cues in the speech of his environment, and that in some way this has resulted in his inability to generate appropriate phonemes and phoneme sequences. Hearing loss, of either short- or long-term duration in young children, is often cited as a causal factor for speech and language disorders. However, there is little direct evidence that indicates what type and degree of hearing disorders disrupt the learning and use of the phonologic level of language.

Intradisorder comparisons

The diagnostician's interpretation of cause–effect relationships relates somewhat to the concept of the normal distribution curve. In order to infer a cause that is more than chance, the diagnostician relies on his knowledge of widely held correlations between causal factors and patterns of disordered behavior (intradisorder comparisons). For example, the diagnostician might interpret Alex's lack of language development as related to a severe bilateral sensorineural hearing loss that was due to the reported maternal rubella because he knows that in a significant percentage of cases of maternal rubella, severe hearing losses result. By relating this patient information to the expected probability he is closer to a more likely cause–effect relationship. However, the diagnostician must keep in mind that when using intragroup disorder comparisons, as with any population–sample comparisons, there is some degree of error. Therefore he must always be parsimonious in drawing his clinical interpretation. The lower the correlations reported (that is, the discrepancies or lack of cause–effect relationships reported in the literature), the more cautious the diagnostician must become. The concept of error due to chance is extremely applicable and indeed necessary in clinical interpretation. It reminds the diagnostician of the limitations of his results, the tentative nature of his diagnosis.

Intradisorder comparisons do form a major framework by which diagnosticians interpret their cause–effect relationships, and the use of the SLPM framework is partially designed to specify more validly and reliably these relationships. A precise and theoretically sound attempt to draw cause–effect relationships for interpretation is the type of work done by Darley et al. (1969a, 1969b, 1975a, 1975b). Based on their work, the diagnostician knowing the patient's neurologic disease could predict the disordered behaviors or, on the other hand, seeing a patient with certain speech behaviors could allow the diagnostician to infer a potential neurologic disease. Of equal importance in their work is the emphasis on interacting, overlapping processing systems responsible for the clusters of speech behaviors seen. That is, because the speech-producing processes have certain neurologic controls in common, speech behaviors tend to cluster. Thus, a particular disease or a particular lesion may lead to a fairly predictable set of disordered speech patterns.

The following is adapted from the clinical report written on Mr. Isadore Alexander, one of the example patients used throughout this book. From these findings interpret the probable causal factor responsible for this speech disorder. Use Dworkin (1978) as an additional resource.

Mr. Alexander was accompanied by his wife but taken alone for clinical testing. His spontaneous speech did not evidence any symbolic comprehension–formulation disturbances (aphasia) but was severely unintelligible and bizarre [Note: Intelligibility and bizarreness are two of the dimensions of dysarthria investigated by Darley et al. (1975). Their articles form the basis for the dimensions observed and evaluated in Mr. Alexander and the conclusions drawn from the evaluation.]

These two dimensions are overall judgments of the speech. Intelligibility relates to how well the listener is able to understand the speech of the patient, and bizarreness relates to the degree to which the speech calls attention to itself. It was possible to understand what Mr. Alexander was saying because in most cases the context of his responses was known and also because a manner of "speechreading" was employed. The examiner visually noted the direction of movement of the articulators and to some extent assumed the speech product because it was distorted by extremely weak articulatory contact and slow rate.

In assessing the speech/voice variation more specifically, the following component dimensions of intelligibility and bizarreness were rated: pitch, loudness, vocal quality, breathing for speech, prosody, and phonetic structure.

Mr. Alexander's pitch level, overall, was somewhat low and monotonous (monopitch). When asked to follow the examiner up and/or down the musical scale on /a/, he demonstrated inability to vary pitch to any great extent.

A significant aspect of loudness was monoloudness; a consistent level of loudness was maintained that was somewhat louder than normal. Significant aspects of vocal quality were severe vocal harshness (a rough, raspy quality), strained-strangled voice, voice stoppages, and hypernasality.

The most prominent feature of breathing for speech was audible inspiration. The prosodic variations were slow rate, short phrases, reduced stress, intervals prolonged, inappropriate silences, and excess and equal stress.

A spontaneous speech sample indicates the prosody variations listed above. "What's the trouble [pause for inspiration] I can't [pause] say [pause] anything [pause] to [pause] her [pause] and she [pause] don't [pause] see." Each pause represents a brief, audible breath intake. Each word is spoken with excessive and equal stress and at the same pitch and loudness level.

Mr. Alexander's phonetic structure variations were characterized primarily by imprecise consonants. That is, the consonant sounds showed slurring, inadequate sharpness, distortions, and lack of crispness. There is clumsiness going from one sound to another. To some extent phonemes were prolonged, especially vowels, which had the effect of distorting the vowels. Specific testing of diadochokinetic rate showed slower than normal rate for all alternating movements of the articulators and repetition of monosyllables such as /kakaka/ and /lalala/. The most markedly slow rate was in production of /kalakala/, which involves moving from a back to a front phoneme. Phoneme substitutions did not involve inappropriate place or direction of articulation, but reduction of force and range, which had the effect of distortion of the phoneme. Voicing of unvoiced phonemes, /b/p/ and /g/k/, tended to occur. Voiceless fricatives either were not produced or were replaced by a plosive, /p/f/. The factor that seemed to underly these phonetic structure errors was that insufficient closure of the velopharyngeal port prevented impounding of air for plosive and fricative production. Indeed, observation of palatal function both in production of sustained /a/ and short, rapid productions of /a/ indicated very little palatal movement. This would also account for the hypernasality.

As testing progressed, Mr. Alexander's speech became slower in rate even than the initial slow rate, and there were more frequent pauses, inappropriate silences, and voice stoppages. Phonation simply ceased and the voice was "squeezed" into a whisper. Even this examiner was exhausted, a seeming reflection of what appeared to be the tremendous effort it increasingly required for Mr. Alexander to communicate.*

Another approach is the work of Shriberg and Kwiatkowski (1982). They have developed a classification system for phonological disorders that relies on establishing causal correlates to the types of phonological disorders they have investigated. They developed elaborate procedures, including weighting of the various factors, for drawing clinical interpretations. Thus, their interpretations are internally consistent. They stem from their orientation to phonological disorders, their system of data collection and analysis, and finally their derivation of the classification system.

Incomplete knowledge base

Intradisorder comparisons are quite useful when the information is available; however, there is still much to be discovered about cause–effect relationships. The variability in patterns of behavior is great; certain causal factors seem to result in any number of behavioral differences. We are just beginning to isolate some of the basic language disorders seen in young children and have hardly tapped their causal bases (Aram & Nation, 1975, 1982). As we learn more about how speech and language are processed by the human being, we will learn more about how causal factors disrupt these processes, resulting in characteristic patterns of speech and language behaviors. Until all the data is in, the diagnostician must use his skills as a problem solver to arrive at the most likely solution to the clinical problem.

Establishing cause–effect relationships is not easy. Diagnosis is not easy, but the diagnostician must strive to understand, to make the best interpretations possible, and to report them with caution. He has an obligation to the profession to continue to seek for reasonable explanations for why speech and language disorders exist, no matter how tentative they may be. Often the findings and interpretations of the diagnostician can point the way for further clinical research. The diagnostician may have arrived at a fairly unique explanation for the disorder he is seeing. He may arrive at an insight about the nature and cause of speech and language disorders that the researcher may use to develop experimental studies– studies that then feed back into the diagnostician's fund of knowledge. For example, a diagnostician may interpret certain phonetic structure errors on the basis of a neurologic disruption of the tongue. However, further study will be required to place this inference by the diagnostician into better perspective. It may be the anatomist, physiologist, neurologist, or speech scientist who provides the necessary data to turn this interpretation–inference into data that may truly demonstrate the relationship and become more usable for future diagnoses.

*Our thanks are extended to Ms. Janet Whitney, speech pathologist, Mt. Sinai Medical Center, Cleveland, OH, for permission to adapt this portion of her clinical report.

Because of the lack of factual and theoretical security for many potential cause–effect interpretations, the diagnostician must exercise care in his explanations. He must carefully consider all the information in order to offer the patient his most reasonable interpretation. And we should not be misled; patients with speech and language disorders want to know "What caused me to talk this way?" The diagnostician should be prepared to respond to the question. Patients are not always satisfied with an explanation that a disorder is present; they often already know that. Nor are they always satisfied that something will be done about it. They have a natural desire to know, and often a high level of anxiety about what caused their disordered behavior. Our clinical interpretations should allow us to respond with a reasonable explanation within our professional boundaries.

Parsimonious interpretations

Parsimonious interpretations are called for. The diagnostician should stick to the best set of data about each patient, information at low levels of abstraction rather than highly theoretical explanations. He must try to interpret on the basis of the factual rather than inferential if at all possible. The diagnostician's intent is to synthesize his information to present the interpretation that fits the data best. What evidence does he have to support his interpretation that Anthony's hypernasality is due to inadequate velopharyngeal closure, that Deli's phonetic errors are due to her short lingual frenum, that Mr. Van Meter's hoarse voice is due to vocal abuse, or that LaVerne's distorted speech sounds are related to his high-frequency hearing loss.

The diagnostician must consider the strengths and weaknesses of all his information. He must remember that some of the tools used may not have provided a typical sample of the patient's behavior. He must be careful not to overemphasize some pieces of data that may support his interpretation in favor of other information that may weaken his interpretive position. As emphasized by Messick (1980), the diagnostician must be concerned with the ethics of test use. He must evaluate the present and future consequences of test interpretation. He must state a case, but unlike a trial attorney he must also present evidence that may weaken his case. The diagnostician is not trying to "win his hypothesis"; he is offering his best reasoning to solve the problem, proposing alternative interpretations if they seem warranted for understanding and treating the patient's problem.

STATES THE DIAGNOSIS

After the diagnostician has completed his interpretation, he undertakes the second task, stating the diagnosis. This task is a formal, succinct statement of his diagnosis. The "statement" may be a mental solidification or may be written explicitly. It expresses the most likely cause–effect relationship, addressing both the speech and language and the probable contributing causes.

This formal diagnostic statement is often used in interprofessional communication and at times may be used directly with the patient. Therefore the diagnostician should work out several ways of stating his diagnosis at various levels of abstraction to suit his communication purposes. Everything that was discussed regarding the statement of the clinical hypothesis in chapter 5 is relevant to the statement of the diagnosis and should be reviewed.

The following serve as examples of various ways a diagnostic statement could be framed for communication with different individuals concerned with Robert's problem. With whom might these statements be used?

1. Robert has a severe phonologic formulation problem. He has not learned the phonologic rule system for producing appropriate phonemes of his language. The causal factors relating to this mislearning are unclear at this time but may have some relationship to long-standing middle ear infections during critical language-learning periods.
2. Robert has great difficulty making sounds. He has not learned how to do this yet.
3. Robert has a severe problem using the sounds of his language. We think he has not learned how to use them because of his significant hearing problems.
4. Robert has a severe language formulation problem on the phonologic level. His phonologic rule system is very rudimentary for his age. We suspect his difficulties are due to his early history of significant middle ear problems that reduced the amount of phonemic information he received at very critical ages. Even though he demonstrates no current auditory processing difficulties, we infer that they existed and resulted in his current processing difficulty.

We are reminded by Johnson et al. (1963) that our diagnosis may only be tentative. The clinical hypothesis from which the diagnostician worked may never be fully verified. The diagnostician is not primarily supporting or rejecting his hypothesis in a manner similar to the experimenter. Instead, he is adding to and subtracting from his original hypothesis that acted as a guide for the diagnostic process. When the process ends, the diagnostician cannot simply say his hypothesis was not supported. Rather, he must come up with a new hypothesis (solution) that better explains the data. Thus while he makes his clinical evaluation in terms of his clinical hypothesis, he is not solely bound to support or reject his most likely hypothesis, a major reason for proposing alternative hypotheses.

Therefore, although the diagnostician must express his findings in a diagnostic statement, this statement does not necessarily imply that the final conclusion has been reached. As the clinical hypothesis is predictive and explanatory, so is the diagnostic statement. Since our major interest is patient concern, our diagnostic statement should reflect the projections the diagnostician will make regarding management proposals. He utilizes his conclusions, his diagnostic statement, to inform the patient, to plan therapeutic objectives, and to make appropriate referrals.

SUPPORTS THE DIAGNOSIS: CLINICAL EVALUATION

The third task, supporting the diagnosis, is a formal support paper for the diagnostic statement, again paralleling the similar task performed in the development of the clinical hypothesis. As a formal support paper, this task draws from literature support, the constituent analysis, and the analysis of the clinical data. This task basically presents the diagnostician's reasoning processes for arriving at his diagnostic conclusion. He "argues" for his position, incorporating, as well, any points that may detract from his position. Rarely will all of the diagnostician's findings relate positively to his diagnosis. Therefore he must make effective use of the negative results; that is, the data that tend to systematically weaken rather than support his position. If the diagnosis is both logically sound and empirically based, then negative results that weaken rather than confirm the diagnosis are valuable for focusing the diagnostician's attention on potential alternative problems.

The task of supporting the diagnosis is taught as a formal presentation of the interpretation of the findings with documentation from the literature. The support paper synthesizes all the information that bears on the patient's problem. The diagnostician offers his best possible explanation, an explanation that may be based as much on inference as it is on fact. The interpretation reflected in the support paper should allow for the logical proposal of management plans, and can also serve as the basis for the clinical evaluation section of the clinical report (see chapter 10).

This last task of clinical interpretation is similar to the final task performed in deriving the clinical hypothesis, that is, evaluating the quality of the clinical hypothesis and presenting a formal support paper. It is recommended that the student review that information.

Example diagnostic support papers

Three examples are now presented to demonstrate the task of supporting the diagnostic statement.

James E. Matkin

For our first example we offer a *clinical hypothesis* support paper for James E. Matkin, a patient project introduced in chapter 4. Even though this support paper was developed for supporting a clinical hypothesis it is presented here to demonstrate how that task is similar to the task of supporting a diagnostic statement.

For the diagnostician the behavioral manifestations of prosody disorders in adults are relatively easy to observe. Therefore many diagnosticians spend their time obtaining many details of the stuttering pattern, the circumstances under which it occurs, the stutterer's attitude toward his disorder, and the effect it has had on his life. The emphasis in the diagnosis is often contemporary; what is happening now when the stutterer attempts to speak. Histories are taken with some interest in how the condition started and developed, but often little use is made of this information for deriving a causal hypothesis from a historical viewpoint or for developing and selecting tools for causal assessment. Conflicting theories exist about the causes of stuttering, and this seems to have led to a behaviorally oriented view of stuttering at the expense of understanding causal factors.

In keeping with the theme developed in this book, we see a need for diagnosticians to strive to uncover the potential cause of the stuttering in each patient they see. These clinical attempts may lead to a better view of causation for stuttering. Presentation of this hypothesis derivation support paper is not meant to represent our position on causation of stuttering, but rather represents the task of supporting a cause-effect relationship from the literature.

• *Clinical hypothesis.* James Matkin has a disfluency disorder (characterized by repetitions, prolongations, and blocks) due to a constitutional deficiency in motor coordination of the speech production processes that is still present. In addition, verbal and nonverbal speech modifiers, various covert reactions (situation/word fears), and a self-concept centering around the disfluency disorder may be present due to conditioning processes throughout his life.

• *Clinical hypothesis support.* As could be seen in the constituent analysis, the number of substantial constituents from which to make causal inferences about James Matkin's stuttering are limited. Therefore the hypothesis I have formulated is primarily based on my funds of knowledge with respect to the disorder of stuttering.

The primary causal factor to which I attribute James' disfluency is that of a constitutional deficiency in motor coordination of the speech production processes. By the term constitutional I mean the physical makeup of the individual that contributes to the person he is or will become. All of us have constitutional differences in the many abilities we possess. Some of us are less adept at certain activities than others. I hypothesize that James' constitutional makeup has not allowed him to develop the intricate, precise motor coordinations necessary for normally fluent speech.

It has been found that substantially more males than females stutter. Van Riper (1971) reviewed the literature on the subject and concluded that in general the ratio of male stutterers to female stutterers was from three or four to one. Many attempts have been made to explain this difference with little definitive results except that the difference definitely occurs in all cultures. Van Riper (1971) suggests that the difference reflects a less stable "neuromuscular control system for speech in the male" in the early years that may mature over time. Dr. Charlotte Avila, a pediatric neurologist at Metropolitan General Hospital, states that males are constitutionally inferior in many respects to females and cites the more frequent occurrences of childhood illnesses, speech and language problems, and higher mortality rates in males as examples of this belief. It would appear that just by virtue of being a male James stood a greater chance of having a disfluency disorder.

Another fact that substantiates the notion of a constitutional basis to stuttering is that stuttering tends to occur through successive generations in families. Studies supporting this view include that of Andrews and Harris (1964), Nelson et al. (1945), Wepman (1939), and Kidd et al. (1978). Even though James did not report any familial incidene of stuttering, these findings tend to support a constitutional factor involved in stuttering.

It has long been observed in the literature that most stuttering begins in early childhood. Andrews and Harris (1964) reported that more of their subjects had an onset at 4 years of age than at any other age. This coincides with James' report of stuttering for as long as he could remember. In posing a constitutional deficiency in James' motor coordination for speech, however, it is necessary to assume that his disfluencies were present from the onset of speech. It has been found by Berry (1938) that of 500 stutterers, 72% began to stutter within the first year after speech began. In Aron's 1958 study, reported by Van Riper (1971), 9 out of 16 parents reported that stuttering began at speech onset. Perkins (1977) states that judgments of sound and syllable disfluencies are usually made when language has context. This statement would tend to explain why age of onset is often reported between 3 and 4 years of age, for this is the time when sentence length and structure is expanding rapidly.

Of further interest is the fact that spontaneous recovery occurs in so many of these children. The exact percentage of children cited as recovering varies with individual studies. Andrews and Harris (1964) report that out of 27 children in a large population of children followed from birth to 15 years of age who had stuttered at least 6 months or more 80% had recovered. Sheehan and Martyn (1970) interviewed a large sample of college students during the course of several years and found 147 who had stuttered at some point in time. The authors reported that spontaneous recovery had taken place in 80% of these subjects. Dickson (1971) studied an elementary and junior high school population, 9% of which had reported to have stuttered at some time. Approximately 55% of these children had recovered spontaneously. Wingate (1964) also looked at a population of college students who had reportedly stuttered at some point and found that 73% of them recovered in adolescence. I interpret these findings as support for a constitutional deficiency in stutterers. For example, it is possible that motor coordination of the speech processes reaches its peak at different ages in all of us. While the majority of us acquire this ability during early childhood, it may be that many of these stutterers reached their peak coordination at later points of maturation. Quite some time ago Steer (1937) commented on this point. He felt that stuttering might well be a function of maturation of the speech mechanism used in speaking, and adults who stuttered were arrested in development of the speech mechanism.

Evidence that stuttering may come from motor incoordination of certain of the speech production processes comes from several sources. The first notable effect that is relevant to the hypothesis is the rhythm effect. Bloodstein (1950) conducted a questionnaire study of the events that would or would not facilitate fluency and found that speaking in time to various rhythmic activities was often cited as creating a significant reduction in stuttering. Fransella and Beech (1965) conducted a study in which stutterers were asked to say each word or syllable of a word list in time with a rhythmic metronome (the authors ruled out distraction as a cause by having the subjects listen carefully to an arrhythmic beat while reading material similar to the above). The rhythmic condition significantly reduced stuttering, and since there was no effect from the arrhythmic listening condition, it was felt that distraction did not account for the effect. Brady (1969), however, found that speaking in time to an arrhythmic metronome was nearly as effective in eliminating stuttering as speaking in time with a rhythmic metronome when one syllable per beat was produced. Bloodstein (1972) explains the rhythm effect in terms of syllabification and rhythm combined. He states that in reducing speech into syllabic units there is in turn a simplification in motor planning. Bloodstein (1972) further suggests that substantial decreases in stuttering while on delayed auditory feedback can be explained in terms of the simplification of motor planning due to a slower rate of speech. Wingate (1969) attributes this effect to the fact that the individual must emphasize intentional vocalization to produce stress patterns centering on the syllable. This same explanation is given by Wingate (1969) to explain the effects of singing and choral speaking on stuttering. Bloodstein (1950), among others, has reported that stutterers become fluent when singing and also when speaking in unison with one or more persons on either the same or different material (choral speaking). One last condition that reduces stuttering significantly is shadowing (Cherry & Sayers, 1956). In all of these conditions Wingate (1969) emphasizes the point that continuity of speech production is present.

Wingate (1969) states that support for his hypothesis comes from studies on phonation and articulation in stutterers. It has been found that initial sounds in words or syllables are stuttered on more than later sounds, and that final sounds are never stuttered (Froeschels, 1961). In addition, the first words of sentences tend to be stuttered on more frequently than later words in nearly all studies on the subject (Van Riper, 1971). Wingate (1969) attributes these points to the fact the "soundmaking" has been initiated after these first sounds and thus induces continuity of phonation. Adams and Reis (1971) tested 14 stutterers on their phonation abilities. They had the subjects read two passages, one composed of all voiced sounds and the other of a combination of voiced and voiceless sounds. They found significantly less stuttering and more rapid adaptation of the all-voiced passage. The authors say this supports the hypothesis of a positive relationship between frequency of stuttering and the frequency with which phonatory adjustments must be made. The authors infer that the repetitions and prolongations exhibited by their subjects were a reflection of their difficulty in initiating, maintaining, and coordinating phonation with articulation in order to make fluent phonetic transitions. Stromstra's spectrographic findings, reported by Perkins (1977), showed repetitions and prolongations of stuttering children were often associated with abnormal, abrupt termination of phonation and that in those children exhibiting this trait, stuttering still existed 10 years later.

A study by Brenner et al. (1972) looked at stutterers' ability to recite 10-syllable sentences from memory after conditions of silent rehearsal, aloud rehearsal, lip rehearsal, whispered rehearsal, and no rehearsal. Aloud rehearsal yielded significantly fewer stutterings than any other condition. The authors state that vocalization is the only distinguishing feature between these conditions and therefore stutterers must have trouble coordinating phonation and articulation. They suggest that aloud rehearsal facilitates coordination of these functions, and they attribute the adaptation phenomenon to this fact. Finally, Wingate (1967), in explaining the stutterer's increased difficulty with longer and more unfamiliar words (Soderberg, 1966), suggests that these words are more difficult because of their difficult or unfamiliar motor plan.

Early studies dealing with breathing irregularities fit well with the incoordination of speech production processes hypothesis. It is interesting to note that one study (Starbuck & Steer, 1953) found that the irregularities in the respiration of stutterers during speech decreased with adaptation in successive readings. As Brenner et al. (1972) explained adaptation as being due to rehearsal of articulatory and phonatory coordinations, so can this adaptation be explained as rehearsal of the coordination of the breathing for speech subprocess with the other subprocesses of speech actualization.

While I advocate the hypothesis that James' disfluencies per se are the result of an inherent constitutional weakness, there is reason to believe that operant conditioning may play a considerable role in the secondary mannerisms (verbal and nonverbal speech modifiers) so often associated with the disorder of stuttering. Brutten and Shoemaker (1967) recognize the application of instrumental conditioning principles to the secondary mannerisms found in stuttering. When an operant (a nonverbal speech modifier) is emitted and followed by reinforcement (a chance termination of a block), there is a greater likelihood of that response occurring again. Wischner (1952) talks about the operation of instrumental avoidance behaviors to avoid stuttering (although he states reinforcement is through the attendant anxiety reduction). Most of the research on the role of operant conditioning deals with the involuntary disfluencies per se and not the secondary mannerisms. However, as reported by Van Riper (1971), Webster did find that in one of his two subjects the word "wrong" used as contingent reinforcement during stuttering moments served to decrease "voluntary" stuttering behaviors (verbal/nonverbal speech modifiers).

In addition to the preceding, it has been found that many stutterers have fears of certain situations or certain words. Van Riper (1971) reviews the literature and concludes that stuttering will increase in situations containing high communicative importance. Some studies have shown that stutterers will stutter less when alone than when in groups of two or more (Porter, 1939). Also, several investigators have found significant relationships between the degree of expectancy to stutter on certain words and the stuttering on them (Knott et al., 1937; Johnson & Ainsworth, 1938). These effects can be accounted for in terms of learning theory—the more these situations or words are paired with stuttering, the more the stutterer will fear them.

Finally, it has been found by Rahman (reported by Van Riper, 1971) that the only real difference between a group of stutterers and their controls in his study was in the real self-concept relating to social interaction. The ideal self-concepts were the same in general. As reported by Van Riper (1971), Nelson found that stutterers tended to perceive themselves primarily in terms of their speech. These findings are in close agreement with James' statements concerning the effects stuttering has had on his social and persoal life. These are difficult to find support for in the literature other than in statements of common sense. It is quite understandable that the stutterer's self-concept would be affected by his disorder, and therefore it is necessary to include this as an important aspect of the total problem.*

This support paper on James Matkin, completed in 1975, demonstrated extensive use of the literature to derive a clinical hypothesis. What changes in the support paper might occur from the use of the following references: Zimmerman, (1980a, 1980b, 1980c), Zimmerman, Smith, and Hanley, (1981), and Kidd, Heimbach, Records, Oehlert, and Webster (1980)?

Traci Newman

The second example presents a clinical evaluation of test results in a manner that might appear in a clinical report. Test results are presented first. The constituent analysis from which the hypothesis was derived is not presented.

• *Testing and observation.* Traci Newman was seen on June 16 and June 30, 1983. On the first date, the Peabody Picture Vocabulary Test (PPVT), the Templin–Darley Screening Test of Articulation, a speech mechanism examination, and an audiometric test were administered. It was requested that Traci return for a dual speech and hearing assessment on June 30. On this date, further audiometric testing was done. Traci's speech and language abilities were also further investigated with pictures to elicit spontaneous speech, and six subtests of the Illinois Test of Psycholinguistic Abilities (ITPA).

On the Peabody Picture Vocabulary Test (Form B) that was given to test vocabulary comprehension, Traci achieved a vocabulary age of 2 years, 8 months as compared to her chronological age of 5 years, 8 months.

On the 50-item Templin–Darley Screening Test of Articulation, Traci produced five correct responses. The mean number of correct responses for 5-year-old girls is 40.6, and the cutoff point of inadequate performance is 31 correct items. Analysis of whole-word responses on the test showed the following pattern.

1. All stops were correctly produced in initial and medial positions but were sometimes omitted in a final position.
2. Substitutions or omissions of fricatives always occurred—the most frequent substitutions were /p/f, t/s/, and /t/ʃ/.
3. The two affricates, /tʃ/ and dʒ/, were not produced but were substituted for by various sounds.
4. Of the four sounds /l/, /w/, /j/, and /r/, the first two were usually produced, the third always had a substitute, and the fourth was produced correctly in the initial position only.
5. Nasal sounds were produced in appropriate positions, with /n/ and /ŋ/ usually omitted in a final position.

---

*Our appreciation is extended to Mrs. Karen Wolf for permission to adapt this material. Mrs. Wolf developed this support paper in 1975 while a graduate student in the Department of Speech Communication, Case Western Reserve University, for a course in diagnosis–evaluation of communication disorders.

6. The "r-colored" vowel had no coloring.

7. In consonant clusters, blends of /s/ plus one or more consonants always had the /s/ omitted; blends of a consonant plus /r/ were usually produced as the consonant plus /w/; and a consonant followed by /l/ was usually produced correctly.

Attempts to modify the phonetic production using integral stimulability techniques resulted in some change from /p/ to /f/; /v/ was not produced; /θ/ could be approximated; and /ʃ/ and /s/ were not produced even with strong stimulation.

Little spontaneous speech (consisting mainly of naming) was elicited with situational pictures. During the administration of the Illinois Test of Psycholinguistic Abilities, a few spontaneous comments were produced; those that were longer than one word consisted mainly of vowels with many of the consonants omitted.

On the six subtests of the Illinois Test of Psycholinguistic Abilities that were given, the following age level scores were obtained: auditory reception, 3.3; visual reception, 4.1; visual sequential memory, 6.2; auditory sequential memory, 4.2; visual association, 2.4; verbal expression, 3.10.

A speech mechanism examination revealed no difficulty in producing movements with the articulators. Diadochokinetic rate was difficult to assess since Traci would not produce the syllables more than a few times.

The first audiometric testing found a pure tone air conduction threshold of 43 dB in both ears when the average was taken of 500, 1,000, and 2,000 Hz. Pure tone bone conduction thresholds with masking ranged from 5 to 15 dB in both ears. The second audiometric test found a pure tone air conduction average of 28 dB in the right and 27 dB in the left ear, with a masked bone conduction average of 8 dB in both ears. The speech reception threshold for the right ear was 20 dB and for the left it was 15 dB, with 100% discrimination at 50 dB. The examiners noticed that it was necessary to raise the loudness of their voices more on the first day Traci was seen than on the second.

Traci's responses to test stimuli were very softly spoken when she was first seen. She was a shy, quiet, well-behaved child who attended to the examiners but made no attempts to speak spontaneously. The second time she was seen, Traci was still highly cooperative but offered only a few spontaneous remarks toward the end of the testing session.

• *Clinical evaluation.* Traci is a child with a language disorder that is severe and is complicated by visual, hearing, and environmental problems. The omission and substitution of consonants made Traci difficult to understand in what little speech she produced that was more than a one-word response.

Tests of comprehension, integration, and formulation of language (utilizing both visual and auditory channels) indicated language performance on an age level much lower than Traci's chronologic age. However, all of these scores may not be completely indicative of her ability. When the Peabody Picture Vocabulary Test was administered, the examiner had to say the stimuli very loudly and more than once to elicit any response. Also, on the Illinois Test of Psycholinguistic Abilities, the examiner felt that Traci did not always understand the task in spite of repeated instructions; this was particularly true of the visual association subtest. On the one subtest—visual sequential memory—where Traci quickly understood what was expected of her and eagerly performed, the score was more commensurate with her chronologic age.

Even though the test results may not be a maximal reflection of Traci's ability, the language scores are so much lower than the norms for children of her age that it is doubtful that she will be able to achieve much success in verbal tasks when she enters the first grade in September.

Whether the lack of normal development in language was caused or merely complicated by respiratory infections and ear infections with resultant conductive hearing loss is difficult to determine.

Katherine Compardo

As a third example we now present an abbreviated clinical evaluation on our demonstration patient, Katherine Compardo who demonstrates a severe language formulation disorder on all levels of language. The characteristics of her disorder would lead us to call it childhood aphasia, and in her case the concept of accompanying apraxia seems warranted. If this diagnosis is on target, the potential cause would reside in cerebral dysfunction that has significantly affected the language processing areas needed for formulating language.

Interestingly, Katherine exhibits a less comprehensive childhood aphasia than typically seen in that her comprehension and integration skills seem relatively intact. Her understanding of language as reported by the mother and as observed during testing appear to be appropriate for her age. However, because it was difficult to maintain Katherine's attention to comprehension tasks, definitive test results are not available. More testing is needed to gain greater security regarding the level of her comprehension and integration abilities.

It is Katherine's language formulation skills that are obviously quite limited for her age. This, of course, was the mother's report and was verified in the diagnosis. She has only a few words that are intelligible; the remainder of her speech output consists of certain stereotyped sound combinations. Other than this, she uses "gestures" to communicate. She uses nothing we call a sentence, and children of her age, 27 months, should be talking in more complex sentence structures.

In Katherine's case we feel that her limited output cannot be explained just by calling it aphasia. She is having significant difficulty using the speech musculature. There may be some question about a concomitant dysarthria indicated by drooling and difficulty keeping food in her mouth, but there is little other evidence for this type of motor speech disorder. If dysarthria were the basis for her problem, we would expect more speech production output than we are seeing. Instead, we find it more useful to consider that Katherine has an accompanying apraxia, that is, difficulty with voluntary control of the speech musculature for speech programming and production. She has little ability to control the use of the speech mechanism on command or in imitation even though we see similar behaviors performed involuntarily, for example, tongue protrusion. When she is asked to repeat speech sounds and words, there is some minimal modification but during testing it was negligible. If this "additional" component to the aphasia is present, it would better explain the severe limitations she demonstrates. Thus, beyond her limitations of creating messages, she seems unable to program the motoric sequences needed to put speech sounds together.

Conditions such as Katherine's are characteristic of children who have been described as expressive aphasics and/or apraxics—a condition associated with cerebral dysfunction. In Katherine's case the suspected cerebral dysfunction is apparently congential since no evidence is present to indicate any brain damage after birth. The only evidence currently available to support cerebral dysfunction as a causal factor is Katherine's history of language development, her current disorder of language, and the observations made of the use of the speech mechanism. Other than this, she demonstrates only mild behavioral signs that are sometimes used as indicative of cerebral dysfunction—the slight general incoordination and slow motor development, the distractibility, and the inability to attend to a directed task for a long period of time. These characteristics, however, all must be viewed in relationship to Katherine's age and level of maturation.

Even though additional information is needed we feel it is important at this time to consider Katherine as severely deviant in language formulation on all linguistic levels as a concomitant of childhood aphasia and apraxia.

SUMMARY

At this sixth step of the diagnostic process the diagnostician offers his clincial interpretation, his diagnosis of the speech and language disorder and its probable causes. It is here that the diagnostician must pull together all that has gone before, using his funds of knowledge and problem-solving skill to arrive at his diagnosis. He achieves his clinical interpretation of all the data through a process very similar to the development of the hypothesis. He uses all the information available prior to the contact with the patient as well as the new information collected during the interview and testing sessions. This step marks the culmination of the diagnostician's application of his professional skills.

1. He interprets the results of all the information. This is the thinking process behind his diagnostic statement in which he synthesizes the information available and arrives at the most likely delimitation of the speech and language disorder and its probable causes.
.2 After thinking through his interpretation, the diagnostician states the diagnosis. This becomes a succinct, formal statement of the patient's disorder and the causes.
3. He finally offers a clinical evaluation supporting the diagnosis. Here the diagnostician offers his support or position for the diagnosis. He documents how he arrived at the diagnosis.

Having interpreted the data and formulated the diagnosis, the diagnostician next will draw conclusions based on that diagnosis. This problem-solving road to diagnosis should lead to the best management of the problem. If the diagnostician has been unsuccessful in finding a best answer, he must begin again, adjusting his procedures and using his mistakes to discover a better answer to the problem.

PATIENT PROJECTS

For each of the patients you have been following throughout this book we offer a diagnostic statement. Match this statement to the work you have done. At this time prepare a support paper for the diagnostic statements provided here.

William Gafford

Reverend Gafford has a severe voice problem characterized by low pitch, hoarseness, pitch breaks, and limited pitch range. The vocal characteristics are related in part to his current bilateral contact ulcers, but more importantly they are related to the vocal abuse that brought on the ulcers. The vocal abuse is characteristic of his habitual, occupational forceful use of the phonatory mechanism, using too low a habitual pitch, achieving loudness by tightening the muscles of the laryngeal area, and using hard glottal attacks. The condition is aggravated by constant throat clearing.

Isadore Alexander

Mr. Alexander presents a severe neuromuscular speech disorder that has its basis in impaired neurologic functioning affecting all speech production processes. Strong evidence from the characteristic speech pattern suggests amyotrophic lateral sclerosis as the basis for the disorder.

Derek Park

Derek Park has an articulation–resonation processing disorder resulting in deviant phonetic structure. His phoneme production is characterized primarily by hypernasality and nasal emission along with numerous other phoneme distortions. This disorder results rather directly from inadequate velopharyngeal closure and deviant dentition secondary to a repaired cleft of the primary and secondary palates.

James E. Matkin

Mr. Matkin manifests a prosody disorder characterized currently by prolongations, circumlocutions, and word modifiers. He also presents associated secondary mannerisms that assist him in maintaining the flow of speech, and he evidences extreme tension in the speech musculature during his difficult speech periods. The onset of this disorder was in early childhood and has developed to its current status.

Marie Abadie

Marie Abadie demonstrates a nonfluent (Broca's) aphasia characterized by slow labored speech, lack of inflection, and lack of many functor words, particularly auxiliary verbs, word endings, and tense markers. This aphasia resulted from a cerebrovascular accident subsequent to the ligation of a left internal carotid artery aneurysm.

Karen Twigg

Karen has a language disorder involving principally the phonologic and semantic levels of both comprehension and formulation which contribute to a reading and written language disorder, all resulting from a progressive sensorineural hearing loss.

STUDY QUESTIONS

1. What cause–effect relationships seem to be the most difficult to interpret? All reported literature that is directed toward discovering patterns of speech and language behavior related to specific causal factors is relevant to this question. For example, what do the following articles offer for helping professionals interpret cause–effect relationships: Bentin, Silverberg, and Gordon (1981); Curtiss, Prutting, and Lowell (1979); Davis and Blasdell (1975); Kamhi and Johnston (1982); Siegel-Sadewitz and Shprintzen (1982).
2. Case studies reported in the literature often are presentations of rare diagnostic circumstances. These studies, however, provide insights for use in more general diagnostic situations— they often present information related to processing disruptions. For example, what do the following example reports offer for diagnostic use: Aronson (1971); Chesson (1983); Fisher and Logemann (1970); Garstecki et al. (1972); Golper, Nutt, Rau, and Coleman (1983); Kent and Netsell (1975); Weinberg et al. (1975)?

Chapter 10

Conclusions: patient management

This seventh, and final step of the diagnostic process is the "pay-off" for the patient. The diagnostician must now offer a solution; he must fulfill the purposes of diagnosis discussed in chapter 1. He must present his conclusions about the nature of the speech and language disorder, its causes, and what might be done about it. The diagnosis is not completed until the diagnostician translates his findings into a management plan for the patient. When this step is completed, it is hoped that everyone will go home knowing what was done, what was said, and what is going to happen later. To conclude the diagnosis, the diagnostician performs four basic tasks.

1. First, he determines the management plan to be proposed to the patient.
2. Second, he holds an interpretive conference to discuss his findings and potential management plan.
3. Third, he writes reports for those who are to receive them.
4. Fourth, he completes any administrative follow-up necessary to assure that action is taken and completed.

When all these tasks are completed, the diagnostician can consider the diagnosis as finished. Sometimes this closure is achieved within a few days; at other times it may take some months before the plans for management have been carried out.

DETERMINES THE MANAGEMENT PLAN

In order to determine the management plan, the diagnostician can proceed in the decision making process by asking himself four interrelated yes/no questions (Nation, 1982).

1. Can the patient change his disordered speech and language behavior?
2. Is speech and language therapy necessary for change?
3. Are referrals needed?
4. Are services available?

Depending on his answers to these questions, he proceeds to think through various management alternatives appropriate to the disorder, its causes, and the personal characteristics of the patient. He develops a definitive plan of action to offer to the patient during the interpretive conference. To do this, the diagnostician draws information from his general knowledge of disordered speech and language, his own expertise in treating various disorders, and his experience with health-related services available in the community.

Can the patient change?

Can the aphasic patient alter his language performance? Can the hypernasal child develop nonnasal speech production? Can the adolescent stutterer become fluent? Will the young child "outgrow" his phonologic errors? The diagnostician must know from his interpretation of the data what the prognosis for change in behavior might be. At times this prognostic information can be based specifically on his test results; the patient was able to modify his behavior. At other times he will have to make prognostic judgments based on prior experience with patients who have demonstrated similar disorders or on the basis of what the literature tells him can be done with problems of this type. From this information the diagnostician should be able to answer the question: "Can the patient change his speech and language disorder?"

Of special significance to the diagnostician are the specific prognostic tools he has available that give direct evidence about a patient's ability to change. Work such as that by Van Demark et al. (1975) illustrates this point. They studied the ability of three measures of velopharyngeal competency to predict the need for further surgical management of the palate. Their interest was to reduce the instance of unnecessary speech therapy and indecision regarding the form of management needed. As a single measure, the best predictor of need for secondary palatal surgery of the three clinical tools studied was the articulation score from the Iowa Pressure Articulation Test (Morris et al., 1961; Templin & Darley, 1969). The best overall predictor was the articulation score in combination with the lateral x-ray rating.

Prognostic information is fundamental in choosing among the various management possibilities and planning their sequence. The diagnostician needs to know what procedures are required to effect a change. No recommendations, no matter how assiduously carried out, will be of any value if the patient cannot or will not change. Just because a problem exists does not always mean that something can be done about it.

For example, 28-year-old Paxton, with an estimated IQ of 30, may very well be severely limited in his use of speech and language, but how likely is it that a change will result from direct therapy? Even if some improvement in communication (possibly through using a nonverbal system) may be brought about, does the amount of change justify the time and expense invested? Would a management plan other than therapy be more appropriate to this patient's total needs and possibly bring about as much improvement as direct speech therapy? Few speech–language pathologists work in settings that can make therapy available to everyone, regardless of the probable prognosis. The diagnostician must determine who can benefit the most from therapy. At times prognostic decisions eliminate some patients from therapy considerations; Those who have a low probability of change may be excluded from consideration if the degree of change would not offset time and money considerations. At the other extreme, some patients with a very favorable prognosis may not need special intervention.

The diagnostician's attitude about treatment for different types of speech and language disorders is crucial to the prognosis question. Since the diagnostician makes the recommendations, patients may receive treatment based only on his particular beliefs. For example, if a certain diagnostician does not believe that aphasics benefit from language therapy, will he recommend it? Treatment recommendations based on prognostic data, however, should make this diagnostician assume an attitude other than his own. Even if he does not believe aphasics improve significantly enough to warrant treatment, he should realize that other professionals do and make his recommendations based on other information rather than just his own bias. Patient concern should be his interest.

Mr. Carl Baldwin, 45 years of age, has been a severe stutterer since childhood. Between the ages of 22 and 37 years, he has attempted therapy four different times with four different therapists using various methods for changing his stuttering. You have just seen him for diagnosis and now must decide if he is a candidate for therapy. Answer this first yes/no question: "Can the patient change?" On what would you base your answer?

Prognosis for better speech and language behavior is dependent on many factors, but one of the most important is the cause of the speech and language disorder. If the diagnostician is to predict changes in speech and language behavior, he has to view disorders in reference to their causal bases and not just the behavioral manifestations. Based on causal factors, the diagnostician knows that certain speech and language disorders are more amenable to change than others. For example, with children having developmental speech and language disorders the diagnostician may be on safe ground in prognosticating considerable improvement, and even for some completely normal speech and language behavior. Maturation in these children contributes considerably to the changes seen in speech and language. However, if the child is deaf or severely retarded, the prognosis will be far different.

Likewise, we know that adult aphasics can make changes in their speech and language, but they seldom achieve complete recovery of their premorbid skill level. Rather, recovery is dependent to a great extent on the site and extent of the cerebral lesion and the resulting pattern of language deficits and concomitant physical, psychological, and emotional problems. Physical processing causal factors relevant to prognosis are many, including the localization and extent of the lesion, status of the disease (static or progressive), and associated pathologies.

Prognosis also depends on other causal variables that affect either speech and language input or physical processing. For example, the age, intelligence, education, general health, emotional status, and motivation of the patient as well as the attitude and resources of the family all affect the degree of improvement that can be expected. Insight into the patient's personal characteristics and general attitude about changing his disorder is also vital in determining if change can occur (Conture, 1982).

Dr. Darrell Cook, speech pathologist at the Cleveland Hearing and Speech Center, offfers the following remarks regarding his assessment of prognostic variables for patients who stutter.

Three variables that I believe I can begin to assess during the first interview have to do with the following matters: (1) acceptance of responsibility for change, (2) willingness to take risks in therapy interactions, and (3) awareness of patterns of avoidance and escape behaviors.

In regard to the first variable, I look for statements such as 'I understand that there's a machine that will make me stop stuttering,' or 'My boss says I can't get ahead in the company unless I stop talking this way,' or 'She/he (referring to wife/mother, brother/boss, etc.) makes me stutter.' Although there may be a grain of truth in each of these statements, I think that the person who is perceptive enough to see how he fits into the picture, in terms of what he does, how he feels, and how he must alter his behavior in order to modify the speech pattern, is the person who will probably be better able to accept clinical suggestions designed to alter his way of speaking.

In regard to risk taking, I usually have a more positive feeling about the patient who will readily go along with an attempt at trying various therapy techniques with a minimum of overt resistance (that is, saying, 'I don't see what good *that* will do!'), my assumption being that the patient who does this has already put himself 'into the hands' of a therapist and already perceives that the unlearning of the escape/avoidance behaviors entails a certain amount of openness, willingness to experiment, etc.

In regard to the third variable, self-awareness, I sometimes find that patients come to the first interview already sensitized to how they stutter. To be sure, where this level of understanding has not been reached, it must be taught. But where it is in evidence in a patient not previously experienced in therapy, I believe it represents some level of ability at looking at the self objectively. If so, it would be a significant contributor to change. (Personal communication, 1975)

As more and more questions are asked about accountability for health services, the diagnostician must develop greater prognostic awareness. Speech–language pathology has long been concerned with prognosis, but little has been done to develop measures that are predictive of change in speech and language behavior as a result of therapeutic intervention (Nation, 1982). The diagnostician needs to be able to predict what management plan will best facilitate change, that is, bring about the best prognosis. Is therapy the best plan alone or in conjunction with other treatment plans? For example, while the resonance and phonetic structure characteristics of a child with velopharyngeal insufficiency may be anticipated to improve, the diagnostician must decide which therapeutic plan will allow for maximal improvement. How much can be accomplished with speech therapy alone? At what point should surgical intervention intercede? Therefore, if the diagnostician answers yes to this prognosis question, he must organize the information that indicates the patient can change for discussion with the patient and his family and for later use in writing his clinical report. If he answers no to the prognosis question, he must be prepared to discuss why a speech and language therapy plan is not offered when a known disorder exists.

Is therapy necessary for change?

If the diagnostician answers yes to the treatment question, he must be prepared to tell the patient that therapy is needed, why it is needed, what can be expected from it, how often it may be needed, the length of the sessions, and even perhaps some of the tasks the patient may be required to do. The objectives of the therapy should be proposed. If the patient is a child, the parent's role in the therapeutic process should be made explicit, especially if parental counseling is to be incorporated into the therapeutic plan.

Approaches to therapy have been proposed, both of a general nature (applicable to many types of disorders) and of a specific nature (therapeutic techniques for a specific set of symptoms) and can be found in many books currently in use. For example, the disorder of stuttering seems to have lent itself to a wide range of treatment considerations, ranging from strict operant conditioning approaches for modifying specific bits of behavior to the psychiatric approach intended to help the stutterer understand the psychosexual and interpersonal basis for his stuttering behavior. The diagnostician must weigh these various alternatives to treatment against what he knows about the effectiveness of each approach, as well as what he knows about his patient as a person. Our profession is asking more sophisticated questions about the treatment process (Nation, 1982; Miller, Yoder, & Schiefelbush, 1982); the diagnostician must continually keep abreast of new information about treatment of speech and language disorders for incorporation into management planning.

Once it is determined that the patient can change his behavior and that therapy is needed, the diagnostician must work out his proposed therapy plan before offering it to the patient. He also must be well versed in alternative plans. For example, not all problems of phonetic structure, phonology, or stuttering are treated alike. He must be able to propose and recommend the best treatment plan for the specific patient. His plan may consider such factors as when to start, individual or group therapy, the number of times and length of sessions per week, the sequence of events needed including referrals, and the involvement of any members of the family. He may suggest a "wait-and-see" approach in cases where he feels maturation may be effective, putting the patient in a "holding pattern" and recommending periodic reevaluations to assess again whether direct therapy is needed. This wait-and-see question arises quite frequently over certain problems seen in young children, frequently over the young child whose parents feel he stutters. For example, there is evidence that children do "outgrow" their stuttering or nonfluent speech patterns (Sheehan & Martyn, 1970; Young, 1975).

The diagnostician should plan the objectives of therapy and what changes might be expected if the therapeutic recommendations are carried out. He must make the patient and family aware of their commitment for achieving the objectives of the proposed therapeutic plans. What is the outcome to be? Will it be complete eradication of the speech and language disorder; will it be movement toward more acceptable speech production; will it be movement toward increased interpersonal communicative abilities; will it allow the patient to achieve his social and vocational objectives? How realistic are the recommendations made by the diagnostician in relationship to the personal goals of the patient and his family? Are the hopes and expectations of the family the same as the diagnostician's view of what can be done about the disorder? Will they be ready to pursue the plans of action that are needed?

Therapy recommendations go far beyond the statement that therapy is needed. If an appropriate contract is to be established for treatment, the diagnostician must develop the beginnings of the contract as realistically as possible. The patient must not develop unrealistic expectations on the basis of recommendations made. A contract entered into unrealistically is bound to result in failure, the diagnostician cannot deliver or the patient cannot succeed. Thus, the diagnostician must specify in his recommendations what is likely to be achieved and what cannot be accomplished. For example, he may be able to improve the intelligibility of a child with inadequate velopharyngeal closure, but he may not be able to decrease the amount of hypernasality.

At times, at the conclusion of the initial diagnostic session, the diagnostician has little definitive information on which to base a diagnosis. He may be left with an alternative hypothesis, little information due to problems in carrying out his diagnostic plan, or a series of suspicions, hunches, and guesses. Therefore, before instituting a particular treatment plan, he may recommend regular sessions designed primarily to uncover more information about the cause–effect relationship rather than as a treatment program. He must plan clearly what the intent of these sessions will be, what procedures he would like to follow to obtain the information of interest. These procedures can be therapeutic as well as diagnostic and have been referred to as "diagnostic therapy."

If the diagnostician, however, answers no to the treatment question when a problem is present, he will have to tell the patient why therapy may not be warranted. Perhaps his evaluation of the prognostic question or the referral question provides his answers; that is, prognosis is too poor, or service is required elsewhere.

Are referrals needed?

As a part of management planning the diagnostician must consider referrals to other professionals who will help in the diagnosis and treatment of the patient. Referrals to adjunct services are pursued for two basic reasons. First, referrals are often considered when the diagnostician needs more information about causal factors. For example, if the diagnostician feels the speech and language disorder may be related to neurologic disease, he refers the patient for neurologic testing. Second, referrals are made if other professionals are needed in the treatment program. For example, a patient may benefit from psychotherapy in addition to, or instead of, speech therapy.

Referrals are made for psychological, neurologic, social work, educational, and other specialized services. Within these broad categories of services are embedded many specialists to whom referrals can be made. Because of these multidisciplinary needs, the diagnostician must have a broad knowledge of what specialties and agencies can assist in the management of a speech and language disorder. He must have access to the facilities in his community that can provide these services as either adjuncts to his own treatment or as primary treatment services. For example, Kenneth has a severe language disorder related to suspected mental retardation. The problem is exacerbated by parents who do not understand why Kenneth behaves as he does, and who feel guilty about his condition. To confirm his suspicions of mental retardation, the diagnostician referred the child to a psychologist for intelligence testing. Together with the psychologist, a management plan was formulated that included seeing Kenneth for language therapy, placing him in a special preschool for retarded children, and providing counseling for the parents by the psychologist. Many management plans involve joint rather than unilateral decisions. When several professionals are involved, the management plan needs to specify who does what and when. Only then can the treatment program be efficiently coordinated.

If the diagnostician answers yes to the referral question, he and the patient will want to know to whom to refer, how to refer, and what to expect from the referral source. He will have to explain the referral to the patient and family in a way that they will be willing and able to follow through. If the referral is essential to understanding the problem and its cause, the referral should be stressed as needed before therapy begins or as soon after as possible. If the referral is to another specialty thought more suitable for the patient's problem, then again, immediate referral is essential since the patient may not be seen for speech and language therapy.

The diagnostician must make intelligent, informed referrals for these needed services. He must be well trained in recognizing what makes a specific referral the logical and correct thing to do. A referral should never be based on "it seems like a good idea." It should be made on the basis of positive, objective, and logical information. Therefore the diagnostician must know (1) when to refer for services, (2) to whom to refer, (3) what to expect from the referral, and (4) how to interpret the results obtained.

The chart on the following page provides some basic information around each of these topics. The student should think through each of these topics for each potential referral source he might choose, as it relates to the various types of speech and language disorders.

At certain times immediate referrals may not be too helpful and, in fact, may be premature. When causal factors are obscure, and no longer operating, and the diagnostician is assured that therapy can proceed without confirmation from another specialty, he may delay a referral until he feels more certain about its need. For example, if minimal cerebral dysfunction is suspected, even though little evidence has accrued, this might not be the best time to suggest a referral. It might be better to wait until the patient responds to a therapy program— often a suspected brain-injured child is a rambunctious child who can be settled down during the therapy sessions. Or if the diagnostician feels the family is not ready to pursue a referral, he may not make an immediate referral. For example, the parents of a child just diagnosed as severely deviant in language development may not be ready to accept the

Referral topic	Comments
1. Referral for type of service	For example, the neurologic examination.
2. Criteria for referral—when to refer	This section should include the various types of behavior observed, tests used, and any results of the diagnosis that indicate the need for the referral. For example, (a) the level of speech and language development could be indicative of mental retardation; (b) drooling, a sign of a more generalized motor dysfunction; and (c) ooververbalization, a sign of emotional disturbance.
3. To whom referral should be made	From the preceding criteria, this may be self-evident, but not always. For example (a) for mental retardation, signs of emotional disturbance, or school failure, you may choose among the psychologist, the psychiatrist, or the educational specialist; or (b) for a child suspected of learning disabilities or minimal cerebral dysfunction, you may opt to refer to a pediatrician, a neurologist, a pediatric–neurologist, etc. Generally, in each community you will discover who works best with the various problems you see.
4. What to expect	Generally a report or telephone call should be forthcoming, depending on the reporting practices of the referral. You should work toward obtaining the tests and observations made and how they were interpreted by the referral source. For example, what is done to determine intelligence?
5. Interpretation of results obtained	The interpretation of the information obtained should be done by the professional referred to; that is, if the referral was to determine intellectual abilities, this interpretation will be done. At times the referral person may relate his findings to the speech and language disorder. However, it is the task of the diagnostician to determine how the findings assist him in understanding the speech and language disorder and planning appropriate management.

diagnostician's suspicions of mental retardation. Therefore he may not make an immediate recommendation for psychological referral to the parents. He can pursue the referral once the child enters therapy for the language disorder and he has established a better relationship with the parents.

If the diagnostician answers "no" to the referral question, there is no referral planning necessary following the diagnosis unless the patient asks for a "second-opinion" referral. In this case the diagnostician is obligated to assist in this process.

The following patients were seen for diagnosis in a community speech and hearing agency. A basic diagnostic statement is provided. From this statement, consider an overall management plan including any referral needs.

1. Mrs. Garfinkel has severe aphasia (Group IV on the Minnesota Test for Differential Diagnosis of Aphasia), resulting from a cerebrovascular accident 3 months ago.

2. Four-year-old David Hayes has severely unintelligible speech related to an extremely short lingual frenulum.

3. Five-year-old August Hatten has a severe phonologic disorder possibly precipitated by temporary hearing losses associated with chronic middle ear infections since an early age. Habit strength and association with an older brother who also has an articulation disorder are both considered as maintaining factors.

4. Mary Weiss has a severe speech production problem. There is little ability to initiate phonation or control the speech production mechanism. This disorder is directly due to the brain injury she sustained in an automobile accident.

5. Geoffrey, aged 4 years, 3 months, has a severe articulation problem accompanied by moderate to severe hypernasality and nasal emission resulting from inadequate velopharyngeal closure subsequent to a repaired cleft lip and palate.

6. James Catlow, aged 23 years, has an excessive high-pitched voice due to failure of the voice to change during puberty, at times referred to as "mutational falsetto."

Are services available?

Many agencies providing speech and language services are unable to schedule immediate therapy for all patients who need it. There may be extensive waiting lists; in some school systems, many children in the lower grades are automatically, by policy, excluded from service; in a rehabilitation unit priority may be given to the patient with the more complicated problems.

When the demands exceed the supply, the agency must provide ways of assisting the patient whose problem has been diagnosed until such time as the therapeutic plan can be implemented. The sensitivity and policies of the agency become extremely important during this time, keeping in touch with the patients who are on waiting lists, giving them appropriate times when service may be implemented, and finding ways to assist them while they are waiting for direct services. At times home programs or group programs can be of some assistance in the interim.

Besides the services available in his own agency, the diagnostician must know the "nitty–gritty" of obtaining other needed community services. There are many practical interagency "in's and out's" he will need to learn with each specialty and agency. He must know what services and personnel are available and the quality, flexibility, location, and expense of the specific service. He must be able to mesh the requirements of the specific service agency with the patient. Can the patient afford the service? Can he get there at the times the service is offered—usually between 9:00 A.M. and 5:00 P.M.?

Unfortunately, adjunct professional services are sometimes limited within the community in which the diagnostician works. If the community has a wide range of health and educational services available it is fortunate, and the patient can probably get what is needed. However, in many instances the diagnostician is functioning in a limited-resource community. In these cases the recommended management alternatives may not exist, and the choices made by the diagnostician will need to be altered. For example, there may be no special classes for the child with a significant learning disability accompanying his speech and language disorder. Therefore the diagnostician cannot refer to a special class unless the family is willing and able to send the child to a special school away from home or they are willing and able to move to a location where the services are available. When services considered important are not available, the diagnostician must work out alternatives best suited to the circumstances of his community. There may be options available, although some of these may not be optimal.

HOLDS AN INTERPRETIVE CONFERENCE

As part of concluding the diagnostic process, the diagnostician will need information and skills that allow him to communicate his findings effectively. He must be able to transmit his information to the patient in an interpersonal interaction, the interpretive conference.

Communication of the diagnostic findings to the patient is vital. None of us, for example, likes to leave a physician's office without an explanation of our illness or disease, its cause, and a plan for treatment. Understanding of the problem fosters cooperation and trust. There is little likelihood that persons will act on advice if they do not understand and accept the information given them. The importance of communicating the diagnostic information to the patient cannot be stressed too strongly.

Conferencing versus counseling

Emerick (1969), Marshall and Goldstein (1969, 1970), and Bangs (1982) are among the few who have written about the actual imparting of diagnostic information. Most of the literature in our area concentrates on parental counseling (Derman & Manaster, 1967; Sander, 1959; Webster, 1977; Wood, 1948) and is directed toward helping parents understand the speech and language problems presented by their child while the child is undergoing therapy. For example, Webster (1977) discusses various counseling techniques for parents of children with speech and language disorders. Her emphasis is on helping parents work through their communication problems with the child to prevent interpersonal difficulties from occurring because the significance of the disorder is not understood. A resource book helpful for understanding the counseling process with parents of the ill and handicapped has been compiled by Noland (1971), and Webster's (1977) work is also particularly helpful.

Conferencing shares with counseling the goal of helping patients define and cope with the facts of their problem. However, we see a distinction between the two processes. Counseling, for us, implies a process in which the person is helped to verbalize, explore, and alleviate his feelings regarding the communication problem, the emphasis here being the feelings of the person counseled. Thus, for us, counseling is a longer, more introspective process requiring considerable interpersonal commitment by all parties involved. Very little counseling, in this sense, can be achieved on a one-shot basis with a virtual stranger.

The interpretive conference, in contrast, emphasizes the transmission of information from the diagnostician to the patient for the purpose of arriving at a management plan. The interpretive conference is an interpersonal interaction; thus, all that has been said regarding interpersonal relations during the interview applies equally here. As well, many counseling techniques are useful during the interpretive conference just as they were during the interview. Just as the interview was used to gather information about the problem, its causes, and what has been done about it, so the interpretive conference is used to impart information about the diagnostician's findings: the nature of the problem, its potential causes, and his proposed solution for it.

Purposes of conference

During the interpretive conference the diagnostician will want to accomplish at least two purposes. First, he aims to provide the patient with a clear understanding of the speech and language problem and its probable causes. Second, he wants to explore the available management alternatives with them so that together they can decide on a management plan. In the interpretive conference the diagnostician and the patient become a team, working toward understanding the nature and cause of the speech and language problem in order to effect an appropriate management plan—one with which everyone concerned can work comfortably with the knowledge that if it is put into effect, the patient can make modifications in this speech and language behavior.

At the outset the diagnostician has to determine when to hold the interpretive conference. Is he to do it immediately following the diagnostic session, or will he schedule a separate appointment for the conference? There is no rule to apply to this situation. It depends solely on the complexity of the problem and the diagnostician's need for time. When the conference can be held at the end of the session, do so; when it cannot, inform the patient that you need to go over the results and if possible make an immediate appointment for the interpretive conference.

Plan of action

In imparting his diagnostic findings, the diagnostician must have a plan of action. He can begin by summarizing the areas that were evaluated in a very general sense. "During the time we tested Don, we were looking at how well he understands and uses words and sentences." Then the diagnostician can mention the patient's strengths, perhaps areas of relatively high performance, or, if appropriate, behavior that facilitated testing. In any event, try to relate something positive about the testing session. "Our tests showed that Carol hears well. She is able to use her tongue, lips, and jaw very well to make speech sounds." Or "Don really worked hard during the session, even though some of the things I asked him to do were frustrating for him."

Following this general picture of strengths and weaknesses, continue into a description of the speech and language disorder, giving specific examples and possibly explaining specific test results. For example, "You remember the test on which Carol named pictures. That test showed us that she is not able to make all of the speech sounds that most 5-year-old girls make." After the detailed description of the disorder, the diagnostician will then want to resummarize the major points.

After describing the speech and language disorder, the diagnostician can then proceed to address the probable causes. Patients and their families usually seek a statement of cause. They may feel that a specific cause will relieve them of the responsibility for the problem or that a discovery of cause will indicate an immediate method of treatment to correct the disorder. In the discussion of causation the diagnostician can encourage the patient to review his own attempts to account for the speech and language problem. While the diagnostician's statements surrounding the topic of cause and effect must be as accurate as possible, attitudes and comments should be directed more toward allowing the patients an opportunity to bring out into the open their own thoughts on the subject, rather than simply presenting them with detailed causal information (Rheingold, 1945).

If the explanation offered by the patient seems reasonable and constructive, the diagnostician should encourage exploration, leading to an accurate representation of causal factors. If the patient's explanation is so divergent as to suggest misconception of the cause, then the diagnostician must discourage their belief and develop another approach to causation.

Causal factors

Often implicating causal factors is a very sensitive subject in that it tends to precipitate more stress for the family. Revealing that the child's speech and language problem may be due to mental retardation, brain damage, or emotional disturbance may serve only to create anxiety and needless fears and adverse home reactions. Of course, if the child has not been examined or assessed by a psychologist, neurologist, or other medical personnel previous to the speech and language diagnosis and the diagnostician suspects causation that may require referrals or additional testing, then he has to work through the need for a referral. "We would like Don to be seen by the Mental Development Center for further testing so that we can get a better idea of his abilities in areas other than speech and language." "We would like to make an appointment for Carol to see a neurologist so that we can obtain additional information about some of the difficulties she is having moving her tongue. Once we have this information, it will help us in planning a therapy program for her." If the parent asks, for example, "Is Don mentally retarded?" then it is necessary to give the parent an honest and direct answer. "Most of Don's skills and behavior seem to be around the 2- to 3-year age level." If a previous diagnosis of mental retardation has been made and has been interpreted to the family, then refer to these findings. However, in discussing causal factors, it is important to be aware of the parent's conception of the terms used. Frequently parents' knowledge about similarly diagnosed persons is the basis for their reactions to and acceptance of certain labels. For example, one mother, because of her severely retarded brother, considered all retarded children incapable of attaining any social or intellectual maturity. Her experience has lead her to consider "retarded" to be synonymous with "vegetable."

You have just seen Arthur, the son of Mr. and Mrs. Gregory Schwartz. Arthur is now 5 years old, but in all the testing and observation you did he performed at about the 3-year level. You also know, as reported by the psychologist, that Arthur is mentally retarded, a reliable reported IQ of 60. The parents do not yet know this, and the psychologist has recommended they not be told at this time. Apart from how you might handle that information, consider how you would discuss your findings with the parents. How will you discuss causal factors in response to their questions?

Many times it is not possible to report definitive causal factors. In such instances we find the concept of historical and contemporary causation a particularly useful way in which to approach a discussion of causal factors. For example, the diagnostician might say, "Carol does not produce many of her sounds clearly because she is having difficulty making her tongue move as she would like it to"—contemporary causation. Or "We are not sure exactly why Carol is having this difficulty with her tongue"—historical causation. Also, in interpreting causation, the diagnostician must keep in mind the multiple nature of causation, serial causation, direct and indirect interactions, and the other perspectives on causation previously discussed. Translated into layman's terms, such perspectives are useful for the interpretive conference.

Imparting information

Of particular importance in the interpretive conference is how the diagnostician imparts information (Bangs, 1982). The patient, family members, or others came to the diagnostician in order to gain understanding and help with the speech and language problem. They are entitled not only to an evaluation, but also a clear, concise explanation of the diagnostic findings. The amount of information given during the interpretive conference varies depending on many variables, particularly the personal characteristics of the patient. The information may vary from specific test findings to only a general impression of the problem. Whatever is given must be presented clearly and concisely—the patient must not be overwhelmed with information he cannot or does not want to handle at this time. The information of prime importance to impart is who is going to do what, when, and where.

It is often said that "comprehension precedes expression" in the acquisition of language. The same holds true for the diagnostician in the conference. Diagnostic information cannot be imparted in a comprehensible manner until it is thoroughly understood by the diagnostician. Too frequently, professional jargon replaces understanding. Everyday the diagnostician uses terms such as phonologic, motor programming, disinhibition, and minimal brain dysfunction. What he must understand is that most patients do not understand what these words mean. The diagnostician needs a clear, down-to-earth means of expressing these concepts. In a sense, he must be a "walking thesaurus" capable of clarifying and interpreting processes, products, and causal factors that may not be readily understood by others.

The following example illustrates the significance of the diagnostician's use of terminology in regard to parental understanding of diagnostic information. During a particular conference session, diagnostic findings were given to the mother of a child. The diagnostician was quite thorough in his description of the child's problem, and his diagnosis seemed quite appropriate: "Devin has a severe language formulation problem that is particularly evident on the phonologic level. His problem seems to represent developmental verbal apraxia that is probably part of the more general minimal brain damage that has been reported by the neurologist, Dr. Moore." After giving this diagnosis, the diagnostician asked the mother if she had any questions; the mother responded that she did not. Fortunately, the diagnostician then added, "Now tell me what you will tell you husband about your child's problem when you go home." The mother's reply was quite inadequate, and after stumbling over a few sentences, she said, "I don't know." The diagnostician in this situation may have a clear understanding of the problem but did not use words that transmitted information to the mother.

The diagnostician must keep in mind how much of the information the patient can absorb, how technical his terminology can be. He must develop a way of talking that allows patients to understand and act. Patients will want to know if the diagnostician saw the problem they saw, if it is a significant problem, if it can be changed, why it is there, and what they can do about it. The diagnostician must have some knowledge of the attitudes and beliefs of the patient and his family if he is to present information they will use—an advantage gained by holding an interview prior to this time. For example, a mother who believes her son stutters because he was in a car accident—"he began to stutter after that"—

may not be ready to accept any other explanation, especially one that includes an interpretation of her attitude toward the child following the auto accident. The diagnostician may have discovered her interactions with the child seemed based on guilt (she was responsible for the auto accident), and he may consider these interactions as the more significant variables. In his interpretive conference with this mother, the diagnostician may have to deal with causal factors on one level in the interpretive conference, using later counseling sessions to explore the mother's attitudes and feelings about her son's stuttering and the role she may be playing in its development.

Some diagnosticians find the use of a summary or profile form to be a useful device for making the information clear. A written summary for the parents aids in transmitting information and also provides them with basic information for future reference. For example, a mother who goes home from the diagnosis and is asked by her husband, "What did they tell you?" will then have the summary available for discussion. A summary form can aid the diagnostician in conveying the whole picture and also can aid the person receiving the information in retaining the whole picture. In educational and psychological assessment the use of summary profiles for charting information are quite common. Salvia and Ysseldyke (1981) provide information that can be adapted to speech–language pathology.

Management decisions

Beyond imparting diagnostic findings, the major purpose of the interpretive conference is to arrive at management decisions. The diagnostician enters the interpretive conference with a proposal for future steps to be taken, having considered prognostic factors, management alternatives, and practical considerations. The diagnostician brings recommendations as to what he thinks would be the best plan and why. He offers a tentative solution to the problem. However, he tries to do this from the perspective of the patient's total concerns and problems. For example, one patient may be primarily concerned about his medical and physical treatments and consider speech a very low priority. Another may have a strong desire to improve his speech despite the fact that the speech disorder is very minimal.

The diagnostician comes only with a proposal. During his interpretive conference, any number of changes in the plan may take place, depending on the reactions of the patient to the plan, or ability to carry out the proposed plans. Thus the diagnostician must get used to having his optimal plans altered by the practicalities inserted by patients. If patients are involved in the decision, they will be more likely to follow through and feel the plan is appropriate for them. At times the points that need to be reconciled are minor. Perhaps the time for initiating therapy does not fit in exactly with their other plans or the patient would prefer to try to find a therapist closer to his home than those suggested. At other times there may be a considerable discrepancy between what the patient believes or is ready to hear and what the diagnostician recommends. An example would be a child referred by his teacher because his speech is unintelligible to her, but the parents feel the child will "outgrow" the problem. The diagnostic findings, however, reveal a significant problem. In this case the diagnostician must help the parents understand the degree of the problem before they will be able to accept therapy as a needed solution. The diagnostician must know how to work this through in his interpretive conference.

In another instance the diagnostician may purposely recommend an alternative plan, paving the way to a more appropriate management solution. For example, Mrs. Guncik seemed to fear the possibility that her daughter Dorathy was retarded. However, she denied such feelings and rejected such a possibility. The diagnostician, however, also suspected retardation. Because he felt the parents would not follow through with a referral for psychological testing, he recommended immediate language therapy and parental counseling to help the parents understand Dorathy's problem. From this management plan hopefully would evolve a more appropriate treatment plan for Dorathy—a combination of professionals trained to work with all aspects of the retardation.

In still other instances, the diagnostician may alter his original plan for direct therapy during the interpretive conference. Early during the conference he may hold his recommendations for direct therapy while he assesses the family's understanding of the problem, what they may be able to carry out, and on this basis alter his original plan—an on-the-spot change that may serve the needs of all concerned better than direct therapy. This type of change is frequently considered when the problem seen has a strong maturational component—the child may well grow out of many of the speech and language behaviors given appropriate amounts and types of stimulation at home.

For example, Judi, 4 years of age, was seen for a stuttering problem. Her parents had been concerned since she was 2 years of age and had been advised to ignore it. However, the speech difficulty persisted and they brought Judi for diagnosis. Judi exhibited significant disfluencies in the form of rapid repetitions of sounds, words, and phrases, usually occurring at the beginning of an utterance. She became increasingly disfluent if asked to answer questions quickly or when not given a chance to respond. If the diagnostician ignored her, her verbal attempts to attract his attention were filled with nonfluencies. During the conference the diagnostician worked to help the parents understand Judi's specific difficulties, assessing their sensitivity to the problem and judging their ability to follow through with suggestions for creating easier communicative situations. Because of the parent's responses, the diagnostician made the decision to help them develop a program at home with periodic conferences to check on the progress being made. With other parents less able to understand and provide the desired environment, the diagnostician would have recommended a different management strategy, probably direct therapy accompanied by parent counseling. The point is that in the interpretive conference the diagnostician must make judgments about parents, their understanding of the problem, and their ability to follow through with general and specific management proposals. This requires finely tuned insight into patients and their families.

The following dialogue is an example of an interpretive conference with Mrs. Russo, whose 5½-year-old son, Jack, has just been seen for a speech and language diagnosis. Evaluate the diagnostician's comments and approach in terms of the information reported, the appropriateness of the language used, and the sensitivity to the mother. What aspects would you emulate? What would you change? Keep in mind that many of the points discussed are related to a number of questions and comments posed by the mother in the history form and the interview.

D: We want to share with you what we did with Jack and to try to help you understand what kinds of problems he is having with speech and language. What I would like to do now is give you the findings of our testing with Jack, and then we can discuss the next steps we want to take. Please stop me at any time if you do not understand what I am saying or if you have additional questions. My first purpose is to help you understand Jack's problem as we see it. This will be our first step in working together on his problems. Roughly, what we did was give him a number of tests that helped us to find out how he is understanding and using language. What we generally found was that Jack's understanding and use of language is at about the 2- or 3-year level.

Sometimes we see children whose understanding is at one level and their expression is at another level. This was not true for Jack. Both his understanding and his expression were at about the same level. We also gave him some other tests to see how well he can produce different kinds of sounds—the types of sounds that we use in words. He had a minor problem with making the different sounds correctly, but for the most part, he is able to produce the correct sounds in easy situations.

Mrs. R: Well then, why do I have trouble understanding him?

D: Sometimes in conversational speech his ability to produce sounds is not as good as his use in single words. The test we gave him used single words, but he does not maintain his level of intelligibility when the words are together in everyday conversational speech. Although in conversation his speech is difficult to understand, in comparison to his other language skills, his ability to produce all the different sounds in single words was really relatively good. But we will also be concerned about working to improve his ability to make sounds correctly in connected speech. The nice thing we know is that he is very, what we call, stimulable. That is, I say a sound and he can sometimes imitate it back to me. If I say /p/ and he says /p/ after me, that is a favorable sign meaning that he can change the way he makes his sounds and with some help will be able to produce them all by himself.

We did attempt to look at how Jack lifted his tongue and produced the motor movements for speech but, as you know, Jack just had a tooth out and was not too anxious to have us looking in his mouth. But the fact that he can produce so many sounds, that is, his articulation is relatively good, indicates to us that he is probably able to use his tongue correctly and is having no problems lifting it or moving it. For example, he can make the t, d, n, and l sounds that require him to put his tongue tip to the top of his mouth like this (demonstration).

So, essentially, what we see is that Jack's ability to understand and use both single words and connected speech is what we would expect from a child of about 2 to 3 years of age.

I thought you might be interested in looking at some of the language tests that we gave Jack to show you briefly the kinds of things we did and the kinds of tasks Jack had problems with.

In terms of his understanding of language, the first thing we looked at was his ability to understand single words, like a vocabulary test. We would say one word and he would have to point to it (Mrs. Russo shown the Peabody Picture Vocabulary Test). For instance, on this page we would say ball and he would point to it. Here we presented him with one single word—usually this kind of task is easier for children to do than to understand longer sentences. On this test he scored at about the 2½-year age level. Then we gave Jack a second test where the language becomes longer and he has to listen to connected speech and choose the correct picture (Mrs. Russo shown the Assessment of Children's Language Comprehension). For example, the phrase "horse standing," requires Jack to listen to both parts—if he listens to just the last word, he might point to "bird standing." The speech continues to get longer and longer. All through this test he was well below the 3-year level.

In terms of his use of speech, we had him name pictures to see what level his expressive vocabulary was (Mrs. Russo shown the Vocabulary Usage Test). For example, he would see a picture like this, and we would say "This is a ____." Jack would have to fill in the right words for what he saw in the picture. Here we were looking at his expressive vocabulary and on this test he scored at the 2½-year age level.

Then we listened to his conversational use of speech. Here we found that he used two words together and occasionally three words. This is not what we would expect of a 5-year-old child. Again, it is more like a 2- or 3-year-old child. Do you have any questions so far?

Mrs. R: Jack does seem quite slow for his age, but will he ever catch up or will he always be slow?

D: We can never really predict when a child is as young as Jack how much progress he will make. We do know that he is going to change, that he is going to learn more. How much we cannot be sure. I would expect his ability to produce sounds is going to show quite a bit of improvement since we know that he is able to produce them correctly with help. Now in terms of the level of his understanding and use of language, we are really not sure how far he may go. Most children by 5 years of age have acquired most of their basic sentence structure. So since Jack has been slow all along, he should continue to put more words together. It will not be like catching up with children who do not have problems, but he will be able to understand and say more than he can now.

Mrs. R: I knew Jack was slow but never wanted to find out why. I was afraid he was retarded.

D: I did want to talk with you about the reason for Jack's slow use of speech and language. There are a number of factors to consider. One of these factors is a possible hearing problem. But you have never noticed a problem with hearing, and we did not suspect any when we were working with Jack.

You just mentioned another major factor why children are slow, like Jack, in developing speech and language. You indicated that you were afraid Jack was retarded. That is a factor we will want to look at carefully with Jack—his general level of mental growth. Here are some things we may want to look for. Are all skills at one level, or are speech and language skills reduced more than his other skills? In other words, we are interested in whether Jack is having more problems with language than with other nonlanguage areas—for example, his ability to put puzzle pieces together, his ability to color, his ability to do selfhelp activities such as dressing and undressing—things that do not require speech and language. What we will want to assess are the other areas of mental growth; language is only one area. Sometimes we find children where this is the only problem; sometimes there are children who have problems in a number of areas. So this is an additional area where we would like to do some more testing. We would like to schedule Jack for a more thorough psychological evaluation—to see if just his speech and language are reduced or if other areas are also at a lower level.

• Note: At this point the diagnostician and Mrs. Russo have information about some of Jack's overall abilities and skills beyond speech and language. A decision here could be made to work through with Mrs. Russo some of that information, depending on how Mrs. Russo is reacting and how much she might need or want to know at this time rather than waiting for a referral. In interpretive conferencing, the diagnostician has to decide how much to reinforce a possible causal factor.

Mrs. R: Will you do this, or will I go somewhere else?

D: It could be handled either way. We have a clinical psychologist here to do psychological testing, or we could refer you elsewhere. What would you prefer?

Mrs. R: Either way.

D: I think it would be best then for us to do it. We have all the information here, and after testing is completed it would be easier for all of us to get together.

Mrs. R: Will you be placing Jack in speech therapy now?

D: I think we will wait to decide that. There are a number of things we might do, but first we should have the results from the psychologist. After testing is finished, you, the psychologist, and I will work out the best plan for Jack. I know that you are anxious to get started, so let's go down to the scheduling office and work out a time that you can bring Jack for the psychological testing. If possible, it would be a good idea for your husband to come.

The following is a partial set of diagnostic findings on Lee Newton, aged 5 years, 5 months. Two hypothetical Mrs. Newtons are described. From this information, consider what might be the major differences in your approach to the interpretive conference with these two mothers.

Mrs. Newton I

Mrs. Newton is a middle-class housewife who is concerned about her adequacy as a mother. Mr. Newton tends to blame his wife for Lee's impulsive, occasionally unmanageable behavior, claiming that if she knew how to manage him, Lee would not have all of his current problems. She fears that Lee may be retarded and is very concerned about the "cause" of his behavior and language problems; however, she attempts to present Lee in the most favorable light and to minimize his difficulties. Although Mr. Newton makes an adequate salary to support his family, the family has felt the effects of inflation and has not had much money for nonessentials. While willing to do whatever is necessary for Lee, Mrs. Newton is worried about the cost of the evaluation and possible therapy, about which she has no information.

Mrs. Newton II

Mrs. Newton is a lower-class mother who communicates her information and impressions about Lee through a "restricted language code." While she knows Lee is not "stupid," she has little knowledge of other factors contributing to speech and language functioning. While her understanding of Lee's problem is limited, she very much wants to do whatever is best for him.

Partial diagnostic findings

- Templin–Darley Screening Test of Articulation: raw score—25 correct; norm—34.7; cutoff—31.

  Errors: /w/r and d/ð/ initially and medially; /w/l, b/v, f/θ/ initially; /f/θ/ in the final position; /w/ substituted for /r/ and /l/ in /spr, br, tr, kr, gr, fr, θr, skr, ʃr, pl, kl, fl, and spl/.

  Additional errors: noted in spontaneous speech—/s/t and t/s/ inconsistently in the initial position; /d/l/ in medial positions.

  Stimulability: /d, t, and θ/ produced correctly in nonsense syllables but not words; /v, l, and r/ not produced correctly.

- Peabody Picture Vocabulary Test: 2 year, 9 month age level (chronological age is 5 years, 5 months).

- Preschool Language Profile: pointed to four body parts (24 months); obeyed five of seven simple commands (24+ months); correctly identified eight pictures (21 months); comprehended three of five prepositions (32 months); comprehended two of five questions (39 to 42 months); pointed to two of four pictures that answered questions (less than 36 months); expressively named four of four objects (30 months); named six of ten picture objects and pointed to two others (30 months); responded to pictures with one or two words; on the action agent test answered eight of twenty questions (3-year-old answers 60% to 70% correctly); told sex (30 to 36 months); named one of four colors (norm for all four is 5 years of age).

- Hearing Testing: audiometric screening test attempted at 15 dB from 250 to 8000 Hz; ring-drop toy used as a conditioning device, but responses obtained in this manner were erratic; thresholds varied as much as 50 dB; however, Lee did respond to several low-intensity tones at most frequencies, when became restless after 15 to 20 minutes, testing discontinued.

Recommendations

1. Additional nonverbal psychological testing.
2. Social service referral to learn more about management factors at home.
3. Additional hearing testing.

WRITES HIS REPORTS

Other than the interpretive conference, the diagnostician's major form of communication is a written report. The report serves as a "permanent" record to be used by various individuals involved with the patient. These written reports take many forms from short summary letters to elaborate clinical reports containing much detailed information.

The style and format of the report may vary depending on the person to whom it is written. The professional's *clinical report*, as a part of the agency records, will be used by the professional who sees the patient for services. This clinical report is usually quite detailed, specifying all components of the diagnosis that occurred and the recommendations made. This same report may be sent, as well, to certain of the referral sources, generally another professional involved with the patient. At other times separate reports, usually much shorter, are sent to the referral source or other professionals. Abbreviated reports or short letters often become the primary means of reporting between experienced professionals who have knowledge of each other's work and rely on one another to be informed and objective.

Other types of written reports are also used. Sometimes a summary report is given to the parents of the child seen. This summary report may be completed at the time of the interpretive conference, giving the parent present information to share with the absent parent, or they may use the report in further contacts they make with teachers, their physician, and so forth. At times, letters are written to the parents following the diagnostic session summarizing the findings and emphasizing the management plan that was worked out. This type of follow-up communication again serves as a record for them and gives them assurance that the diagnostician is still involved with them. Thus, there are many ways to write reports, each facilitating communication in different ways. What is written on a medical chart in a hospital may vary significantly from the comprehensive clinical report written in a community speech and hearing agency. Many factors go into the decisions regarding the style and format of reports; however, the report must communicate the diagnostician's findings clearly.

Because of the many purposes of writing reports, the diversity of settings in which diagnosticians work, the many different referral sources, and the policies and practices about report writing dictated by agencies, specifying how to construct reports is difficult. However, guidelines can be offered. Generally, regardless of the format of the report or to whom it is written, it will include information about the statement of the problem, what was done in the diagnostic session, an interpretation of the findings, and what is to be done about the problem. Following these general guidelines, a number of formats for structuring clinical reports have been offered (Emerick & Hatten, 1979; Johnson et al., 1963; Knepflar, 1976; Sanders, 1979; Tallent, 1980).

Clinical report writing should follow quite naturally the steps of the diagnostic process. As the researcher must communicate his findings through a well-reasoned research report, so the diagnostician must develop a well-reasoned clinical report. To this end, we believe that report writing can best be taught by learning how scientific papers are written; an article in a professional journal serves a parallel purpose to a clinical report. The report should indicate clearly the process the diagnostician has gone through to arrive at the diagnosis he is reporting. If the diagnostic process has been well thought out, the report will also be. If the diagnostician has developed a clear perspective about his patient, it will be reflected in his report.

The diagnostician must develop a report-writing style that allows each reader to find what he wants quickly. But there may be many readers for each report or the need to write a number of different reports for each patient. There is a point of practicality that must be entertained; that is, how many reports can a diagnostician be expected to write for any given patient seen for services? Therefore, we advocate the use of a single, rather comprehensive clinical report that can be readily adapted for various involved individuals but whose primary use is within the diagnostician's agency. This comprehensive clinical report serves as a resource document about the patient at the time he was initially seen. We believe it is essential that students in training be taught this method of report writing before moving on to others.

The format that we are presenting is not unlike other formats; however, we are tying the sections of the report to the steps of the diagnostic process, indicating the general nature of the information to be included within each section. The sections should stand relatively independent from each other; that is, each section can be read as a separate unit. The most vital component of this report is the clinical evaluation section. This section should provide a complete summary of the diagnostician's interpretation of the problem and his reasons for his diagnosis. It can be written in a deductive fashion, stating the diagnosis and then how and why it was arrived at. Once it is clearly written, it serves as a practical device in that it can be sent as it is to certain individuals or easily adapted for others.

The following is a suggested format for constructing a clinical report. The heading titles are suggestive, and exactly how information is ordered and discussed in each section depends on the patient and the type of problem. Some sections could be collapsed into larger units if needed. At the left are indicated the steps of the diagnostic process from which information is applicable to each of the sections of the report.

Following this format a clinical report becomes similar to a research article. If presented this way, the report allows the reader to make judgments about the nature and quality of the diagnosis that took place. The reader can review the information presented, make his own interpretations, accept or reject the diagnostician's conclusions, or ask for more information. A report written this way does not demand that the reader be accepting of the diagnostician's findings, only that he give careful consideration to how the diagnostician went about the diagnosis and how he arrived at his interpretation of the data. A clinical report of this type is an open communication rather than a closed communication. It is open to other interpretations; it does not unequivocally state this is the disorder, and this is what should be done about it. The clinical report should invite other considerations; it should open doors for clinical interpretation and new insights, rather than close the avenues of further communication. Our interest is patient concern, not unchallenged diagnoses.

Steps of the diagnostic process	Sections of the clinical report
Constituent analysis	Section I: Identification information
	This is usually prescribed in standard form by the agency and includes such items as name, address, and agency number.
Constituent analysis	Section II: Statement of the problem
	This is the patient's, not the diagnostician's, statement of the problem as well as any that have come from the referral sources. The information here gives the reader a clear idea of how people involved with the patient have viewed the problem and the sequence of events that led to the referral. Keep in mind that the reason for referral and the statement of the problem may not be the same, and different sources report them differently. What is wanted in this section is a clear statement of how the problem is seen and how the patient came to you.
Constituent analysis Clinical hypothesis	Section III: Background history
	This section can become quite lengthy depending on what information is included. What is used comes from information available prior to the diagnosis as well as certain information gathered during the interview. Basically, the history information that is most directly relevant to the problem should be included. The information should be ordered by topic and sequence—it is time-dimension reporting. It can be structured according to such topics as presented on the children's case history questionnaire or any topics suitable

continued.

Steps of the diagnostic process	Sections of the clinical report
	to the patient. A guideline for inclusion is to use that information that will be needed for the clinical evaluation. Remember that this information has been used to derive the clinical hypothesis, which included a determination of the significance of the information. Thus information in this section can be presented in light of its relevance to the overall clinical problem as long as *all* relevant information is presented. This comment is not meant as a license for including only that which supports your conclusions; it is a license for pertinency. Generally, the diagnostician's hypothesis is not included in a report as we have previously discussed. But a case could be made for including it in some instances, and if so, it would most logically appear at the end of the history section, perhaps as stated in the following example: "This history led us to believe that Mr. Goldstein was exhibiting a severe dysarthria related to his diagnosed neurologic disease, multiple sclerosis."
Clinical design Data collection Data analysis	Section IV: Testing and observation This section would include all the procedures that were used, the results of the procedures, and the analysis of the data—the objectification of what took place during the diagnostic session. This, too, could become quite a lengthy section depending on how much was included and how it is structured. We recommend basic information be provided in the report and not all the details of the analysis. The emphasis should be summary analyses rather than reporting all the raw data, again depending on the nature of the problem. This section could be ordered test by test in the sequence in which they were given; however, this would be a test-oriented report rather than a patient-oriented report. Instead, we suggest ordering the testing under umbrella headings and reporting appropriate information within these headings regardless of the sequence in which they occurred unless, of course, sequential reporting is indicated. We would recommend using a processing system for ordering the results. The broad heading of reception, comprehension, integration, formulation and production could be used as needed. Within each, the tools that are appropriate could be discussed, reporting the results in product and behavioral correlate terms. In this section a general statement of the patient's reactions to the diagnostic session could be included. It can be placed at the beginning of the section so the reader gets immediate knowledge about the effects of the patient's behavior on the test results.
Clinical interpretation	Section V: Clinical evaluation In this section the diagnostician draws together all the information into a summary interpretation. He presents his diagnostic interpretation and offers his support from the history and his testing. This can be done in a deductive manner, starting out with a diagnostic statement and then providing the evidence for the diagnosis. The

continued.

Steps of the diagnostic process	Sections of the clinical report
	criteria for this section is: can it stand alone and be read as a "report"? We consider this section to be the most vital of all the sections; it requires considerable writing skill.
	Section VI: Diagnostic statement
	This section is included only for the convenience of the reader. It can be located quickly to obtain an immediate statement of the diagnostician's findings.
Conclusions	Section VII: Recommendations
	This section states as succinctly as possible the management proposal for the patient, including any practical considerations for carrying out the management plan. It should not be just a statement of what the diagnostician recommends but rather it should let the reader know who is to do what, when, and where.

In Appendix V, we have amplified this material by providing examples of information that might be included in each section of the clinical report. We have also included samples of reports written to parents that have been adapted from the clinical report. Keep in mind that these examples are out of context of the remainder of the report.

The diagnostician can teach by the reports he writes. In providing detailed information, the diagnostician can teach other interested professionals something about speech and language beyond the specific patient's problem. Other professionals cannot evaluate the importance or validity of the diagnostician's findings if they know little or nothing about his area of expertise. To illustrate the teaching function of a clinical report, we can draw a reverse example. If a diagnostician receives a report from a physician who says that the electroencephalograph (EEG) findings were normal and stops there, the diagnostician learns little. He would have to find out the meaning of these findings. If the physician has included information about how abnormality is determined and what abnormal findings may mean in terms of brain function, brain injury, and so forth, he then has taught the speech–language pathologist something useful about the profession of neurology. The diagnostician can do the same thing. When he says that speech is deviant, he says little. When he says speech behavior varies from normal in the following ways——he says much more and provides the physician with a broader view of abnormal speech. Many examples could be provided about the teaching role of clinical reports.

We have found professional report writing to be among the most difficult skills to teach. It seems as if some students have the knack and others do not. However, writing reports helps to develop problem-solving discipline. By having to commit himself on paper, the student is forced to think through his interpretations carefully. Even if report writing will later become abbreviated, we feel it is important for students to first develop the skill of writing detailed clinical reports. If he initially learns to write thorough, exacting reports, he can always reduce their length when he becomes accomplished in the diagnostic process and has established himself as a diagnostician.

If report writing is difficult, it may stem from one of two reasons. First, and often the case, is that the diagnostician has not yet developed a clear perspective on the patient and second, that he truly has difficulty writing. In the first instance we would suggest going back over the information and clarifying it until the perspective develops and can be conveyed in written form. In the second instance the only recommendation that can be made is hard work, self-criticism, and write, write, write.

We do offer the following resources as assistance. We mentioned previously that learning how research articles are constructed and written is an important guide to clinical report writing. The article by Forscher and Wertz (1970) can serve as a useful guide. Several other sources are helpful. Hammond and Allen (1953) give extensive information about report writing geared for psychologists and Tallent (1980) for special education. Their ideas and suggestions are equally relevant to the speech–language pathologist. They discuss the tediousness of report writing, and how it can be combatted. A report-writing handbook for students and clinicians has appeared (Knepflar, 1976).

Two other articles, besides being interesting and humorous, provide specific information on report-writing style. Moore (1969) and Jerger (1962) demonstrate via specific examples the poor writing seen in research literature and clinical reports with general rules for correcting these examples. Their emphasis is on clarity and brevity—two aspects of style everyone should hold on to.

One additional general comment about report writing seems unavoidable. The diagnostician must be sure to edit and proofread the final copy once it is typed. This last step, although tedious, serves as a fresh look at what has been written and corrects any number of errors that may occur in the typing process.

COMPLETES ADMINISTRATIVE FOLLOW-UP

In chapter 3 the administrative aspects of the diagnostic process including follow-up were discussed. The diagnostician basically has two roles to play in follow-up. First, he must make sure that all management decisions are carried out or, if not, why they will not be followed through. Second, he will have some function to play in record keeping, of which his clinical reports are one part.

The diagnostician's job is not completed until he knows the final disposition of his patient. This means careful and consistent follow-up. Once again, setting demands often dictate the nature of follow-up responsibilities. If the therapy recommended is done in the same setting as the diagnosis and by the staff member who has done the diagnosis, then it is a matter of scheduling the patient for therapy as soon as the professional has an opening in his schedule. If there is a long waiting list, the diagnostician should feel obligated to refer the patient elsewhere if other services are available. If this is not feasible nor desired by the patient, the diagnostician must make the patient aware of how long he may have to wait for therapy services. In the meantime the diagnostician might put the patient on a once-a-month visit to do a quick check of progress, offering suggestions for things to do while waiting. A periodic telephone call may also help patients during this waiting period. Many patients are lost because contact by the agency is not forthcoming.

The diagnostician should keep a log of each patient seen and the disposition of the patient. Even if scheduling in the agency is done by the administrative support personnel, the diagnostician must be the one who keeps in professional contact until the patient is scheduled. If the patient is scheduled with other staff members in the agency, the diagnostician must be available for consultation and assistance in the scheduling and interpretation of the management plan he has proposed.

More follow-up difficulty is encountered when referrals to other agencies are required. If it is a referral to another agency for therapy, the diagnostician may have to convince the agency to accept the patient without undergoing a second diagnostic process. In communities where the professionals have developed a working relationship based on mutual respect for one another's work this is readily accomplished. Unfortunately, however, many agencies refuse to start the therapy process with a patient diagnosed at an outside agency. In this case, if the diagnostician refers outside for therapy, he must follow through with his recommendation. If possible, he may want to talk directly with the personnel of the outside agency to arrange a time. He should, at least, alert the agency that the patient may be calling for an appointment. He should have obtained permission from the patient to forward the diagnostic information along with his letter of referral. It is the obligation of the agency to which the patient is referred to let the diagnostician know they have accepted and scheduled a patient; however, this is not always done. We feel the diagnostician who has not received such a confirmation should check with the agency referred to so he can know and record in his clinical records the final disposition of the patient.

If therapeutic recommendations are being withheld until an examination is made by another professional to whom the patient has been referred, it is important for the diagnostician to keep on top of the progress made in completing these recommendations. Besides making the purpose of the referral clear to the patient, the diagnostician must make sure that the agency or professional he refers to understands his purpose in making the referral. As with all referrals, the diagnostician should make direct contact with the professional via telephone, referral letter, and reports. He must let the patient know how to go about getting seen by the professional to whom he has been referred. Again, many patients are lost to therapy because of long delays that occur in this process. They may lose patience with the process and give it up as not being worth it.

Record-keeping systems vary significantly in different settings, ranging from basic notations on charts about the predominant symptoms and causes to complex data retrieval systems maintained over the time period the patient is seen. In general practice the records kept are the clinical report followed by a series of log notes recording the day-to-day therapy activities and progress made. This system fulfills the professional's first responsibility, getting the information down accurately for later use by himself or other professionals.

Record keeping, however, forms the basis of much needed research about clinical problems. Therefore, we recommend that each setting in which the diagnostician works develop and maintain a standard, and yet flexible, record-keeping system devised for easy recording and retrieval of information for both clinical and research purposes. The data accumulated during the diagnostic process and the clinical report can serve as the basis for recording data in master data files to facilitate retrieval.

An extensive discussion of data retrieval systems is beyond the scope of this book, but we want to point out some information of interest to the reader. We have moved full blast into the computer age, and as computers are adapted to clinical functions, most of us will become involved in some way with retrieval systems based on computer technology. Several systems of data recording have been reported (1) for general clinical use (Elliott & Vegely, 1971; Elliott et al., 1971), (2) specific to a type of causal disorder, for example, cleft lip and palate (McCabe, 1966), and (3) directed to recording details from a specific test (Van Demark & Tharp, 1973).

Time, personnel, and costs currently prohibit the extensive use of highly complex computerized systems for most settings. But computers are not the only means to record adequate information for retrieval. The intent to keep such information is the primary ingredient for any record-keeping system. Data summary sheets can be utilized to transfer the information collected during the diagnostic process.

In developing the system the diagnostician must begin with a set of objectives that guide his creation of the system. His objectives for the system lead him to consider the amount and type of information to include. Rees et al. (1969) presented a standardized data-recording system to meet the needs of public school clinicians working in the Los Angeles area. The descriptions they provide for setting up their system, although not complex, are similar to systems set up for computers. Regardless of the method of storage and retrieval, the system must have a set of objectives, a system for reducing and recording the data, and a system for facilitating use by the various people who will be using it—either as recorders, storers, transmitters, receivers, or interpreters.

SUMMARY

In this last step of the diagnostic process the diagnostician should be able to fulfill the purposes of diagnosis. All that has gone on before this point has allowed him to delineate the speech and language disorder and to achieve some level of understanding of the causal factors involved. Now he must translate his diagnosis into feedback and payoff for the patient. In summary, the final step of the diagnostic process involves four tasks:

1. The diagnostician will *determine a management plan.* In doing this he needs to know if the patient can change his speech and language disorder with or without direct speech and language therapy. He plans for any referrals that are needed to fulfill the management plan, considering what services are available throughout the community in which he works.

2. Armed with a management plan, the diagnostician then *holds an interpretive conference,* during which he discusses his diagnostic findings and works out the management plan with the patient, including any practical alterations that are needed.

3. The diagnostician then *writes his reports,* the number and type varying with his work setting and special needs for communicating his concerns about the patient. At the very least he will write a clinical report for the agency in which he works, for self-recall, or later use by other professionals.

4. Finally, the diagnostician will need to *complete his administrative follow-up,* seeing to it that all management plans are worked out and appropriate paperwork and record-keeping completed.

KATHERINE COMPARDO

Management plan and interpretive conference

Develop your management plan for Katherine Compardo and consider how you would impart this information in the interpretive conference. In your management plan a referral to a pediatric neurologist should be included. Consider the following questions in your planning: Does she need therapy to change her level of language abilities? How will you explain Katherine's disorder and its causes? How much information do you feel Mrs. Compardo will be able to handle? Could you just describe the language behavior and make the referral? Will you schedule language therapy without the results of the referral?

Consider two approaches for your conference: first, an approach where you describe speech and language of aphasic children; second, an approach where you want causal information to come from the referral.

At this time you may be interested in what such a referral might tell you. We are including here an example of a report that might have been received from the pediatric neurologist. What additional information will it give Mrs. Compardo? This information is provided now for your understanding of what to expect from a referral; the information cannot be used during your interpretive conference with Mrs. Compardo, since it would not yet be available to you.

I saw Katherine Compardo on November 4, 1983. This 2-year, 8-month-old girl has a major problem with delayed speech and a secondary problem of poor gait. According to Mrs. Compardo, her language development is significantly delayed. She still does not talk in more than a few single words or two-word phrases, and the only one she uses consistently is "Here, Ma." Most of the rest of her speech is an occasional portion of a word, and the mother can name maybe six or eight such words and that is the sum extent of expressive language. Mother states she understands everything including two-stage commands. And yet, she does not seem to understand too well in conversation, though one cannot be absolutely sure about this. However, single objects are fairly well understood. She knows more than four body parts, recognized many objects in excess of 50 by name, but still does not point to objects in books. She has poor concentration and does not play for long. She sits close when watching TV and seems to enjoy it.

She was born following a full-term pregnancy. The mother was in labor 3½ hours and had a normal delivery under spinal anesthesia. Birth weight was 8 pounds. Sucking and swallowing were normal, and she was nursed for 3 months. She walked at 14 months. Mother keeps going back to the fact that the child did not cry right from the beginning, that she babbled and cooed little, and that at 3 to 4 months her laugh was most peculiar and unusual. There is no other significant language disability in this family.

Physical examination showed a pleasant-looking youngster with head circumference of 47 cm. The child was irritable and would not concentrate on anything for long. I did not hear any language except a few noises. During periods when she was more friendly, she would look at me, copy all my gestures, mimic facial grimacing, and copy my examination. It is quite clear that this child understands a good deal more by the visual route than any other. With language, she was able to comprehend a fair amount, carry out one-stage commands, and point to some objects, but she soon lost concentration. Her play was repetitive with little concentration and not much imagination. She would carry the doll around and throw it about without any apparent awareness of what she was doing with it.

The eye movements are full, and funduscopic examination was normal. The discs and maculae are unremarkable. Hearing is grossly normal and was not tested further. There is no facial asymmetry. She has no difficulty protruding her tongue and licks a lollipop without much problem. Her motor strength seems unimpaired, the reflexes are symmetric, and plantar flexion is normal.

The mother had a question about an additional problem, namely, poor gait for which she has seen an orthopedic surgeon. I noticed some toeing-in but no serious difficulty here.

This child has a very definite and significant expressive and probably receptive language disorder. I think she would fall into the category of what I would call "moderate developmental language delay" (receptive and expressive aphasia being less good terms for this). There is nothing evident in the neurologic examination that accounts for this. We will schedule an EEG and look into it. Speech therapy plus nursery school are going to be very important for this young lady. The speech pathologist indicated to me in a conversation that comprehension is apparently age level. There is a question on their part about apraxia, but I think that most of what she is showing now represents the expressive language difficulty. There is no doubt that the observation of possible apraxia could be relevant, because as the years go by, we do find that many of these children do show other disorders of learning including significant sensory disorders and perceptual disorders as well as some motor difficulties that are easier to examine at that time. I will let you know the result of the EEG and will also be discussing the management further with the speech pathologist. I thank you for the referral.

Report writing

Now that all the information has been considered for Katherine Compardo, the student should plan and write a clinical report. Since a referral has been recommended for Katherine, we would suggest that a parental letter (report) and a referral letter also be written. These we have found to be especially useful when follow-up beyond therapy is indicated.

PATIENT PROJECTS

The student should now develop management plans, interpretive conference approaches, clinical reports and follow-up for each of the demonstration patients used throughout this book.

STUDY QUESTIONS

1. Develop a list of variables that have been considered as important prognostic indicators for the following speech and language disorders: stuttering in adults, phonologic/phonetic structure problems in elementary school children, adult aphasics, laryngectomees, "aphasic" children, and adults with voice disorders not associated with pathologic conditions.

2. The student should return to the discussion about tools and procedures that provides information about "prognosis for change." What, actually, do these tools tell us? Do they predict overall change in the disorder? Do they predict success in amount of change? Are they related to recovery curves for specific speech and language tasks? How much can we predict from these tools about the overall ability of a patient to alter his disorder? How much do the tools tell us, and how much does our knowledge about the disorder and its causes tell us?

3. Are there any speech and language disorders where you would not expect the patient to change? What are the many variables that have to be considered to answer this prognosis question, such as the effects of maturation, length of time the problem has existed, the severity of the disorder, and its causal basis?

4. Nation (1982) has discussed the concept of speech–language pathology services including the need to develop a cohesive model to guide the treatment process for speech and language disorders. What conclusions did he arrive at regarding the state of the art in our profession?

5. Dreher and Baltes (1973) recommended the use of bibliotherapy as an adjunct to treatment of speech and language disorders. They provide an annotated list of materials they feel will be useful. Can reading materials be developed and distributed to patients and their families as part of the recommendations given for management of the speech and language problem? Review the materials presented by Dreher and Baltes as an initial source of such information.

6. Bangs (1982) recommends the use of summary analysis charts in parent conferencing. The profile charts she discusses with the parents cover the specific areas of testing given the children before and during placement in their treatment program. Can a procedure similar to this be established for routine use in diagnosis of different types of speech and language disorders? How would you do this for children who stutter, have voice problems, or have phonologic disorders?

7. One of the first things diagnosticians should do when they arrive in a new community, on a new job, is to develop a resource book on available community services including the exact name, address and telephone number of the agency; the types of services generally and specifically provided; and the personnel of major contact. As a project, do this for your local hospital. What departments exist in the hospital that may provide you with services or that may refer patients to you for services?

8. Pannbacker (1975) draws on the articles by Jerger (1962) and Moore (1969) in her discussion of diagnostic report writing. What further insights does she offer?

Administrative forms

REQUEST FOR SERVICE

Date_____

Service requested for _____ Birth date _____

Address _____ Phone _____
     (Street)   (City)   (State)   (Zip)

Requested by (referral) _____ Relationship _____

Address of referral source _____ Phone _____

Responsible relative: Name _____

                  Address _____

Address for appointment _____

What seems to be the problem? (Remarks) _____

_____

_____

Any previous evaluations or therapy at (agency name)? Yes _____ No _____

                              Recorded by_____

....

Correspondence record (Please initial each entry.)

	Date sent	Date returned
Acknowledgment, patient history, release forms	_____	_____
Follow-up acknowledgment letter	_____	_____
Letters to other sources (name and address)		
_____	_____	_____
_____	_____	_____
_____	_____	_____
_____	_____	_____

Scheduled for diagnosis: Date _____ Time _____ Diagnostician _____

Appointment letter sent: Date   _____

ACKNOWLEDGMENT OF REQUEST FOR SERVICE

Date_____

To   _____

 _____

 _____

Dear_____:

We have received a request for an appointment for _____ at the Hearing and Speech Center.

In order for our evaluation to be most effective, past history information is needed. We are enclosing a client history form. Please fill it out carefully to the best of your knowledge. The enclosed release forms, which allow us to obtain information from appropriate professional people or agencies (doctors, hospitals, etc.), also need to be signed.

Since we can schedule only a limited number of people, a prompt return of the history and release forms will allow us to give you an earlier appointment. Please use the enclosed self-addressed envelope for your completed forms.

Sincerely,

_____

FOLLOW-UP ACKNOWLEDGMENT LETTER

Date _____

To _____

  _____

  _____

Re _____

  _____

  _____

Dear _____:

On _____ we received a request for a diagnosis for _____ . On _____ history and release forms were sent. These forms need to be completed and returned to our agency before we can schedule an appointment.

If you still desire an appointment, complete the forms and return them to the Hearing and Speech Center by _____. If we do not receive the forms by this date, we will assume that you do not wish to have an appointment at this time. Enclosed please find an extra set of forms for your use.

Sincerely,

_____

CHILDREN'S SPEECH, LANGUAGE, AND HEARING HISTORY

Our evaluation of your child's speech, language, and hearing problems will depend on information about his past history. Fill out the form as completely as possible and return in the enclosed envelope. If there are any items you do not fully understand, put a check mark in the left margin and we can discuss them when you come for your appointment.

Date_____

Person completing this form _____ Relationship to child _____

I. IDENTIFICATION

Name _____ Birth date _____ Sex_____ Age_____
Address _____ Phone_____
Mother's name _____ Address _____ Age_____
Father's name _____ Address _____ Age_____
Referred by _____ Address _____
Family doctor _____ Address _____
Child's pediatrician_____ Address_____

II. STATEMENT OF THE PROBLEM

Describe as completely as possible the speech, language, and hearing problem.
_____
_____
_____

When was the problem first noticed? _____
_____

How has the problem changed since you first noticed it?_____
_____

What has been done about it? Has this helped? _____
_____

What do you think caused the problem? _____
_____

Are there any family members or relatives who have or had speech, language, or hearing problems? _____

Continued.

CHILDREN'S SPEECH, LANGUAGE, AND HEARING HISTORY—Cont'd

III. SPEECH, LANGUAGE, AND HEARING HISTORY

How much did your child babble and coo during the first 6 months? _____
When did he speak his first words? _____ What were the child's first few words? _____
_____

How many words did the child have at 1½ years?_____ When did he begin to use two-word sentences? _____
Does he use speech? Frequently_____ Occasionally_____ Never_____
Does he use many gestures? (Give examples if possible.) _____
_____

Which does the child prefer to use? Complete sentences _____ Phrases _____
One or two words _____ Sounds _____ Gestures _____
Does he make sounds incorrectly?_____ If so, which ones? _____
_____

Does he hesitate, "get stuck," repeat, or stutter on sounds or words? _____
If so, describe. _____
How does his voice sound? Normal_____ Too high_____ Too low_____
Hoarse_____ Nasal_____
How well can he be understood? By his parents _____ By his brothers and sisters and playmates_____ By relatives and strangers_____
Did your child ever acquire speech and then slow down or stop talking? _____
_____

Does he imitate speech but not use it? _____
How well does he understand what is said to him? _____
_____

Does your child hear adequately?_____ Does his hearing appear to be constant or does it vary? ____ Is his hearing poorer when he has a cold? ____
Has your child ever worn a hearing aid? _____ Which ear? _____
How long? _____ Hours per day? _____ Does it seem to help him?

NOTE: If the child has a hearing aid, please bring it and the earmold along with you when you come in for your appointment.

Continued.

CHILDREN'S SPEECH, LANGUAGE, AND HEARING HISTORY—Cont'd

Check these as they apply to your child.

	Yes	No	Explain: give ages if possible
Cried less than normal amount			
Laughed less than normal amount			
Yelled and screeched to attract attention or express annoyance			
Head banging and foot stamping			
Extremely sensitive to vibration			
Very alert to gesture, facial expression, or movement			
Shuffled feet while walking			
Generally indifferent to sound			
Did not respond when spoken to			
Responded to noises (car horns, telephones) but not to speech			
Difficulty using tongue			
Difficulty swallowing			
Talked through nose			
Mouth breather			
Tongue-tied			
Difficulty chewing			
Drooled a lot			
Food came out nose			
Constant throat clearing			
Difficulty breathing			
Large tongue			
Difficulty moving mouth			

Continued.

CHILDREN'S SPEECH, LANGUAGE, AND HEARING HISTORY—Cont'd

IV. GENERAL DEVELOPMENT
A. Pregnancy and birth history

Total number of pregnancies _____ How many miscarriages, stillbirths? _____
Explain. _____
Which pregnancy was this child? __ Length of pregnancy? __ Was it difficult? __
What illnesses, diseases, and accidents occurred during pregnancy? _____
Was there a blood incompatibility between the mother and father? _____
Age of mother at child's birth _____ Age of father at child's birth _____
What was the length of labor? _____ Were there any unusual problems at birth
(breech birth, Caesarean birth, others)? If so, describe._____

What drugs were used? __ High or low forceps? __ Weight of child at birth? __
Were there any bruises, scars, or abnormalities of the child's head? _____
Any other abnormalities?_____

Did infant require oxygen?_____ Was child "blue" or jaundiced at birth?_____
Was a blood transfusion required at birth? _____
Were there any problems immediately following birth or during the first 2 weeks of
the infant's life (health, swallowing, sucking, feeding, sleeping, others)? If so, describe.

At what age did infant regain birth weight? _____

B. Developmental

At what age did the following occur? Held head erect while lying on stomach__
Rolled over alone _____ Sat alone unsupported _____ Crawled _____ Stood
alone ___Walked unaided ___ Fed self with spoon ___ Had first tooth ___
Bladder trained _____Bowel trained _____ Completely toiled trained:
Waking ___ Sleeping ___ Dressed and undressed himself ___ What hand
does he prefer? _____ Has handedness ever been changed? _____ If so,
at what age? How would you describe your child's current physical development?

Continued.

CHILDREN'S SPEECH, LANGUAGE, AND HEARING HISTORY—Cont'd

V. MEDICAL HISTORY

Is your child now under the care of a doctor?_____ Why?_____

Is he taking medication?_____ Type? _____ Why? _____

At what ages did any of the following illnesses, problems, or operations occur? Please indicate how serious they were.

	Age	Mild	Mod.	Severe		Age	Mild	Mod.	Severe
Adenoidectomy					Heart problems				
Allergies					High fevers				
Asthma					Influenza				
Blood disease					Mastoidectomy				
Cataracts					Measles				
Chickenpox					Meningitis				
Chronic colds					Mumps				
Convulsions					Muscle disorder				
Cross-eyed					Nerve disorder				
Croup					Orthodontia				
Dental problems					Pneumonia				
Diptheria					Polio				
Earaches					Rheumatic fever				
Ear infections					Scarlet fever				
Encephalitis					Tonsillectomy				
Headaches					Tonsillitis				
Head injuries					Whooping cough				

Has the child ever fallen or had a severe blow to the head? _____ If so, did he lose consciousness? _____ Did it cause a concussion? _____ Did it cause Nausea _____ Vomiting _____ Drowsiness _____ Describe any other serious illnesses, injuries, operations, or physical problems not mentioned above. _____

_____

What illnesses have been accompanied by an extremely long, high fever?_____

Temperature _____ How long did the fever last? _____

Which of the above required hospitalization?_____

Where was the child hospitalized? _____ For how long?_____

Who was the attending physician? _____

Continued.

CHILDREN'S SPEECH, LANGUAGE, AND HEARING HISTORY—Cont'd

VI. BEHAVIOR

Check these as they apply to your child.

	Yes	No	Explain: give ages if possible.
Eating problems			
Sleeping problems			
Toilet training problems			
Difficulty concentrating			
Needed a lot of discipline			
Underactive			
Excitable			
Laughs easily			
Cried a lot			
Difficult to manage			
Overactive			
Sensitive			
Personality problem			
Gets along with children			
Gets along with adults			
Emotional			
Stays with an activity			
Makes friends easily			
Happy			
Irritable			
Prefers to play alone			

How do you discipline your child? _____

What are the child's favorite play activities? _____

Continued.

CHILDREN'S SPEECH, LANGUAGE, AND HEARING HISTORY—Cont'd

VII. EDUCATIONAL HISTORY

Did child attend day care or nursery school? _____ Where? _____ Ages _____
Kindergarten? _____ Where? _____ Ages _____
School now attending _____ Address _____
Grade he is now in _____ Grades skipped _____ Grades failed _____
What are his average grades? _____ Best subjects _____ Poorest _____
Is the child frequently absent from school? _____ If so, why? _____
How does child feel about school and about his teacher? _____
_____

What is your impression of your child's learning abilities? _____
_____
_____

Has anyone ever thought he was a slow child? _____
_____

Describe any speech, language, hearing, psychological, and special education services that have been performed including where this was done. How often was your child seen in this service? _____
_____
_____

Continued.

CHILDREN'S SPEECH, LANGUAGE, AND HEARING HISTORY—Cont'd

VIII. HOME AND FAMILY INFORMATION

Father's occupation _____ Last grade completed in school_____
Mother occupation _____ Last grade completed in school_____

Brothers and sisters:

Name	Age	Sex	Grade in school	Speech, hearing, or medical problem
1.				
2.				
3.				
4.				
5.				
6.				
7.				
8.				

Are there any other languages spoken in the home? _____ If so, by whom and how often?_____

Home and neighborhood (check all that apply): Residential_____ Business area _____ House _____ Rural _____ Above average _____ Housing development _____ Excellent condition _____ Apartment area _____ Average _____ Crowded _____ Suburban_____ Number of rooms?_____ Members of household other than family?_____

Primary source of income (check the appropriate blanks): Salary _____ Hourly wages _____ Commission _____ Welfare _____ Profits and fees _____ Savings and investments_____ Other_____

Please add any additional information you feel will help us in understanding your child and his problem: _____

_____

_____

_____

_____

_____

_____

_____

_____

_____

PATIENT HISTORY: APHASIA

Our evaluation of your speech and language difficulties will depend on information about your past history. Fill out the form as completely as possible and return in the enclosed envelope. No appointment is given until the form has been returned and evaluated.

NOTE: *All information given is kept confidential.*

Date _____

Person completing this form _____

Relationship to patient_____

I. IDENTIFICATION

Name_____ Sex_____ Age_____

Address _____ Phone_____
　　　　　(Street)　　　(City)　　　(State)　　(Zip)

Birth date_____ Birthplace _____
　　　　(Month)　(Day)　(Year)

Referred by _____

Address _____ Phone_____
　　　　　(Street)　　　(City)　　　(State)　　(Zip)

II. PERSONAL AND FAMILY HISTORY

Marital status: Single__Married__Separated__Divorced__Widowed__Remarried__

Spouse's name _____Address _____
　　　　　　　　　　　　　　　　　　　　　　　　(Street)　(City)　(State)

Spouse's occupation _____

Children:

Name	Age	Living		Address
		Yes	No	
1.				
2.				
3.				
4.				
5.				

Do you have brothers and sisters? Number_____ List ages_____

Continued.

PATIENT HISTORY: APHASIA—Cont'd

III. MEDICAL HISTORY

When did the illness or accident occur? Date _____
Describe the illness or accident: _____
_____

Were you unconscious? ____ Paralyzed? ____ Did you have convulsions? ____
If yes, describe. _____
How soon were you seen by a physician? _____
Physician's name _____ Address _____
Were you hospitalized? _____ If yes, how long? _____
Name of hospital _____ Address _____
If not hospitalized, describe how you were cared for._____
_____

Are you now under a physician's care?_____ If yes, for what reason?_____
_____

Physician's name _____ Address _____
Are you now taking medication? _____ Name and dosage _____
Are you responsible for taking your medication? _____
Your health before this illness or accident was: Excellent__ Average__ Fair__ Poor__
Before this illness or accident have you ever had a: Heart condition? ____ High
blood pressure? ____ Previous strokes? ____ Seizures? ____ Fainting spells? ____
Describe any other serious illnesses, accidents, and operations you have had.

When	Problem	Where hospitalized	Attending physician
1.			
2.			
3.			
4.			
5.			

Describe any visual problems you have. _____
_____ Glasses? Yes_____ No_____
Describe any hearing problems you have. _____
_____ Hearing Aid? Yes_____ No_____
Please give information below about any of the following services you have had.

	Date or dates	Person/agency	Address
Speech/language examination			
Speech/language therapy			
Hearing examination			
Psychological testing/ counseling			
Vocational counseling			
Physical therapy			
Occupational therapy			

Continued.

PATIENT HISTORY: APHASIA—Cont'd

IV. EDUCATIONAL HISTORY

University

Circle highest grade completed: 1 2 3 4 5 6 7 8 9 10 11 12   1 2 3 4
Graduate school degree? Yes ___ No ___ Area of university study or specialization.

_____

Describe any other education or special training. _____

_____

_____

V. EMPLOYMENT HISTORY

Last occupation _____ How long? _____
Employer _____
Address _____
               (Street)   (City)   (State)   (Zip)
Are you still employed? _____ What present employment arrangement do you
have with your employer? _____

_____

Describe briefly the type of work you were doing in your past occupations. ____

_____

Check here if you are a housewife. _____ What are your primary sources of
income? (Check all the appropriate blanks.) Salary _____ Hourly wages _____
Commission _____ Savings and investments _____ Profits and fees _____ Public
welfare _____ Other (Please give details). _____

_____

_____

_____

VI. SPEECH AND LANGUAGE HISTORY

In what country have you lived most of your life? _____ What is
your native language? _____ What other languages do you speak,
understand, read, or write? _____ What languages
other than English do you speak at home? _____ When
did the present speech difficulty begin? _____ What was your
speech like at that time? _____
How has it changed? _____

_____

Describe any speech problems you had before this illness or accident. _____

_____

_____

_____

_____

_____

Continued.

PATIENT HISTORY: APHASIA—Cont'd

VI. SPEECH AND LANGUAGE HISTORY—Cont'd

The following items are very important for helping us plan our test procedures so as to keep the time spent in evaluation at a minimum. Please check as carefully as possible those items you can and cannot do.

I CAN   I CANNOT

Language and Speech

I CAN	I CANNOT	
_____	_____	Indicate meaning by pointing or gesture
_____	_____	Say a word if I write it first
_____	_____	Repeat words spoken by others
_____	_____	Articulate sounds
_____	_____	Say words
_____	_____	Say short phrases
_____	_____	Say short sentences
_____	_____	Talk without using "roundabout" way of getting meaning across
_____	_____	Speak with relative fluency
_____	_____	Be easily understood
_____	_____	Relate a story read or seen on television
_____	_____	Carry on a telephone conversation

Comprehension

I CAN	I CANNOT	
_____	_____	Understand single spoken words
_____	_____	Understand simple spoken sentences
_____	_____	Understand conversational speech with one person
_____	_____	Understand conversational speech with several persons
_____	_____	Follow radio or television speech
_____	_____	Understand spoken directions
_____	_____	Recognize objects
_____	_____	Understand the use of these objects
_____	_____	Understand everything I listen to

Reading

I CAN	I CANNOT	
_____	_____	Read signs with understanding
_____	_____	Read numbers with understanding
_____	_____	Read single words with understanding
_____	_____	Read newspaper headlines with understanding
_____	_____	Read magazine articles with understanding
_____	_____	Read books with understanding
_____	_____	Tell time

Writing

I CAN	I CANNOT	
_____	_____	Copy numbers, letters, or words
_____	_____	Write my name by myself
_____	_____	Write single words by myself
_____	_____	Write short sentences by myself
_____	_____	Write personal letters by myself
_____	_____	Write creatively by myself

PATIENT HISTORY: APHASIA—Cont'd

VII. DAILY BEHAVIOR

I CAN   I CANNOT

Orientation

I CAN	I CANNOT	
_____	_____	Remember past events
_____	_____	Remember events relative to my accident or illness
_____	_____	Remember recent events
_____	_____	Find my way about my home town
_____	_____	Find my way about a strange town

Daily living

I CAN	I CANNOT	
_____	_____	Do simple arithmetic
_____	_____	Dress myself
_____	_____	Tie shoes
_____	_____	Tie necktie
_____	_____	Handle all bathroom needs by myself
_____	_____	Shower myself
_____	_____	Shave myself
_____	_____	Handle money
_____	_____	Plan my own activities
_____	_____	Go shopping alone
_____	_____	Answer the telephone

Walking

I CAN	I CANNOT	
_____	_____	Walk unaided by myself
_____	_____	Walk with leg brace
_____	_____	Walk with cane
_____	_____	Rise to a standing position from a seated position without assistance
_____	_____	Seat myself from a standing position

Eating

I CAN	I CANNOT	
_____	_____	Eat unassisted
_____	_____	Eat with special eating utensils

Using hands

I CAN	I CANNOT	
_____	_____	Use both hands easily for all tasks
_____	_____	Use right hand easily for all tasks
_____	_____	Use left hand easily for all tasks
_____	_____	Open doors easily by myself

Were you right- or left-handed before the present illness or accident?
Right_____   Left_____

Continued.

PATIENT HISTORY: APHASIA—Cont'd

VII. DAILY BEHAVIOR—Cont'd

Check those hobbies and interests that apply to you.

Reading

____ Books
____ Magazines
____ Newspapers

Music

____ Play instrument
____ Listening
____ Going to concerts
____ Other_____
       (Specify)

Sports

____ Baseball
____ Football
____ Basketball
____ Hockey
____ Golf

Writing

____ Letters
____ Other_____
       (Specify)

Interests

____ Gardening
____ Cooking
____ Sewing
____ Fishing
____ Boating
____ Traveling, Sights
____ Painting
____ Other_____
       (Specify)

How many hours per day do you watch television?_____

VIII. HOME

Housing (Please check.): House ____ Apartment building ____ Apartment over a business _____ Other (Please describe.) _____

How many rooms? _____ Members of household other than family? _____

Neighborhood (Check all that best describe your neighborhood.):
Residential ____ Business ____ Poor ____ Rural ____ Above average ____
Crowded ____ Average ____ Run-down ____ Excellent ____ Suburban ____
Tenement_____ Housing development_____

Please date and sign these release forms that allow the Hearing and Speech Center to obtain appropriate information from other professional persons or agencies.

Authorization to obtain information

I hereby authorize _____
(Source from whom information is to be obtained)

to release information regarding _____to the Hearing
(Name of patient)

and Speech Center.

Signed _____ Date_____
(By the patient or responsible relative)

Authorization to obtain information

I hereby authorize _____
to release information regarding _____to the Hearing
and Speech Center.

Signed _____ Date _____

Authorization to obtain information

I hereby authorize _____
to release information regarding _____to the Hearing
and Speech Center.

Signed _____ Date _____

Authorization to obtain information

I hereby authorize _____
to release information regarding _____to the Hearing
and Speech Center.

Signed _____ Date _____

REQUEST FOR INFORMATION

Date_____

To   _____
          _____
          _____
          _____

Dear _____ :

_____ has requested an evaluation at the Hearing and Speech Center for_____ In order for our evaluation to be complete, no appointments are given until pertinent history has been obtained. It has been suggested that you would be able to give us helpful information. Please provide us with information in the areas checked below:

____Birth history   ____School adjustment
____General development   ____Behavioral problems
____Health history   ____Physical therapy
____Operations   ____Emotional adjustment
____Physical defects   ____Psychological evaluation
____Occupational therapy   ____Psychometrics
____Vision   ____Speech and hearing problems
____ENT examination   ____Vocational guidance
____Neurologic examination   ____Other_____

Enclosed please find a signed authorization allowing you to send us the desired information.

Sincerely,

_____

SCHEDULING FORM

Name _____ Birth date_____ Age_____ Center No._____
    (Last)   (First)

Address _____ Phone _____ Agency No._____

_____ CBR No._____

Assignment by _____Date _____

Suggested schedule

Problem _____

_____

Staff, group, or program _____

Days_____ Times _____Reeval:Month _____
Year_____Notations _____

_____

_____

_____

Management decision (check)
Add _____
Reevaluation _____
Change _____
Transfer-reschedule _____
Drop-reschedule _____
Drop-closure _____
Drop-close-reeval_____

Routing (date and initial)
Dept. office (A-R)_____
Scheduling _____
Dept. office (T-D) _____
Scheduling (DCR) _____

Current schedule

	Staff	Days	Times	I	G
1.					
2.					
3.					
4.					
5.					

New schedule

	Staff accepting	Days	Times	I	G	Beg. date
1.						
2.						
3.						
4.						
5.						

APPOINTMENT LETTER: INFORMATION FOR CHILDREN

Date_____

To _____

_____

_____

Dear_____ :

_____ has been scheduled for an evaluation at the Hearing and Speech Center on _____ . This appointment time has been set aside for you alone; however, if for any reason you are unable to keep the appointment, please let us know a day or so in advance so we can use the time for someone else. On the day of your appointment please arrive on time since we have a lot to do in the 1½ hour evaluation. Although we try to complete our evaluation in one appointment, there are times when we have to ask that you return for a second visit.

Oftentimes children and their parents do not know what to expect from their visit here. While here, a Speech-Language Pathologist will be testing your child's speech and language abilities. The tests used require the child to name pictures; to repeat words, sounds, and sentences; to talk about pictures, etc. He will also be asked to listen carefully to instructions so we can find out how well he understands speech and language. We sometimes will do an examination of your child's mouth. Here we are interested in how the tongue, jaw, lips, etc. are used in speech. This examination is in no way painful for the child. If indicated, we often give your child a hearing test using an audiometer and earphones. This is an easy task for most children requiring them to listen carefully to different tones and then let us know if he hears them. Sometimes this testing is done in a special soundproof room.

Like most of us, children are afraid of the unknown. They are more relaxed and cooperative when they know ahead of time where they are going and what they will be doing. This is where part of the parent's work comes in. The following are general guidelines of what some parents have found helpful, although preparation should fit your particular child.

1. Tell him he is coming to the center.
2. Tell him that most children have fun.
3. Tell him it is a place very much like school. This is especially helpful for children under 5 years of age who have older brothers and sisters in school; however, a suggestion like this would not be helpful for a child who hates school.
4. Tell him about our special rooms for testing and our tests.
5. Be sure he understands there is nothing in our evaluation that will hurt in anyway.

If we can be of further assistance in helping you prepare your child or answer any questions, please call me at the center. We are looking forward to meeting you and your child.

Sincerely,

_____

RELEASE FORM

Authorization is given to the Hearing and Speech Center to release information concerning

Name _____   Date _____
Address _____   Birth date _____
_____

to the following persons or agencies:

1. Name _____
   Address _____
   _____

2. Name _____
   Address _____
   _____

3. Name _____
   Address _____
   _____

Signed _____
Relationship to patient_____

NOTE: Reports may be sent *only* to the sources listed above. Requests for reports made by other sources must be accompanied by a separate release form.

Patient Projects

REQUEST FOR SERVICE: William Gafford
Speech and Hearing Clinic
2897 Berkshire Road
Chile, Ohio 12142

Area code 216
321-3981

Date   *October 17, 1983*

Service requested for   *Reverend William G. Gafford*   Birth date   *2-18-1937*

Address   *173 E. 86th St. Chile, Ohio 12142*   Phone   *321-0214*
          (Street)   (City)   (State) (Zip)

Requested by (referral)   *Drs. G. Gershon and L. Lefkoff*

Relationship   *Ear, Nose, and Throat Specialists*

Address of referral source   *Parkway Medical Center*   Phone   *368-2381*

Responsible relative: Name   *Mrs. Tillie Gafford*

          Address   *Same*

Address for appointment   *Same*

What seems to be the problem? (Remarks)   *Hoarse voice from ulcers on my vocal cords.*
When I was young, my voice never changed until my professor told me to lower it. Two years ago my
throat started to bother me and I got hoarse. I had an operation and it was better, but now it feels like
something is in my throat all the time.

Any previous evaluations or therapy at SHC?   Yes _____   No   ✓

                    Recorded by   *Matkin*

- -

Correspondence record (Please initial each entry.)

	Date sent	Date returned
Acknowledgment, patient history, release forms		
Follow-up acknowledgment letter		
Letters to other sources (name and address) *Called Gershon and Lefkoff following call*	*10-17-83*	*10-19-83*
from Rev. Gafford. They will send a referral letter.		

Scheduled for diagnosis: Date   *10-19-83*   Time   *9:00*   Diagnostician   *Seligman*

Appointment letter sent: Date _____

REFERRAL LETTER: William Gafford

October 19, 1983

Dorothy M. Aram, Ph.D.
Speech and Hearing Clinic
2897 Berkshire Road
Chile, Ohio 12142

Dear Dr. Aram:

We have seen Rev. William Gafford on several occasions for complaints of hoarseness, aphonia, and laryngeal pain. Rev. Gafford is plagued with recurring hoarseness that we feel is secondary to vocal abuse. After prolonged speaking, he has developed contact ulcerations on the posterior aspect of the vocal cords. We have treated these ulcerations with vocal rest and they do improve. However, we are referring him for voice therapy in the hope that recurrence of the contact ulcers can be prevented by removing the cause and establishing better speaking habits.

We would appreciate a report of your evaluation. Should you need more information, please feel free to contact us.

Sincerely yours,

Gerald Gershon, M.D.
Lewis Lefkoff, M.D.

GG/LL:val

CONSULT NOTES: Isadore Alexander

Department of Otolaryngology
University of Hospitals
923 Spaight Road
Loami, Illinois 82233

Identification information   Date: September 20, 1983

Name: Isadore Alexander
Address: 147 Orton Court
　　　　　Loami, Illinois 82233
Birth date: August 4, 1915
Age: 68

Consult notes

I saw Mr. Alexander today on referral from Dr. William Fowles who saw him on recommendation from Dr. Lee Uransky. Mr. Alexander's chief complaint was hoarseness. Findings were negative.

IMPRESSION: Functional dysarthria
COMMENT: I advise speech therapy for Mr. Alexander.

Jarius Lambert, M.D.

LETTER OF INFORMATION: Isadore Alexander

William Fowles, M.D.
Practice Limited to Otolaryngology
Loami Medical Building
1523 West Monroe Street
Loami, Illinois 82233

September 25, 1983

Dear Dr. Eichelberger:

My only contact with Mr. Alexander was very brief. I saw him on June 15, 1983, on referral from Dr. Uransky. Mr. Alexander complained of hoarseness and blurred speech. I could find no laryngeal pathology, although I did hear the hoarseness and the blurred speech. I did a hearing test that was essentially negative, a slight loss in the high frequencies. I did not feel equipped to handle this man's complaint, so I referred him to Dr. Lambert at University Hospitals.

Sincerely,

William Fowles, M.D.

LETTER OF INFORMATION: Isadore Alexander

Lee Uransky, M.D.
Practice Limited to Neurology and Neurosurgery
Loami Medical Building
1532 West Monroe Street
Loami, Illinois 82233

September 25, 1983

Dear Dr. Eichelberger:

I am pleased to hear that Mr. Alexander is being seen for speech services. I had recommended that to him when I saw him on May 20, 1983, but did not feel he would follow through. When I saw him, his voice was hoarse and he exhibited a bizarre speech pattern. His speech was slow with little affect. My neurologic examination was negative, and I felt this man was demonstrating a functional speech disorder perhaps secondary to some organic mental changes. His personality and anxiety about his condition led me to suspect some possible psychiatric implications. I referred him to Dr. Fowles for further consultation.

Sincerely,

Lee Uransky, M.D.

LETTER OF INFORMATION: Derek Park

September 22, 1983

Mr. Maurice Posch, M.A.
Iles Elementary School
1818 So. 14th Street
Springfield, Illinois 82233

Dear Mr. Posch:

Derek Park was born June 10, 1978, with a left complete cleft lip and palate following a full-term pregnancy. The repair of the lip was performed on July 12, 1978.

On July 12, 1979, a bone graft was performed to the anterior cleft area. On November 2, 1979, the cleft palate was repaired.

He was last seen in my office on November 7, 1982. It was my feeling that there was a fair amount of nasal escape.

I would appreciate a report from you after completion of your evaluation.

Very truly yours,

M. Sugarman, M.D.

MS:val

LETTER OF INFORMATION: Derek Park

September 21, 1983

Mr. Maurice Posch, M.A.
Iles Elementary School
1818 So. 14th Street
Springfield, Illinois 82233

Dear Mr. Posch:

When Derek Park last came to the Cleft Palate Clinic, there was an evaluation of his speech. It was generally immature with articulation defects related to this immaturity. His problems with weak and nasally emitted fricatives, however, seem to be the effect of poor velopharyngeal pressure. It is felt that better articulation may be stimulated by intensive speech therapy when Derek starts school.

Although Mr. and Mrs. Park have agreed with our recommendation, it should be noted that in the past we have found Mrs. Park to be somewhat evasive and passively resistive. She does follow through but seems to "hold back."

Please send your report to our Cleft Palate Clinic.

Sincerely yours,

Lois Fry, Ph.D.
Speech Pathologist

LF:val

REQUEST FOR SERVICE: James E. Matkin
Eastern Speech and Hearing Clinic
2661 Coventry Road
Cleveland, Ohio 44106

Area code 216
444-8223

Date   *September 15, 1983*

Service requested for   *James E. Matkin*   Birth date   *7-17-60*

Address   *423 E. 96th St. Cleveland, Ohio   44105*   Phone   *822-1933*
            (Street)   (City)   (State) (Zip)

Requested by (referral)   *Al Butts—BVR*   Relationship   *Vocational Counselor*

Address of referral source   *Room 104—Eastern Speech and Hearing Clinic*

Phone   *444-8223 Ext. 406*

Responsible relative: Name   *Betty Matkin — Mother*

            Address   *Same*

Address for appointment   *Same*

What seems to be the problem? (Remarks)   *Stuttering*

_____

_____

Any previous evaluations or therapy at ESCH?   Yes _____   No _✓__

                                    Recorded by   *Gretchen Redlands*

....

Correspondence record (Please initial each entry.)

	Date sent	Date returned
		Rec'd 9-15-83
Acknowledgment, client history, release forms		*with referral*
Follow-up acknowledgment letter	_____	_____
Letters to other sources (name and address)		
_____	_____	_____
_____	_____	_____
_____	_____	_____

Scheduled for diagnosis: Date   *9-20-83*   Time   *9:00*   Diagnostician   *J. Nation*

Appointment letter sent: Date   *Telephone appointment 9-18-83*

REFERRAL LETTER: James E. Matkin

September 9, 1983

Eastern Speech and Hearing Center
2661 Coventry Road
Cleveland, Ohio 44106

Dear Sirs:

We have accepted James E. Matkin as a client for vocational rehabilitation services. As part of those services, we are requesting a speech evaluation for his stuttering disability.

James has previously worked in a cemetery as a groundskeeper for 3 years and for 3 years as a truck driver for his mother's catering service. We have no other reports available nor has James had any special training for any particular job skills.

We would like a speech evaluation and a request for therapy and amount of therapy if applicable. Enclosed is the history questionnaire completed by Mr. Matkin.

Sincerely,

Al Butts
Vocational Counselor
Bureau of Vocational Rehabilitation
Room 104
Eastern Speech and Hearing Clinic

AB:jen
Encl.: (1)

HISTORY QUESTIONNAIRE: James E. Matkin

Eastern Speech and Hearing Clinic
2661 Coventry Road
Cleveland, Ohio 44106

1. Name of client *James E. Matkin*	Sex *Male*	Date of birth *July 17, 1960*

2. Your address *432 East 96th Street*	Phone no. *822-1933*

3. Where are you employed and for how long?

    Unemployed

4. What is your occupation? (Briefly describe what you do.)

    Driver and maintenance

5. Name and address of person who recommended this center to you

    Mr. Al Butts, Bureau of Vocational Rehabilitation

FAMILY HISTORY

6. Name of wife/husband *None*	His/her occupation

7. Names of children	Age	Sex	Speech problem	Remarks
a.				
b.				
c.				

8. What other relatives have a speech problem? Is it similar to yours?

    None

Continued.

HISTORY QUESTIONNAIRE: James E. Matkin—Cont'd

MEDICAL

---

9. List any serious illnesses, injuries, childhood diseases, and operations. Give dates and length of disabilities. Include any physical handicaps, prolonged fevers, convulsions, after effects, etc.

   Tonsils—5 years old
   Appendix—11 years old

---

10. Describe any past or present hearing problems. This to include any history of hearing loss, ear infections, ear surgery, etc.

    None

---

11. Do you have a medical problem now that may be related to your speech problem? State whether or not you are presently under the care of a physician, and whether you are taking any medication.

    None

---

12. What hand do you use for skills such as writing?	Have you ever changed hands? If so, when and why?
Right	*No*

EDUCATION

13. Schools attended	Where	What grade
a. *Garfield Heights*	*Garfield Heights*	*11*
b		
c.		
d.		

14. Describe your speech problem.

   I have been stuttering for as long as I can remember

Continued.

HISTORY QUESTIONNAIRE: James E. Matkin—Cont'd

---

15. What do you think caused your speech problem?

    I don't know.

---

16. How do you feel your speech problem has affected your social life?

    It is difficult to really have meaningful relationships with people when you have a hard time expressing yourself.

---

17. How do you feel your speech problem has affected your occupation?

    I can't get employment that involves talking to other people.

---

18. If you didn't have a speech problem, how would your life be different?

    I know I would be able to lead a fuller life than what I am now.

---

19. Describe the reaction of people, including your immediate family, to your speech problem.

    They try and act like they don't notice it.

---

20. If you have received previous help with your speech problem, give details such as from whom, when, where, how long, etc.

    None

---

21. What have you tried to do to correct your speech problem?

    I have tried to talk slower.

---

22. Write down any additional informmation you feel will help us in understanding your speech problem.

    It's a bad habit that I have had for as long as I can remember.

Signature: _____

DISCHARGE SUMMARY I: Marie Abadie

Kankakee General Hospital
Kankakee, Illinois 30603

Name: Marie Abadie

Admitted: 4/28/83

Discharged: 5/22/83

Neurology-Neurosurgery

6 West

Diagnosis: Left internal carotid artery aneurysm

Procedures:
1. Clamp application left internal carotid artery
2. Ligation left internal carotid artery
3. Right brachial arteriogram
4. Left carotid arteriogram

Reason for admission: Severe headache and nuchal rigidity

Present illness: This 57-year-old white female tried to change her position to rest her head while watching television but on twisting her body felt a sudden severe pain in her head. The pain radiated down the spine to her back and right thigh. She was grasping and wringing her arms and trying to hold onto something. She was awake until the following morning but remembers nothing. She was seen by her private physician who referred her to this hospital.

Past medical history: Reveals no history of headache, dizziness, hypertension, or trauma. Operations include bilateral exploration for chocolate cyst of the ovaries and subtotal hysterectomy at St. Alexis Hospital in 1963; underwent thyroidectomy for adenoma of thyroid in 1974; allergy to codeine; smoking—history of a package of cigarettes a day for many years.

Physical examination: Reveals an alert, conscious, coherent female who is in no acute distress. She is cooperative and complaining of mild to moderate headache. Her general physical examination including cardiovascular system is entirely normal. Pulses are 2+ and equal with bruits. Neurologically, the patient is alert to time and place. Her cranial nerve examination was entirely normal as was the remainder of the general neurologic examination including her reflexes. The patient does have moderate stiffness in neck flexion and rotation.

Laboratory and x-ray data: Includes hematocrit of 40% and white blood cell count of 12,600 with a normal differential count. Urinalysis and SMA-12 were entirely normal. Chest and skull x-ray films and brain scan were entirely normal.

Hospital course: The patient was placed on bed rest and underwent initial lumbar puncture that revealed grossly bloody fluid. Protein cerebrospinal fluid was 26 mg/100 ml, and sugar was 91 mg/100 ml. The patient underwent a right brachial arteriogram that was entirely normal. (Lumbar puncture opening pressure was 140 mm H_2O.) The patient underwent a right retrobrachial arteriogram that was entirely normal followed in 4 days by left carotid arteriogram that revealed a long, lobulated left internal carotid artery aneurysm. The patient at this time exhibited dilation of her left pupil with slight ptosis on the left, which improved over the next several days. She remained afebrile and had gradual diminution of her headache over the next several days. Her repeat lumbar puncture revealed 13,000 red blood cells and normal pressure. The patient remained perfectly alert with minimum symptoms. On May 11, 1983, she underwent application of a Ferguson clamp to her left internal carotid artery. Some difficulty was encountered in maintaining the clamp's pressure, but the patient evidenced no neurologic difficulty throughout this time. Following the application of the clamp, she states that her diplopia, which had been present for several days, had been resolved. She underwent removal of the clamp and ligation of her left internal carotid artery on May 13, 1983, and postoperatively remained entirely normal afebrile and asymptomatic. She was finally discharged on the ninth day postligation, ambulating with no neurologic deficit. She was discharged on no medication. Follow-up through Dr. White's office.

Discharge diagnoses: As noted above.

Denise Aronson, M.D.

DISCHARGE SUMMARY II: Marie Abadie

Kankakee General Hospital
Kankakee, Illinois 30603

Name: Marie Abadie   Neurology-Neurosurgery
Admitted: 5/23/83   6 West
Discharged: 6/13/83

Diagnosis: 1. Left Cerebrovascular accident
                    2. Left internal carotid artery aneurysm, status postligation of left
                       internal carotid artery May 13, 1983

Procedures: Lumbar puncture

Reason for admission: Sudden onset of aphasia at home.

Present illness: This 57-year-old white female, discharged on May 22, 1983, following successful left internal carotid artery ligation for treatment of left internal carotid artery aneurysm, had experienced a benign postoperative course and was fully ambulatory when discharged. She did well at home on only moderate activity. Having spent a quiet evening asleep, she was noted on the morning of admission to be entirely well but was found that afternoon by her friend lying on the floor unable to speak with a right hemiparesis. She was brought to the hospital immediately.

Past medical history: Please see old chart.

Physical examination: Revealed an alert patient who was trying to sit up. She was very calm; she was gazing to all fields, left more than right; she was not moving her right side, and she seemed to recognize people by smiling. Pulse was 80 and regular. Blood pressure was 160/80 mm Hg; respirations were 60; temperature was 36.5°C. The general physical examination revealed carotids that were 2+ and full. General physical examination was entirely normal and her neurologic examination revealed her mental status to be as stated previously. She was unable to follow commands or to verbalize. Cranial nerves all revealed no response to threat on the right side. The discs were both sharp. Her doll's eye movements were full without nystagmus. There was no ptosis, and her pupils were equal and rapidly reactive to light. She had a decreased corneal reflex on the right. There was normal sensation to pin prick on the face. She had inability to test lower cranial nerves. Motor examination revealed hemiparesis on the right with increased tone, lower extremity greater than upper extremity. Reflexes were 3+ on the right with an 8+ and upgoing toe, normal on the left. Sensory examination revealed bilateral response to pin prick with no motor response on the right side. The patient was gazing 2 to left and disregarding the right. Cerebellar function not tested.

Laboratory and x-ray data Included hematocrit of 35% and white blood cell count 17,000/cu mm. Normal urinalysis. Chest and skull x-rays and brain scan normal. Electrolytes were generally normal.

Hospital course: The patient was placed on bed rest. Lumbar puncture was done with an opening pressure of 110 mm H_2O. Cells revealed 3 to 6 white blood cells, 0 to 1 red blood cells, sugar, protein and culture negative. The sugar was 18 mg/100 ml and protein 15 mg/100 ml. The patient was essentially placed on bed rest over the next several days. It was felt that she had experienced a left cerebrovascular accident related in some way to a stressful social situation. It was later discovered that the patient had been presented with multiple bills and announcement of foreclosure because of her past due mortgage payments. Over the next several days she exhibited normal reflexes with downgoing toes and no ankle clonus and gradual and persistent return of strength on her right side. However, her speech remained with marked deficits in that she had a marked and mixed receptive aphasia and for a full 2 weeks could only respond by saying, "Ah, you." She was able to write her name. She could at times demonstrate full sentences and solve simple problems. She could count by mimicry and she said reasonable sentences; she says "Hello" and "Goodby" and "Thank you." She remained very anxious and was desirous to return home throughout all of her course. She is being transferred to the rehabilitation unit where Dr. Sandy Mayfield will follow her for speech and language services.

Discharge diagnosis: As noted above.

                                                            Denise Aronson, M.D.

SPEECH PATHOLOGY FINDINGS: Marie Abadie

Kankakee General Hospital
Kankakee, Illinois 30603

Name: Marie Abadie   Rehabilitation Unit
Admitted: 6/13/83   3 West
Tested: 6/14/83

This information will be presented as a sequence of tasks used for testing Marie Abadie, pointing out certain features for analysis consideration. This is not to be considered as all the testing and information that was obtained on Ms. Abadie.

A.   Test samples used to measure
     1. Fluency in
     2. Comprehension of   } Semantics, syntactics, and phonemics
     3. Formulation of
     4. Repetition of

B.   The emphasis of the tasks is on verbal output as related to the above processes. The attempt is to discover processing deficits for planning therapy around language processing rather than on specific language products that are deviant.

C.   On all tasks given observations should be made about all processes and behaviors elicited by the task.

D.   Tasks
     1. Fluency measures elicited by two tasks from the Boston Diagnostic Aphasia Examination
        a. Spontaneous speech sample requiring
           (1) General biographical information
           (2) Yes/no response
           (3) Descriptive answers
        b. More confrontation situations in which Marie has to describe or tell a story about a picture that involves a cookie theft. This task should be more difficult since it is tied to a specific stimulus that is unfamiliar information.
        c. Responses to this task
           (1) Rate: slow; generally under 50 words/minute
           (2) Prosody was abnormal—slow and halting
           (3) Pronunciation was abnormal
               (a)   Sounds or syllables have slipped out of sequence, have been deleted, or are entirely extraneous to desired response; but more than half of the response corresponds to more than half of the required word. Use of one phoneme for another or a breakdown in the word structure but the meaning of the word is preserved.
           (4) Phrase length was short, which relates to the slow and halting speech.
           (5) Effort in initiation is noted, and this can be seen in the abnormal prosody and short phrase lengths. Facial grimacing and body movements used as attempts to facilitate speech production.
           (6) Pauses are frequent.
               (a)   According to Boston Diagnostic Aphasia Examination, pauses are more for articulation difficulties
               (b)   Pauses are attempts to correct error or to decide to continue despite errors

Continued.

SPEECH PATHOLOGY FINDINGS: Marie Abadie—Cont'd

D. Tasks—Cont'd

  (c) Pauses result because the patient cannot continue because of difficulty producing the words

  (d) Patient who demonstrates effort to produce words will pause preceding and following phonation

  (e) May be pauses for word finding but mostly for difficulty in initiating proper phoneme

  (7) Word choice was mostly substantive words with grammatical errors noted. More concentration and effort noted when Marie is attempting to use pronouns, tenses, and functor words.

  (8) Up to this point comprehension skills appear intact.

  2. Comprehension task from the *Minnesota Test for Differential Diagnosis of Aphasia*

  a. Semantic: patient points to appropriate letter named

  b. Syntactic

  (1) Identifying three items named serially

  (2) Following directions

  c. Responses to the comprehension tasks

  (1) No errors made

  3. Formulation tasks: a variety of tasks for naming, producing sentences, cloze procedures, describing pictures, etc.

  a. Primary problems seem to center more on the pronunciation of words rather than word-finding problems. Phrase length was short, effort present, syntactical errors seen in tense, pluralization, and use of functor words. Phonemic substitutions present, difficulties with distinctive features and careful use of the articulators noted during speech production. Throughout, her rate is slow; effort and pauses are seen between syllables as she strives to produce the correct sounds. Her naming abilities are good.

  4. Repetition tasks: words, phrases, and sentences with complex phonemic sequences

  a. Most errors produced were in pronunciation and not in remembering what the stimulus was. In the longer sentences she tended to omit syntactic words such as they and of, although all the substantive words were preserved.

  b. Many phonemic errors seen, occurring more frequently on the more complex phonemic sequences such as "Methodist Episcopal" and "My favorite vegetable." More effort and pauses occurred in these instances.

  Sandy Mayfield, Ph.D.

REFERRAL LETTER: Karen Twigg

October 1, 1983

Caroline Ekelman, Ph.D.
Children's Hospital
Carrollton, Georgia 33323

Dear Dr. Ekelman:

I have referred to you Karen Twigg, a nine year old black girl with a high frequency sensorineural hearing loss which appears to be progressive in nature. The family history is positive on both sides for S/N hearing loss. The patient's hearing loss was first identified at age 5 years, but in recent months has become progressively severe. Her most current audiogram is included. She is currently in third grade but has repeated second grade because of difficulty in reading and speech. Although her speech is intelligible, she does have a number of speech sound errors. We are questioning how much of her learning problem is secondary to a possible speech and language deficit. I would like you to (1) evaluate and advise re: speech and language management, and (2) evaluate for hearing aid selection.

Thank you for seeing this young girl and her family.

Edward Worjak, M.A.
Audiologist

EW:jn

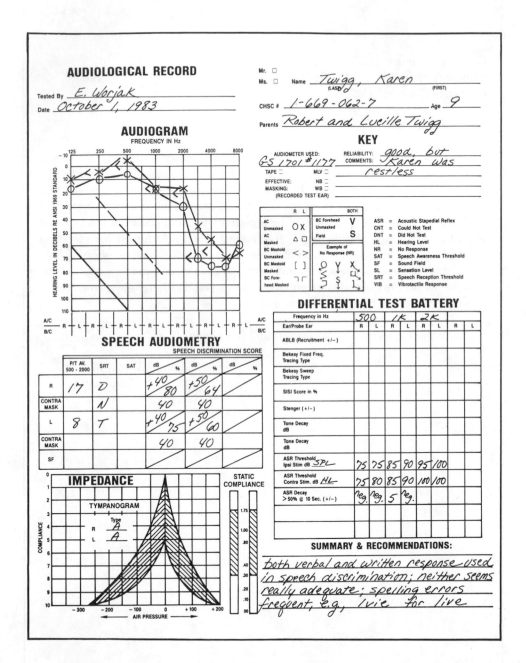

AUDIOLOGICAL RECORD

Tested By *E. Worjak*
Date *October 1, 1983*

Mr. ☐
Ms. ☐   Name *Twigg, Karen*
(LAST)   (FIRST)

CHSC # *1-669-062-7*   Age *9*

Parents *Robert and Lucille Twigg*

AUDIOGRAM
FREQUENCY IN Hz

KEY

AUDIOMETER USED: *GS 1701 #1177*

RELIABILITY: *good, but*
COMMENTS: *Karen was*
restless

TAPE ☐   MLV ☐
EFFECTIVE: NB ☐
MASKING: WB ☐
(RECORDED TEST EAR)

	R	L	BOTH
AC Unmasked	O	X	BC Forehead Unmasked V
AC Masked	△	☐	Field S
BC Mastoid Unmasked	<	>	
BC Mastoid Masked	[	]	Example of No Response (NR)
BC Forehead Masked	⌐	⌐	

ASR = Acoustic Stapedial Reflex
CNT = Could Not Test
DNT = Did Not Test
HL = Hearing Level
NR = No Response
SAT = Speech Awareness Threshold
SF = Sound Field
SL = Sensation Level
SRT = Speech Reception Threshold
VIB = Vibrotactile Response

SPEECH AUDIOMETRY
SPEECH DISCRIMINATION SCORE

	P/T AV. 500-2000	SRT	SAT	dB	%	dB	%	dB	%
R	17	D		+40	80	+50	64		
CONTRA MASK		N		40	40				
L	8	T		+40	75	+50	60		
CONTRA MASK				40	40				
SF									

DIFFERENTIAL TEST BATTERY

Frequency in Hz	500		1K		2K			
Ear/Probe Ear	R	L	R	L	R	L	R	L
ABLB (Recruitment +/−)								
Bekesy Fixed Freq. Tracing Type								
Bekesy Sweep Tracing Type								
SISI Score in %								
Stenger (+/−)								
Tone Decay dB								
Tone Decay dB								
ASR Threshold Ipsi Stim dB *SPL*	75	75	85	90	95	100		
ASR Threshold Contra Stim. dB *HL*	75	80	85	90	100	100		
ASR Decay >50% @ 10 Sec. (+/−)	neg.	neg.	5	neg.				

IMPEDANCE

TYMPANOGRAM

Type
R *A*
L *A*

STATIC COMPLIANCE

SUMMARY & RECOMMENDATIONS:

both verbal and written response used
in speech discrimination; neither seems
really adequate; spelling errors
frequent, e.g., lvie for live

A tool-retrieval source: tests and tools available for designing the diagnosis

Appendix III is a presentation of tests and tools available for measuring (1) various dimensions of speech and language disorders, (2) "causally related" factors, and (3) associated problems that frequently accompany speech and language disorders, and which may also be causally related.

The appendix is designed as an extension of chapters 6 and 7 covering the design of the diagnosis and collection of the clinical data. As discussed in those chapters, selection of appropriate tools for data collection is critical to diagnosis.

We have developed this appendix of testing tools to assist the student with his diagnostic design. Because of the infinite number of tools available, our listing is not exhaustive; rather it is exemplary. Further, we feel the student in training needs to explore many different tools of varying quality, rather than being given a set of tools to use for the different speech and language disorders. This selection and organization should serve as a starting point for the student in training—as the beginning of a tool-retrieval source. As he develops in his diagnostic skill, he can add and delete tools from this everchanging list.

In order to retrieve tools for use in diagnostic design the reader should first consult the Table of Contents of Appendix III to locate the page number of tool sections that may be potentially appropriate for measuring aspects of his cause–effect relationship. Information about the use of each section will be provided there.

A. Speech and Language Tools

The speech and language tools are listed here alphabetically irrespective of their purpose. These tools, coded within the speech and language processing component of the SLPM, measure some dimension of (1) the speech and language product, (2) behavioral correlates, and (3) speech and language processes. A *P* is used to code the primary use of the tool; however, it should be kept in mind that these tools may be useful for other purposes than those coded here. In order to retrieve specific tools the reader can go down the column(s) of interest and locate the tool(s) that may be potentially appropriate for measuring aspects of the cause–effect relationship expressed in the hypothesis. The name of the tool and references are provided to determine the specific relevance of the tool for the patient being seen for diagnosis. Darley (1979) can be used as an evaluation resource for many of these tools and, the September 1981 and 1983 issues of ASHA provide resource guides to multicultural tests and materials.

TOOL-RETRIEVAL TABLE

NAME OF TOOL	Reception Segment	Central Segment	Production Segment	Breathing	Phonation	Resonation	Articulation	Prosodation	Sensation	Perception	Comprehension	Integration	Formulation	Repetition	Sequencing	Motor Control	Voice	Resonance	Phonetic Structure	Prosody	Pragmatic	Semantic	Syntactic	Phonologic
				PHYSICAL PROCESSING SEGMENTS							BEHAVIORAL CORRELATES								SPEECH PRODUCT			LANGUAGE PRODUCT		
Aphasia Clinical Battery 1 — Eggert, G. H. Aphasia clinical battery 1. Chicago: Biolinguistics Clinical Institutes, 1980		P									P	P	P								P	P	P	P
Aphasia Language Performance Scales — Kennan, J., & Brassel, E. Aphasia language performance scales. Murfreesboro, TN: Pinnacle Press, 1975.		P									P	P	P								P	P	P	P
Appraisal of Language Disturbances. Emerick, L. L. Manual for appraisal of language disturbances. Marquette, MI: Northern Michigan University, 1971.		P									P	P	P								P	P	P	P
Apraxia Battery for Adults — Dabul, B. L. Apraxia battery for adults. Tigard OR: C. C. Publications, Inc., 1979.		P	P				P						P		P	P								P
Arizona Articulation Proficiency Scale — Fudala, J. B. Arizona articulation proficiency scale. Los Angeles: Western Psychological Services, 1970.		P	P				P						P			P			P					P
Articulation Testing for Use with Children with Cerebral Palsy — Irwin, O. C. A manual of articulation testing with children with cerebral palsy. Cerebral Palsy Review, 1961, 22, 1-24.		P	P				P						P						P					P

TOOL-RETRIEVAL TABLE—cont'd

NAME OF TOOL	PHYSICAL PROCESSING SEGMENTS								BEHAVIORAL CORRELATES								SPEECH PRODUCT				LANGUAGE PRODUCT			
	Reception Segment	Central Segment	Production Segment	Breathing	Phonation	Resonation	Articulation	Prosodation	Sensation	Perception	Comprehension	Integration	Formulation	Repetition	Sequencing	Motor Control	Voice	Resonance	Phonetic Structure	Prosody	Pragmatic	Semantic	Syntactic	Phonologic
Assessing Language Production in Children Miller, J. F. *Assessing language production in children.* Baltimore: University Park Press, 1981.		P										P	P								P	P	P	
Assessment of Children's Language Comprehension Foster, R., Giddan, J. J., & Stark, J. *Manual for the assessment of children's language comprehension.* Palo Alto, CA: Consulting Psychologists Press, 1973.		P								P		P	P								P	P	P	
Assessment of Intelligibility of Dysarthric Speech Yorkston, K. M., & Beukelman, D. R. *Assessment of intelligibility of dysarthric speech.* Tigard, OR: C. C. Publications, Inc., 1981.		P	P				P								P	P			P					
The Assessment of Phonological Processes Hodson, B. W. *The assessment of phonological processes.* Danville, IL: The Interstate Printers Publishers, Inc., 1980.		P	P				P						P			P			P					P
Auditory Analysis Test Rosner, J., & Simon, D. *Auditory analysis test.* Pittsburgh: Learning Research and Development Center, University of Pittsburgh, 1970.	P								P															

TOOL-RETRIEVAL TABLE—cont'd

NAME OF TOOL	Reception Segment	Central Segment	Production Segment	Breathing	Phonation	Resonation	Articulation	Prosodation	Sensation	Perception	Comprehension	Integration	Formulation	Repetition	Sequencing	Motor Control	Voice	Resonance	Phonetic Structure	Prosody	Pragmatic	Semantic	Syntactic	Phonologic
	PHYSICAL PROCESSING SEGMENTS								BEHAVIORAL CORRELATES								SPEECH PRODUCT				LANGUAGE PRODUCT			
Auditory Behavior Observation Guides McConnell, F., & Ward, P. *Deafness in childhood.* Nashville: Vanderbilt University Press, 1967. Myklebust, H. R. *Auditory disorders in children.* New York: Grune & Stratton, Inc., 1954. Rose, D. E. (Ed.). *Audiological assessment.* Englewood Cliffs, NJ: Printice-Hall, Inc., 1971.	P	P							P	P														
Auditory Comprehension Test for Sentences. Shewan, C. M. *Auditory comprehension test for sentences.* Chicago: Biolinguistics Clinical Institutes, 1980.		P									P													
Auditory Discrimination Test Wepman, J. *Auditory discrimination test.* Chicago: Language Research Associates, 1958.	P									P														
Auditory Memory for Speech Sounds Metraux, R. W. Auditory memory span for speech sounds of speech defective children compared with normal children. *Journal of Speech Disorders,* 1942, 6, 33-36. Metraux, R. W. Auditory memory span for speech sounds: Norms for children. *Journal of Speech Disorders,* 1944, 9, 31-38.	P	P								P				P										P

TOOL-RETRIEVAL TABLE—cont'd

NAME OF TOOL	PHYSICAL PROCESSING SEGMENTS								BEHAVIORAL CORRELATES								SPEECH PRODUCT				LANGUAGE PRODUCT			
	Reception Segment	Central Segment	Production Segment	Breathing	Phonation	Resonation	Articulation	Prosodation	Sensation	Perception	Comprehension	Integration	Formulation	Repetition	Sequencing	Motor Control	Voice	Resonance	Phonetic Structure	Prosody	Pragmatic	Semantic	Syntactic	Phonologic
Auditory Memory Span Test Wepman, J. M., & Morency, A. *Auditory memory span test.* Chicago: Language Research Associates, 1973.	P	P								P				P										
Auditory Pointing Test Fudala, J. B., Kunze, L. H., & Ross, J. D. *Auditory pointing test.* San Rafael, CA: Academic Therapy Publications, 1974.	P									P														
Auditory Sequential Memory Test Wepman, J. M., & Morency, A. *The auditory sequential memory test.* Chicago: Language Research Associates, 1973.	P	P								P				P										
Austin Spanish Articulation Test Carrow, E. *Austin Spanish articulation test.* Boston: Teaching Resources Corp., 1974.		P	P				P									P			P					P
Bankson Language Screening Test Bankson, N. W. *Bankson language screening test.* Baltimore: University Park Press, 1977.		P									P	P	P								P	P	P	
Basic Concept Inventory Englemann, S. *The basic concept inventory.* Chicago: Follett Educational Corporation, 1967.		P									P	P	P									P	P	

TOOL-RETRIEVAL TABLE—cont'd

NAME OF TOOL	Reception Segment	Central Segment	Production Segment	Breathing	Phonation	Resonation	Articulation	Prosodation	Sensation	Perception	Comprehension	Integration	Formulation	Repetition	Sequencing	Motor Control	Voice	Resonance	Phonetic Structure	Prosody	Pragmatic	Semantic	Syntactic	Phonologic
PHYSICAL PROCESSING SEGMENTS									**BEHAVIORAL CORRELATES**								**SPEECH PRODUCT**				**LANGUAGE PRODUCT**			
Basic Language Concepts Test Engelmann, S., Ross, D., & Bingham V. *Basic language concepts test.* Tigard, OR: C. C. Publications, Inc., 1982.		P									P	P	P									P	P	
Berry-Talbott Tests of Language: I. Comprehension of Grammar Berry, M. *Berry-Talbott tests of language: I. Comprehension of grammar.* Rockford, IL: 4322 Pinecrest Road, 1966.		P									P													
Birth to Three Developmental Scale Bangs, T., & Dodson, S. *Birth to three developmental scale.* Hingham, MA: Teaching Resources, 1979.		P									P	P	P								P	P	P	
Boehm Test of Basic Concepts Boehm, A. E. *Boehm test of basic concepts.* NY: Psych. Corp., 1971.		P									P	P										P		
Boston Diagnostic Aphasia Examination Goodglass, J., & Kaplan, E. *The assessment of aphasia and related disorders.* Philadelphia: Lea & Febiger, 1972.		P									P	P	P	P							P	P	P	P
Bowan-Chalfont Receptive Language Inventory Bowan, M. L., & Chalfant, C. C. *Bowan-Chalfant receptive language inventory.* Tigard, OR: Publications, Inc., 1981.		P									P	P										P	P	P

TOOL-RETRIEVAL TABLE—cont'd

Name of Tool	Reception Segment	Central Segment	Production Segment	Breathing	Phonation	Resonation	Articulation	Prosodation	Sensation	Perception	Comprehension	Integration	Formulation	Repetition	Sequencing	Motor Control	Voice	Resonance	Phonetic Structure	Prosody	Pragmatic	Semantic	Syntactic	Phonologic
	Physical Processing Segments								Behavioral Correlates								Speech Product				Language Product			
Bzoch Error Pattern Diagnostic Articulation Test — Bzoch, K. R. Introduction to section C: Measurement of parameters of cleft palate speech. In W. C. Grabb, S. W. Rosenstein, & K. R. Bzoch, *Cleft lip and palate: Surgical, dental, and speech aspects.* Boston: Little Brown & Co., 1971.	P		P			P	P						P			P		P	P					P
Carrow Auditory-Visual Abilities Test — Carrow-Woolfolk, E. *Carrow auditory-visual abilities test.* Hingham, MA: Teaching Resources Corporation, 1981.		P								P	P	P		P										
Carrow Elicited Language Inventory — Carrow-Woolfolk, E. *Carrow elicited language inventory.* Austin, TX: Learning Concepts, 1974.		P									P	P	P	P									P	
Check List of Stuttering Reactions — Johnson, W., Darley, F., & Spriestersbach, D. *Diagnostic methods in speech pathology.* New York: Harper & Row, Publishers, 1963.			P					P					P	P		P				P	P			
Clinical Articulation Profile — Rilla, D., & Hurvitz, J. A. *Clinical articulation profile.* Tulsa, OK: Modern Education Corp., 1983.		P	P				P									P			P					P
Clinical Evaluation of Language Function — Semel, E. M., & Wiig, E. H. *Clinical evaluation of language functions: Examiner's manual.* Columbus, OH: Charles E. Merrill Pub. Co., 1980.		P									P	P	P	P							P	P	P	

TOOL-RETRIEVAL TABLE—cont'd

NAME OF TOOL	Reception Segment	Central Segment	Production Segment	Breathing	Phonation	Resonation	Articulation	Prosodation	Sensation	Perception	Comprehension	Integration	Formulation	Repetition	Sequencing	Motor Control	Voice	Resonance	Phonetic Structure	Prosody	Pragmatic	Semantic	Syntactic	Phonologic
				PHYSICAL PROCESSING SEGMENTS							BEHAVIORAL CORRELATES								SPEECH PRODUCT				LANGUAGE PRODUCT	
The Communication Screen Striffler, N., & Willig, S. *The communication screen: A preschool speech-language screening tool.* Tucson, AZ: Communication Skill Builders, 1982.		P									P	P	P								P	P	P	P
Communicative Abilities in Daily Living Holland, A. *Communicative abilities in daily living.* Baltimore: University Park Press, 1980.		P									P	P	P								P	P	P	P
Communicative Evaluation Chart From Infancy to Five Years Anderson, M., Miles, M., & Matheny, P. *Communicative evaluation chart from infancy to five years.* Cambridge, MA: Educators Publishing Service, Inc., 1963.		P									P	P	P								P	P	P	P
Compton-Hutton Phonological Assessment Compton, A. J., & Hutton, J. S. *Compton-Hutton phonological assessment.* San Francisco: Carousel House, 1978.		P	P				P				P	P	P			P			P					P
Compton Speech and Language Screening Evaluation Compton, A. J. *Compton speech and language screening evaluation.* San Francisco: Carousel House, 1979.		P	P								P	P	P								P	P	P	P

TOOL-RETRIEVAL TABLE—cont'd

NAME OF TOOL	PHYSICAL PROCESSING SEGMENTS								BEHAVIORAL CORRELATES								SPEECH PRODUCT				LANGUAGE PRODUCT			
	Reception Segment	Central Segment	Production Segment	Breathing	Phonation	Resonation	Articulation	Prosodation	Sensation	Perception	Comprehension	Integration	Formulation	Repetition	Sequencing	Motor Control	Voice	Resonance	Phonetic Structure	Prosody	Pragmatic	Semantic	Syntactic	Phonologic
Deep Test of Articulation — McDonald, E. T. *A deep test of articulation.* Pittsburgh: Stanwix House, Inc., 1964.	P		P				P						P			P			P					P
McDonald, E. T. *A screening deep test of articulation.* Pittsburgh: Stanwix House, Inc., 1968.	P		P																					
Del Rio Language Screening Test *English/Spanish* — Toronto, A. S., Leverman, D., Hanna, C., Rosensweig, P., & Maldonado, A. *Del Rio language screening test English/Spanish.* National Education Laboratory Pub., 1975.		P									P	P	P									P	P	
Denver Articulation Screening Exam — Drumwright, A. F. *Denver articulation screening exam.* Denver: University of Colorado Medical Center, 1971.		P	P				P						P			P			P					P
Drumwright, A., Van Natta, P., Camp, B., Frankenburg, W., & Drexler, H. The Denver articulation screening exam. *Journal of Speech and Hearing Disorders,* 1973, 38, 3-14.		P	P							P														
Denver Auditory Phoneme Sequencing Test — Aten, J. *The Denver auditory phoneme sequencing test.* Houston: College Hill Press, 1979.	P	P								P				P										
Detroit Tests of Learning Aptitude — Baker, J. H., & Leland, B. *Detroit tests of learning aptitude.* Indianapolis: The Bobbs-Merrill Co., 1959.		P									P	P	P	P							P	P	P	

TOOL-RETRIEVAL TABLE—cont'd

NAME OF TOOL	Reception Segment	Central Segment	Production Segment	Breathing	Phonation	Resonation	Articulation	Prosodation	Sensation	Perception	Comprehension	Integration	Formulation	Repetition	Sequencing	Motor Control	Voice	Resonance	Phonetic Structure	Prosody	Pragmatic	Semantic	Syntactic	Phonologic
PHYSICAL PROCESSING SEGMENTS →									**BEHAVIORAL CORRELATES** →							**SPEECH PRODUCT** →				**LANGUAGE PRODUCT** →			
Developmental Articulation Profile Tanner, D. C., Mahoney, K. E., & Derrick, G. *Developmental articulation profile*. Tulsa, OK: Modern Education Corp., 1983.		P	P P				P						P			P			P					P
Developmental Articulation Test Hejna, R. *Developmental articulation test.* Ann Arbor, MI: Speech Materials, 1958.		P	P				P						P			P			P					P
Developmental Sequence Scoring and Developmental Sentence Types Lee, L. L. *Developmental sentence analysis.* Evanston: Northwestern University Press, 1974.		P											P			P							P	
Dworkin-Culatta Oral Mechanism Examination Dworkin, J. P., & Culatta, R. A. *Dworkin-Culatta oral mechanism examination.* Nicholasville, KY: Edgewood Press, Inc., 1980.			P P	P	P	P	P									P								
Edinburgh Articulation Test Anthony, A., & others. *The Edinburgh articulation test.* Edinburgh & London: E & S Livingstone, 1971.		P P	P P				P						P			P			P					P
Environmental Language Inventory MacDonald, J. D. *Environmental language inventory.* Columbus, OH: Charles E. Merrill, 1978.		P											P									P	P	

TOOL-RETRIEVAL TABLE—cont'd

NAME OF TOOL	PHYSICAL PROCESSING SEGMENTS								BEHAVIORAL CORRELATES								SPEECH PRODUCT				LANGUAGE PRODUCT			
	Reception Segment	Central Segment	Production Segment	Breathing	Phonation	Resonation	Articulation	Prosodation	Sensation	Perception	Comprehension	Integration	Formulation	Repetition	Sequencing	Motor Control	Voice	Resonance	Phonetic Structure	Prosody	Pragmatic	Semantic	Syntactic	Phonologic
Environmental Prelanguage Battery Hostmeier, D., & MacDonald, J. D. *Environmental prelanguage battery.* Columbus, OH: Charles E. Merrill, 1978.		P											P								P	P	P	
Examining for Aphasia Eisenson, J. *Examining for aphasia.* New York: The Psychological Corporation, 1954.		P	P								P	P	P			P	P					P	P	P
Examining for Harshness Fairbanks, G. *Voice and articulation drill book* (2nd ed.). New York: Harper & Row, Publishers, 1960.					P												P							
Expressive One-Word Picture Vocabulary Test Gardner, M. *Expressive one-word picture vocabulary test.* Novato, CA: Academic Therapy Publications, 1979.		P											P									P		
Fisher-Logemann Test of Articulation Competence Fisher, H. B., & Logemann, J. A. *Fisher-Logemann test of articulation competence.* Boston: Houghton Mifflin Co., 1971.		P	P				P						P			P			P					P
The Fletcher Time-by-Count Test of Diadochokinetic Syllable Rate Fletcher, P. *The Fletcher time-by-count test of diadochokinetic syllable rate.* Tigard, OR: C. C. Publications, Inc., 1978.			P				P								P	P								

TOOL-RETRIEVAL TABLE—cont'd

NAME OF TOOL	Reception Segment	Central Segment	Production Segment	Breathing	Phonation	Resonation	Articulation	Prosodation	Sensation	Perception	Comprehension	Integration	Formulation	Repetition	Sequencing	Motor Control	Voice	Resonance	Phonetic Structure	Prosody	Pragmatic	Semantic	Syntactic	Phonologic
Flowers-Costello Test of Central Auditory Abilities — Flowers, A., Costello, M., & Small, V. *Flowers-Costello test of central auditory abilities.* Dearborn, MI: Perceptual Learning Systems, 1970.	P	P							P	P														
Fluharty Preschool Speech and Language Screening Test — Fluharty, N. B. *Fluharty preschool speech and language screening test.* Hingham, MA: Teaching Resources Corporation, 1978.		P	P				P				P	P	P			P			P			P	P	P
Full-Range Picture Vocabulary Test — Ammons, R. B., & Ammons, H. S. *Full-range picture vocabulary test.* Missoula, MT: Psychological Test Specialists, 1948.		P									P													
Quick Test — Ammons, R. B., & Ammons, C. H. *Quick test.* Missoula, MT: Psychological Test Specialists, 1962.		P									P													
Functional Communication Profile — Sarno, M. T. *Functional communication profile.* New York: New York University Medical Center, Institute of Rehabilitation Medicine, 1963.		P									P	P	P								P	P	P	P
Goldman-Fristoe Test of Articulation — Goldman, R., & Fristoe, M. *Goldman-Fristoe test of articulation.* Circle Pines, MN: American Guidance Service, Inc., 1969.		P	P				P						P			P			P					P

TOOL-RETRIEVAL TABLE—cont'd

Name of Tool	PHYSICAL PROCESSING SEGMENTS								BEHAVIORAL CORRELATES								SPEECH PRODUCT				LANGUAGE PRODUCT			
	Reception Segment	Central Segment	Production Segment	Breathing	Phonation	Resonation	Articulation	Prosodation	Sensation	Perception	Comprehension	Integration	Formulation	Repetition	Sequencing	Motor Control	Voice	Resonance	Phonetic Structure	Prosody	Pragmatic	Semantic	Syntactic	Phonologic
Goldman-Fristoe-Woodcock Auditory Skills Test Battery — Goldman, R., Fristoe, M., & Woodcock, R. *Goldman-Fristoe-Woodcock auditory skills test battery.* Circle Pines, MN: American Guidance Service, 1974.	P	P							P	P														
Goldman-Fristoe-Woodcock Test of Auditory Discrimination — Goldman, R., Fristoe, M., & Woodcock, R. *Goldman-Fristoe-Woodcock test of auditory discrimination.* Circle Pines, MN: American Guidance Service, Inc., 1970.	P	P							P	P														
Grammatical Analysis of Elicited Language Tests — Moog, J. S., & Geers, H. E. *Grammatical analysis of elicited language tests.* St. Louis: Central Institute for the Deaf, 1979.	P	P	P										P										P	
Hannah-Gardner Preschool Language Screening Test — Hannah, E., & Gardner, J. *Hannah-Gardner preschool language screening test.* Northridge, CA: Joyce Publications, 1974.		P	P								P	P	P								P	P	P	P
Houston Test for Language Development — Crabtree, M. *Houston test for language development.* Houston: Houston Test Co., 1963.	P	P									P	P	P								P	P	P	P
Illinois Children's Language Assessment Test — Arlt, P. B. *Illinois children's language assessment test, instruction booklet.* Danville, IL: The Interstate Printers & Publishers, Inc., 1977.	P	P	P				P					P	P			P						P	P	P

TOOL-RETRIEVAL TABLE—cont'd

NAME OF TOOL	Reception Segment	Central Segment	Production Segment	Breathing	Phonation	Resonation	Articulation	Prosodation	Sensation	Perception	Comprehension	Integration	Formulation	Repetition	Sequencing	Motor Control	Voice	Resonance	Phonetic Structure	Prosody	Pragmatic	Semantic	Syntactic	Phonologic
	PHYSICAL PROCESSING SEGMENTS								BEHAVIORAL CORRELATES								SPEECH PRODUCT				LANGUAGE PRODUCT			
Illinois Test of Psycholinguistic Abilities Kirk, S. A., McCarthy, J., & Kirk, W. D. *Illinois test of psycholinguistic abilities* (Rev. ed.). Urbana, IL: University of Illinois Press, 1968.		P									P	P	P	P								P	P	
Interpersonal Language Skills Assessment Blagden, C. M., & McConnell, N. L. *Interpersonal language skills assessment: A test of pragmatic behaviors.* Moline, IL: Lingui Systems, 1983.		P										P									P			
Inventory for Assessment of Laryngectomee Rehabilitation La Borwit, L. J. *Inventory for assessment of laryngectomee rehabilitation.* Tigard, OR: C. C. Publications, Inc., 1981.			P		P											P	P							
Iowa Pressure Articulation Test (see Templin-Darley Tests of Articulation) Morris, H. L., Spriestersbach, D. C., & Darley, F. L. An articulation test for assessing competency of velopharyngeal closure. *Journal of Speech and Hearing Research*, 1961, 4, 48-55.			P			P	P									P		P	P					
Iowa Scale for Rating Severity of Stuttering Sherman, D. *Iowa scale for rating severity of stuttering.* Danville, IL: The Interstate Printers & Publishers, Inc., 1961.			P					P								P				P				

TOOL-RETRIEVAL TABLE—cont'd

NAME OF TOOL	PHYSICAL PROCESSING SEGMENTS								BEHAVIORAL CORRELATES								SPEECH PRODUCT				LANGUAGE PRODUCT			
	Reception Segment	Central Segment	Production Segment	Breathing	Phonation	Resonance	Articulation	Prosodation	Sensation	Perception	Comprehension	Integration	Formulation	Repetition	Sequencing	Motor Control	Voice	Resonance	Phonetic Structure	Prosody	Pragmatic	Semantic	Syntactic	Phonologic
Iowa Scale of Attitude Toward Stuttering — Ammons, R., & Johnson, W. The construction and application of a test of attitude toward stuttering. *Journal of Speech Disorders*, 1944, *9*, 39-49.			P					P								P				P	P			
Iowa Scale of Stuttering Behavior — Johnson, W., Darley, F. L., & Spriestersbach, D. C. *Diagnostic methods in speech pathology.* New York: Harper & Row, 1963.			P					P								P				P	P			
Irwin-Hammill Abstraction Test — Irwin, O. C., & Hammill, D. D. An abstraction test for use with cerebral palsied children. *Cerebral Palsey Review*, 1964, *25*, 3-9.	P	P							P	P	P	P												
Kindergarten Auditory Screening Test — Katz, J. *Kindergarten auditory screening test.* Chicago: Follett Educational Corporation, 1971.	P	P							P	P														
Kindergarten Language Screening Test — Gauthier, S. V., & Madison, C. L. *Kindergarten language screening test.* Tigard, OR: C. C. Publications, Inc., 1978.		P									P	P	P									P	P	
Language Facility Test — Dailey, J. T. *The language facility test.* Alexandria, VA: Arlington Corporation, 1977.		P					P				P	P	P	P					P			P	P	P

TOOL-RETRIEVAL TABLE—cont'd

NAME OF TOOL	Reception Segment	Central Segment	Production Segment	Breathing	Phonation	Resonation	Articulation	Prosodation	Sensation	Perception	Comprehension	Integration	Formulation	Repetition	Sequencing	Motor Control	Voice	Resonance	Phonetic Structure	Prosody	Pragmatic	Semantic	Syntactic	Phonologic
	PHYSICAL PROCESSING SEGMENTS								BEHAVIORAL CORRELATES								SPEECH PRODUCT				LANGUAGE PRODUCT			
Language Modalities Test for Aphasia — Wepman, J., & Jones, L. *Studies in aphasia: An approach to testing; manual of administration and scoring for the language modalities test for aphasia.* Chicago: Education-Industry Service, 1961.		P									P	P	P								P	P	P	P
Language Sampling, Analysis and Training — Tyack, D., & Gottsleben, R. *Language sampling, analysis and training.* Palo Alto, CA: Consulting Psychologists Press, 1974.		P											P									P	P	P
Laradon Articulation Scale — Edmonston, W. *Laradon articulation scale.* Los Angeles: Western Psychological Services, 1963.		P	P				P						P			P			P					P
"Let's Talk" Inventory for Adolescents — Wiig, E. *The "Let's Talk" inventory for adolescents.* Columbus, OH: Charles E. Merrill Publishing Co., 1982.		P									P	P	P								P			
Lindamood Auditory Conceptualization Test — Lindamood, C. H., & Lindamood, P. C. *Lindamood auditory conceptualization test.* Boston: Teaching Resources Corp., 1969.		P								P		P												
Measure of Adaptation of Stuttering — Johnson, W., Darley, F., & Spriestersbach, D. *Diagnostic methods in speech pathology.* New York: Harper & Row, Publishers, 1963.			P					P					P			P				P	P			

TOOL-RETRIEVAL TABLE—cont'd

NAME OF TOOL	PHYSICAL PROCESSING SEGMENTS								BEHAVIORAL CORRELATES								SPEECH PRODUCT				LANGUAGE PRODUCT			
	Reception Segment	Central Segment	Production Segment	Breathing	Phonation	Resonation	Articulation	Prosodation	Sensation	Perception	Comprehension	Integration	Formulation	Repetition	Sequencing	Motor Control	Voice	Resonance	Phonetic Structure	Prosody	Pragmatic	Semantic	Syntactic	Phonologic
Measure of Consistency of Stuttering — Johnson, W., Darley, F., & Spriestersbach, D. Diagnostic methods in speech pathology. New York: Harper & Row, Publishers, 1963.			P					P								P				P	P			
Miami Imitative Ability Test — Jacobs, R. J., Phillips, B. J., & Harrison, R. A stimulability test for cleft-palate children. *Journal of Speech and Hearing Disorders*, 1970, 35, 354-360.			P			P	P							P		P			P	P	P			
Michigan Picture Language Inventory — Lerea, L. Michigan picture language inventory. Ann Arbor, MI: University of Michigan Press, 1958. Wolski, W. The Michigan picture language inventory. Ann Arbor, MI: University of Michigan Press, 1962.		P									P		P									P	P	
Miller-Yoder Test of Grammatical Comprehension — Miller, J. F., & Yoder, D. E. The Miller-Yoder test of grammatical comprehension: Experimental edition. Madison, WI: Department of Communicative Disorders, University of Wisconsin, 1972.		P									P											P	P	

TOOL-RETRIEVAL TABLE—cont'd

Name of Tool	PHYSICAL PROCESSING SEGMENTS								BEHAVIORAL CORRELATES								SPEECH PRODUCT				LANGUAGE PRODUCT			
	Reception Segment	Central Segment	Production Segment	Breathing	Phonation	Resonation	Articulation	Prosodation	Sensation	Perception	Comprehension	Integration	Formulation	Repetition	Sequencing	Motor Control	Voice	Resonance	Phonetic Structure	Prosody	Pragmatic	Semantic	Syntactic	Phonologic
Minnesota Test for Differential Diagnosis of Aphasia — Schuell, H. Differential diagnosis of aphasia with the Minnesota test. Minneapolis: University of Minnesota Press, 1965.		P									P	P	P	P							P	P	P	P
Short Examination for Aphasia — Schuell, H. A short examination for aphasia. Neurology, 1957, 7, 625-634.											P	P	P	P								P	P	P
Muma Assessment Program (MAP) — Muma, J. R., & Muma, D. B. Muma assessment program. Lubbock, TX: Natural Child Publishing Co., 1979.		P									P	P	P								P	P	P	P
Natural Process Analysis (NPA) — Shriberg, L. D., & Kwiatkowski, J. Natural process analysis (NPA): A procedure for phonological analysis of continuous speech samples. New York: John Wiley & Sons, 1980.		P	P				P									P			P					P
Neurosensory Center Comprehensive Examination for Aphasia — Spreen, O., & Benton, A. L. Neurosensory center comprehensive examination for aphasia. Victoria, B.C.: University of Victoria, Department of Psychology, 1969.		P									P	P	P								P	P	P	P

TOOL-RETRIEVAL TABLE—cont'd

NAME OF TOOL	Reception Segment	Central Segment	Production Segment	Breathing	Phonation	Resonation	Articulation	Prosodation	Sensation	Perception	Comprehension	Integration	Formulation	Repetition	Sequencing	Motor Control	Voice	Resonance	Phonetic Structure	Prosody	Pragmatic	Semantic	Syntactic	Phonologic
	PHYSICAL PROCESSING SEGMENTS								BEHAVIORAL CORRELATES								SPEECH PRODUCT				LANGUAGE PRODUCT			
Northwestern Syntax Screening Test Lee, L. Northwestern syntax screening test. Evanston, IL: Northwestern University Press, 1969.	P	P									P		P										P	
Northwestern University Children's Perception of Speech Test AUDITEC of St. Louis: St. Louis, MO: 1980.		P								P														
Ohio Test of Articulation and Perception of Sounds Irwin, R. The Ohio test of articulation and perception of sounds. Pittsburgh: Stanwix House, 1973.			P							P				P		P			P					P
Oliphant Auditory Synthesizing Test Oliphant, G. Oliphant auditory synthesizing test. Cambridge, MA: Educators Publishing Service, 1971.	P	P								P														
Oral Language Sentence Imitation Test and Oral Language Sentence Diagnostic Inventory Zachman, L., Hulsingh, R., Jorgensen, C., & Barrett, M. Oral language sentence imitation test and oral language sentence diagnostic inventory. Moline, IL: Lingui Systems, Inc., 1976.		P											P	P									P	
Oral Reading Sentences for Breathy Quality Fairbanks, G. Voice and articulation drill book (2nd ed.). New York: Harper & Row, Publishers, 1960.			P		P											P	P							

TOOL-RETRIEVAL TABLE—cont'd

NAME OF TOOL	PHYSICAL PROCESSING SEGMENTS								BEHAVIORAL CORRELATES								SPEECH PRODUCT				LANGUAGE PRODUCT			
	Reception Segment	Central Segment	Production Segment	Breathing	Phonation	Resonation	Articulation	Prosodation	Sensation	Perception	Comprehension	Integration	Formulation	Repetition	Sequencing	Motor Control	Voice	Resonance	Phonetic Structure	Prosody	Pragmatic	Semantic	Syntactic	Phonologic
Orzeck Aphasia Evaluation — Orzeck, A. *Orzeck aphasia evaluation manual.* Beverly Hills, CA: Western Psychological Services, 1964.		P									P	P	P								P	P	P	P
Parental Diagnostic Questionnaire: Revised Ed. — Tanner, D. C. *Parental diagnostic questionnaire* (Rev. Ed.). Tulsa, OK: Modern Education Corp., 1983.		P	P					P			P	P	P	P		P				P	P	P	P	P
Parsons Language Sample — Spradlin, J. E. Assessment of speech language of retarded children. The Parsons language sample. *Journal of Speech and Hearing Disorders,* Monograph Suppl., 1963, 10, 8-31.		P									P	P	P								P	P	P	P
Patterned Elicitation Syntax Screening Test — Young, E. C., & Perachio, J. J. *The patterned elicitation syntax screening test.* Tucson, AZ: Communication Skill Builders, 1982.													P										P	
P-B Articulation Test — VanDemark, D. R., Swickard, S. L. A preschool articulation test to assess velopharyngeal competency. *Cleft Palate Journal,* 1980, 17, 175-179.			P			P	P									P		P	P					

TOOL-RETRIEVAL TABLE—cont'd

NAME OF TOOL	PHYSICAL PROCESSING SEGMENTS								BEHAVIORAL CORRELATES								SPEECH PRODUCT				LANGUAGE PRODUCT			
	Reception Segment	Central Segment	Production Segment	Breathing	Phonation	Resonation	Articulation	Prosodation	Sensation	Perception	Comprehension	Integration	Formulation	Repetition	Sequencing	Motor Control	Voice	Resonance	Phonetic Structure	Prosody	Pragmatic	Semantic	Syntactic	Phonologic
Peabody Picture Vocabulary Test — Dunn, L. M. Expanded manual for the Peabody picture vocabulary test. Circle Pines, MN: American Guidance Service, Inc., 1965.		P									P													
Dunn, L. M., & Dunn, L. M. Peabody picture vocabulary test—Revised. Circle Pines, MN: American Guidance Service, Inc., 1981.																								
Perception of Stuttering Inventory — Wooli, C. The assessment of stuttering as struggle avoidance, and expectancy. British Journal of Dis. Comm., 1967, 2, 158-171.		P	P					P								P				P	P			
Phonological Process Analysis — Weiner, F. F. Phonological process analysis. Baltimore: University Park Press, 1979.		P	P				P						P			P			P					P
Photo Articulation Test — Pendergast, K., Dickey, S. E., Selman, J. W., & Soder, A. Photo articulation test. Danville, IL: The Interstate Printers & Publishers, Inc., 1969.		P	P				P						P			P			P					P
Picture Articulation and Language Screening Test — Rodgers, W. C. Picture articulation and language screening test. Salt Lake: Word Making Productions, 1976.		P	P				P						P			P			P					P

TOOL-RETRIEVAL TABLE—cont'd

Name of Tool	Physical Processing Segments								Behavioral Correlates								Speech Product				Language Product			
	Reception Segment	Central Segment	Production Segment	Breathing	Phonation	Resonation	Articulation	Prosodation	Sensation	Perception	Comprehension	Integration	Formulation	Repetition	Sequencing	Motor Control	Voice	Resonance	Phonetic Structure	Prosody	Pragmatic	Semantic	Syntactic	Phonologic
Porch Index of Communicative Ability — Porch, B. E. *Porch index of communicative ability.* Palo Alto, CA: Consulting Psychologists Press, 1967.		P									P	P	P								P	P	P	P
Porch, B. E. *Porch index of communicative ability: Theory and development* (Vol. 1). Palo Alto, CA: Consulting Psychologists Press, 1967.											P	P	P										P	P
Porch, B. E. *Porch index of communicative ability: Administration, scoring, and interpretation* (Vol. 2, Rev. ed.). Palo Alto, CA: Consulting Psychologists Press, 1971.																								
Porch Index of Communicative Ability in Children — Porch, B. E. *Porch index of communicative ability in children.* Palo Alto, CA: Consulting Psychologists Press, 1974.		P									P	P	P								P	P	P	P
Predictive Screening Test of Articulation — Van Riper, C., & Erickson, R. *Predictive Screening tests of articulation.* Kalamazoo, MI: Western Michigan University Press, 1968.		P	P				P									P			P					P
Preschool Language Assessment Instrument — Blank, M., Rose, S. A., & Berlin, L. J. *Preschool language assessment instrument.* New York: Grune & Stratton, 1978.											P	P	P								P	P	P	
Blank, M., Rose, S. A., & Berlin, L. J. *The language of learning.* New York: Grune & Stratton, 1978.											P	P	P								P	P	P	

TOOL-RETRIEVAL TABLE—cont'd

NAME OF TOOL	Reception Segment	Central Segment	Production Segment	Breathing	Phonation	Resonation	Articulation	Prosodation	Sensation	Perception	Comprehension	Integration	Formulation	Repetition	Sequencing	Motor Control	Voice	Resonance	Phonetic Structure	Prosody	Pragmatic	Semantic	Syntactic	Phonologic
Preschool Language Scale — Zimmerman, I., Steiner, V., & Evatt, R. *Preschool language manual.* Columbus, OH: Charles E. Merrill Publishing Co., 1969.		P									P	P	P								P	P	P	P
Preschool Language Screening Test — Fluharty, N. The design and standardization of a speech and language screening test for use with preschool children. *Journal of Speech and Hearing Disorders,* 1974, 39, 75-88.		P	P				P				P	P	P			P			P			P	P	P
Preschool Preposition Test — Aronson, M., & Schaefer, E. Preschool preposition test. In O. G. Johnson & J. W. Bommarito (Eds.), *Tests and measurements in child development: A handbook.* San Francisco: Jossey-Bass, 1971.		P									P													
Procedures for the Phonological Analysis of Children's Language — Ingram, D. *Procedures for the phonological analysis of children's language.* Baltimore: University Park Press, 1981.		P	P				P						P			P			P				P	P
Proverbs Test — Gorman, D. R. *Proverbs test.* Missoula, MT: Psychological Test Specialists, 1956.		P									P	P	P								P	P		

TOOL-RETRIEVAL TABLE—cont'd

Column groups: PHYSICAL PROCESSING SEGMENTS (Reception Segment, Central Segment, Production Segment, Breathing, Phonation, Resonation, Articulation, Prosodation); BEHAVIORAL CORRELATES (Sensation, Perception, Comprehension, Integration, Formulation, Repetition, Sequencing, Motor Control); SPEECH PRODUCT (Voice, Resonance, Phonetic Structure, Prosody); LANGUAGE PRODUCT (Pragmatic, Semantic, Syntactic, Phonologic).

NAME OF TOOL	Reception Segment	Central Segment	Production Segment	Breathing	Phonation	Resonation	Articulation	Prosodation	Sensation	Perception	Comprehension	Integration	Formulation	Repetition	Sequencing	Motor Control	Voice	Resonance	Phonetic Structure	Prosody	Pragmatic	Semantic	Syntactic	Phonologic
Rainbow Passage — Fairbanks, G. *Voice and articulation drillbook* (2nd ed.). New York: Harper & Row, Publishers, 1960.			P	P	P	P	P	P							P	P	P	P	P	P				
Reading Comprehension Battery for Aphasia — La Pointe, L. L., & Horner, J. *Reading comprehension battery for aphasia.* Tigard, OR: C. C. Publications, Inc., 1980.		P									P													
Receptive-Expressive Emergent Language Scale (Reel) — Bzoch, K., & League, R. *Assessing language skills in infancy.* Gainesville, FL: Tree of Life Press, 1971.		P									P	P	P								P	P	P	P
Reynell Developmental Language Scales — Reynell, J. *Reynell developmental language scales: Manual* (Experimental Ed.). Buckinghamshire, England: National Foundation for Educational Research n England and Wales, 1969.		P									P	P	P								P	P	P	
Rhode Island Test of Language Structure — Engen, E., & Engen, T. *Rhode Island test of language structure.* Baltimore: University Park Press, 1983.		P									P	P										P	P	P
Riley Articulation and Language Test — Riley, G. *Riley articulation and language test.* Beverly Hills, CA: Western Psychological Services, 1966.		P	P				P				P	P	P			P			P			P	P	P

TOOL-RETRIEVAL TABLE—cont'd

NAME OF TOOL	Reception Segment	Central Segment	Production Segment	Breathing	Phonation	Resonation	Articulation	Prosodation	Sensation	Perception	Comprehension	Integration	Formulation	Repetition	Sequencing	Motor Control	Voice	Resonance	Phonetic Structure	Prosody	Pragmatic	Semantic	Syntactic	Phonologic
Roswell-Chall Auditory Blending Test Roswell, F. G., & Chall, J. S. *Roswell-Chall auditory blending test.* Planetarium Station, NY: Essay Press, 1963.		P								P					P				P					P
Screening Kit of Language Development Bliss, L. S., & Allen, D. V. *The screening kit of language development.* Baltimore: University Park Press, 1983.		P	P								P	P	P	P								P	P	
Screening Speech Articulation Test Mecham, M., Jex, J. L., & Jones, J. D. *Screening speech articulation test.* Salt Lake City: Communication Research Associates, 1970.		P	P				P						P			P			P					P
Screening Test for Auditory Perception Kimmell, G. M., & Wahl, J. *Screening test for auditory perception.* San Rafael, CA: Academic Therapy Publications, 1969.		P								P														
Screening Test for Developmental Apraxia of Speech Blakely, R. W. *Screening test for developmental apraxia of speech.* Tigard, OR: C. C. Publications, Inc., 1980.		P	P				P	P							P	P			P	P				P
Screening Test of Adolescent Language Prather, E. M., Breecher, S. V. A., Stafford, M. L., & Wallace, E. M. *Screening test of adolescent language.* East Aurora, NY: Slosson Educational Publications, Inc., 1980.		P									P	P	P									P	P	

TOOL-RETRIEVAL TABLE—cont'd

NAME OF TOOL	PHYSICAL PROCESSING SEGMENTS								BEHAVIORAL CORRELATES								SPEECH PRODUCT				LANGUAGE PRODUCT			
	Reception Segment	Central Segment	Production Segment	Breathing	Phonation	Resonation	Articulation	Prosodation	Sensation	Perception	Comprehension	Integration	Formulation	Repetition	Sequencing	Motor Control	Voice	Resonance	Phonetic Structure	Prosody	Pragmatic	Semantic	Syntactic	Phonologic
Semantic Habits Inventory — Nunnally, J. C., Flaugher, R. L., & Hodges, W. F. Semantic habits inventory. In O. G. Johnson & J. W. Bommarito (Eds.), *Tests and measurements in child development: A handbook.* San Francisco: Jossey-Bass, 1971.		P									P	P	P								P	P		
Sequenced Inventory of Communication Development — Hedrick, D. L., Prather, E. M., & Tobin, A. R. *Sequenced inventory of communication development.* Seattle: University of Washington Press, 1975		P								P	P	P	P	P							P	P	P	
Short Term Auditory Retrieval and Storage Test — Flowers, A. *Short term auditory retrieval and storage test.* Dearborn, MI: Perceptual Learning Systems, 1972.		P									P	P	P	P										
Sklar Aphasia Scale — Sklar, M. *Sklar aphasia scale manual.* Beverly Hills, CA: Western Psychological Services, 1966.		P								P	P	P	P								P	P	P	P
Sound Discrimination — Irwin, O. C. *Communication variables of cerebral palsied and mentally retarded children.* Springfield: C. C. Thomas, 1972.	P	P																						
Southern Illinois University Behavior Check List — Brutten, G. J., & Shoemaker, D. J. *Southern Illinois University behavior check list.* Carbondale, IL: Southern Illinois University, 1974.			P					P								P				P	P			

TOOL-RETRIEVAL TABLE—cont'd

NAME OF TOOL	PHYSICAL PROCESSING SEGMENTS								BEHAVIORAL CORRELATES								SPEECH PRODUCT				LANGUAGE PRODUCT			
	Reception Segment	Central Segment	Production Segment	Breathing	Phonation	Resonance	Articulation	Prosodation	Sensation	Perception	Comprehension	Integration	Formulation	Repetition	Sequencing	Motor Control	Voice	Resonance	Phonetic Structure	Prosody	Pragmatic	Semantic	Syntactic	Phonologic
Southern Illinois University Speech Situations Check List — Brutten, G. J., & Shoemaker, D. J. *Southern Illinois University speech situations check list.* Carbondale, IL: Southern Illinois University, 1974.			P					P								P				P	P			
Stephens Oral Language Screening Test — Stephens, I. *Stephens oral language screening test.* Peninsula, OH: Interim Publishers, 1977.		P	P				P						P			P			P				P	P
The Stocker Probe Technique — Stocker, B. *The Stocker probe technique.* Tulsa, OK: Modern Education Corp., 1983.		P	P					P								P				P			P	P
Stuttering Severity Instrument — Riley, G. D. A stuttering severity instrument for children and adults. *Journal of Speech and Hearing Disorders,* 1972, *37,* 314-322.			P					P								P				P	P			
Supplementary Examination for Breathiness — Johnson, W., Darley, F., & Spriestersbach, D. *Diagnostic methods in speech pathology.* New York: Harper & Row, Publishers, 1963.			P		P											P	P							
Supplementary Examination for Nasality — Johnson, W., Darley, F., & Spriestersbach, D. *Diagnostic methods in speech pathology.* New York: Harper & Row, Publishers, 1963.			P			P										P		P						

TOOL-RETRIEVAL TABLE—cont'd

NAME OF TOOL	PHYSICAL PROCESSING SEGMENTS								BEHAVIORAL CORRELATES								SPEECH PRODUCT				LANGUAGE PRODUCT			
	Reception Segment	Central Segment	Production Segment	Breathing	Phonation	Resonation	Articulation	Prosodation	Sensation	Perception	Comprehension	Integration	Formulation	Repetition	Sequencing	Motor Control	Voice	Resonance	Phonetic Structure	Prosody	Pragmatic	Semantic	Syntactic	Phonologic
Templin-Darley Tests of Articulation Templin, M. C., & Darley, F. L. *Templin-Darley test of articulation* (2nd. ed.). Iowa City, IO: Bureau of Educational Research and Service, University of Iowa, 1969.		P	P				P						P			P			P					P
Test of Adolescent Language Hammill, D. D., Brown, V. L., Larsen, S. C., & Wiederholt, J. L. *Test of adolescent language.* Allen, TX: Developmental Learning Materials, 1980.		P									P	P	P									P	P	
Test of Articulation Performance—Diagnostic Bryant, B. R., & Bryant, D. L. *Test of articulation performance—diagnostic.* Austin, TX: Pro-ed, 1983.		P	P				P						P			P			P					P
Test of Auditory Comprehension of Language Carrow-Woolfork, E. *Test for auditory comprehension of language.* Austin, TX: Learning Concepts, 1973		P									P											P		
Test of Early Language Development Hresko, W. R., Reid, D. K., & Hammill, D. D. *Test of early language development.* Allen, TX: Developmental Learning Materials, 1981.		P									P	P	P								P	P	P	P

TOOL-RETRIEVAL TABLE—cont'd

NAME OF TOOL	PHYSICAL PROCESSING SEGMENTS								BEHAVIORAL CORRELATES								SPEECH PRODUCT				LANGUAGE PRODUCT			
	Reception Segment	Central Segment	Production Segment	Breathing	Phonation	Resonation	Articulation	Prosodation	Sensation	Perception	Comprehension	Integration	Formulation	Repetition	Sequencing	Motor Control	Voice	Resonance	Phonetic Structure	Prosody	Pragmatic	Semantic	Syntactic	Phonologic
Test of Language Development Newcomer, P., & Hammill, D. D. *Test of language development.* Austin, TX: Empiric Press, 1977.		P								P	P	P	P	P							P	P	P	
Test of Language Development—Primary Newcomer, P. L., & Hammill, D. D. *Test of language development—primary.* Austin, TX: Pro-ed, 1982.										P	P	P	P	P								P	P	
Test of Language Development—Intermediate Hammill, D. D., & Newcomer, P. L. *Test of language development—intermediate.* Austin, TX: Pro-ed, 1982.											P	P	P									P		
Test of Listening Accuracy in Children Mecham, M.J., Jex, J.L., & Jones, J.D. *Test of listening accuracy in children.* Provo, UT: Brigham Young University Press, 1969.		P								P														
Test of Syntactic Abilities Quigley, S. P., Steinkamp, M. W., Power, D. J., & Jones, B. W. *Test of syntactic abilities.* Beaverton, OR: Dormac, Inc., 1981.		P									P		P										P	

TOOL-RETRIEVAL TABLE—cont'd

NAME OF TOOL	PHYSICAL PROCESSING SEGMENTS								BEHAVIORAL CORRELATES								SPEECH PRODUCT				LANGUAGE PRODUCT			
	Reception Segment	Central Segment	Production Segment	Breathing	Phonation	Resonance	Articulation	Prosodation	Sensation	Perception	Comprehension	Integration	Formulation	Repetition	Sequencing	Motor Control	Voice	Resonance	Phonetic Structure	Prosody	Pragmatic	Semantic	Syntactic	Phonologic
Tina Bangs Language Scale Bangs, T. E. Evaluating children with language delay. *Journal of Speech and Hearing Disorders*, 196-, *26*, 6-18.		P									P	P	P								P	P	P	
Bangs, T. E. *Language and learning disorders of the pre-academic child.* New York: Appleton-Century Crofts, 1968.												P	P									P	P	
Token Test DeRenzi, E., & Vignolo, L. A. The token test: A sensitive test to detect receptive disturbances in aphasia. *Brain*, 1962, *85*, 665-678.		P									P													
Spellacy, F., & Spreen, O. A short form of the token test. *Cortex*, 1969, *5*, 390-397.																								
Revised Token Test McNeill, M., & Prescott, T. *Revised token test.* Baltimore: University Park Press, 1978.		P									P													
Token Test for Children DiSimoni, F. *Token test for children.* Boston: Teaching Resources Corp., 1978.																								
Toronto Tests of Receptive Vocabulary (English/Spanish) Toronto, A. S. *Toronto tests of receptive vocabulary (English/Spanish).* Austin, TX: Academic Tests, 1977.		P									P													

TOOL-RETRIEVAL TABLE—cont'd

NAME OF TOOL	PHYSICAL PROCESSING SEGMENTS								BEHAVIORAL CORRELATES								SPEECH PRODUCT				LANGUAGE PRODUCT			
	Reception Segment	Central Segment	Production Segment	Breathing	Phonation	Resonation	Articulation	Prosodation	Sensation	Perception	Comprehension	Integration	Formulation	Repetition	Sequencing	Motor Control	Voice	Resonance	Phonetic Structure	Prosody	Pragmatic	Semantic	Syntactic	Phonologic
Total Dysfluency Index Johnson, W., Darley, F., & Spriestersbach, D. *Diagnostic methods in speech pathology*. New York: Harper & Row, Publishers, 1963.			P					P								P				P				
Utah Test of Language Development Mecham, M., Jex, J., & Jones, J. *Utah test of language development*. Salt Lake City: Communication Research Associates, 1967.		P									P	P	P								P	P		P
Vane Evaluation of Language Scale Vane, L. *Vane evaluation of language scale*. Brandon, VT: Clinical Psychology Pub. Co., 1975.											P	P	P								P	P		
Verbal Language Development Scale Mecham, M. *Verbal language development scale*. Circle Pines, MN: American Guidance Service, Inc., 1958.		P									P	P	P								P	P	P	
Vocabulary Comprehension Scale Bangs, T. E. *Vocabulary comprehension scale*. Boston: Teaching Resources Corporation, 1975.		P									P											P	P	
Vocabulary Usage Test Nation, J. E. A vocabulary usage test. *Journal of Psycholinguistic Research*, 1972, *1*, 221-231.		P											P									P		

TOOL-RETRIEVAL TABLE—cont'd

NAME OF TOOL	PHYSICAL PROCESSING SEGMENTS								BEHAVIORAL CORRELATES								SPEECH PRODUCT				LANGUAGE PRODUCT			
	Reception Segment	Central Segment	Production Segment	Breathing	Phonation	Resonation	Articulation	Prosodation	Sensation	Perception	Comprehension	Integration	Formulation	Repetition	Sequencing	Motor Control	Voice	Resonance	Phonetic Structure	Prosody	Pragmatic	Semantic	Syntactic	Phonologic
Washington Speech Sound Discrimination Test Prather, E. M., Miner, A., Addicott, M. A., & Sunderland, L. *Washington speech sound discrimination test.* Danville, IO: Interstate Printers and Publishers, Inc., 1971.		P								P														
Weiss Intelligibility Test Weiss, C. E. *Weiss intelligibility test.* Tigard, OR: C. C. Publications, Inc., 1982.			P				P									P			P					P
Western Aphasia Battery Kertesz, A. *The Western aphasia battery.* New York: Grune & Stratton, 1982.		P									P	P	P	P							P	P	P	
Woodcock Language Proficiency Battery Woodcock, R. W. *Woodcock language proficiency battery.* Hingham, MA: Teaching Resources Corporation, 1982.		P									P	P	P	P							P	P	P	
Word Intelligibility by Picture Identification Ross, M., & Lerman, J. *Word intelligibility by picture identification.* Pittsburgh: Stanwix House, Inc. 1971.		P								P														
The Word Test Jorgensen, C., Barrett, M., Huisingh, R., & Zachman, L. *The word test.* Northridge, CA: Lingua Press, 1981.		P									P	P	P									P		

B. Causally Related Tools

Tools which directly or indirectly measure causal factors have been organized in terms of the segment of the speech and language processing component affected: Audiologic Tools are grouped under the Auditory Reception Segment; Cognitive–Mental Development–Intelligence Tools, General Development Tools, and Social and Psychological Adjustment, and Behavior Rating Tools are included within the Central Language–Thought Segment; finally Motor Performance Tools are listed under the Speech Production Segment. Salvia and Ysseldyke (1981) can be consulted for details on many of these tools as can Lezak (1976).

1. Reception Segment

AUDIOLOGIC TOOLS*

Procedure	Conductive	Cochlear	Eighth nerve	Brainstem	Cortical	Functional
Behavioral response						
Pure-tone air and bone conduction thresholds	X	X	X	X	X	X
Spondee thresholds	X	X	X	X	X	X
Speech discrimination in quiet	X	X	X	X	X	X
Alternate Binaural Loudness Balance (ABLB)		(recruitment)	decruitment)			
Monaural Loudness Balance (MLB)		X	X			
Short Increment Sensitivity Index (SISI)			(high level)			
Tone decay		X	X			
Bekesy (conventional)	Type I	Type II	Type III,IV			Type V
Critical-Off Time (COT)			X			
Lengthened-Off Time (LOT)						X
Bekesy Comfortable Loudness (BCL)			X			
Bekesy Ascending-Descending Gap Evaluation (BADGE)						X
Forward-backward tracings			X			
Brief-tone audiometry		X	X			
Aural Overload Test		X				
Frequency DLs		X				
Performance-Intensity Function (PI-PB)			X			
Synthetic Sentence Identification with Ipsilateral Competing Message (SSI-ICM)			X	X		
Synthetic Sentence Identification with Contralateral Competing Message (SSI-CCM)					X	
Speech-in noise				X	X	
Binaural fusion				X		
Rapidly alternating sentences				X		
Masking Level Differences (MLDs)				X		
Mid-plane balancing				X		

Procedure	Conductive	Cochlear	Eighth nerve	Brainstem	Cortical	Functional
Chocholle Test				X		
SWAMI Test				X		
Competing Sentence Test					X	
Filtered Speech Test					X	
Staggered Spondaic Word Test (SSW)					X	
Competing Environmental Sounds (CES)					X	
Time Altered Speech (compression and expansion)					X	
Rush Hughes Speech Discrimination Test					X	
NU No. 6 Competing Message Test					X	
Auditory pitch pattern perception					X	
Dichotic digits, syllables, etc.					X	
Spondee threshold and pure-tone discrepancy						X
Stenger Test						X
Shadow Curve						X
Delayed Auditory Feedback (DAF)						X
Doerfler-Steward Test						X
Lombard Test						X
Swinging (Shifting) Story Test						X
Electrophysiologic response						
Immittance measurements						
Tympanometry	X					X
Acoustic reflex thresholds	X	X	X	X		X
Static compliance	X					
Stapedial reflex decay			X			
Acoustic reflex latency test			X	X		
Eustachian tube function tests (Pressure-swallow testing, Valsalva, Toynbee, etc.)	X					
Auditory evoked response potentials						
Electrocochleography (ECoG)	X	X	X			X
Brainstem Auditory Evoked Potentials (BAEP)	X	X	X	X		X
Cortical Auditory Evoked Potentials					X	X
Electrodermal audiometry						X

*Prepared by Craig Newman, Department of Communication Sciences, Case Western Reserve University, Cleveland, OH.

2. Central Segment

a. COGNITIVE–MENTAL DEVELOPMENT–INTELLIGENCE TOOLS

Assessment in Infancy: Ordinal Scales of Psychological Development

Uzgiris, I. C., & Hunt, J. *Assessment in infancy: Ordinal scales of psychological development.* Urbana, IL: University of Illinois Press, 1975.

Dunst, C. J. *A clinical and educational manual for use with the Uzgiris and Hunt scales of infant psychological development.* Baltimore: University Park Press, 1980.

Bayley Scales of Infant Development*
    Bayley, N. *Bayley Scales of Infant Development*. New York: Psychological Corporation of America, 1969.
Cattell Infant Intelligence Scale*
    Cattell, P. *The measurement of intelligence of infants and young children*. New York: The Psychological
        Corporation, 1947.
Chicago Non Verbal Examination
    Brown, A. W., & Stein, S. *Chicago Non Verbal Examination*. New York: The Psychological Corporation, 1936.
Columbia Mental Maturity Scale
    Burgemeister, B., Blum, L., & Lorge, I. *Columbia Mental Maturity Scale*. New York: Harcourt Brace Jovanovich,
        1953.
Goodenough–Harris Drawing Test
    Goodenough, R. L., & Harris, D. V. *Goodenough–Harris Drawing Test*. New York: Harcourt Brace Jovanovich,
        1963.
    Harris, D. *Children's drawing as measures of intellectual maturity*. New York: Harcourt Bruce Jovanovich, 1963.
Hiskey-Nebraska Test of Learning Aptitude
    Hiskey, M. *Hiskey-Nebraska Test of Learning Aptitude*. Lincoln, NB: University of Nebraska Press, 1966.
    Hiskey, M. S. *Nebraska test of learning aptitude for young deaf children*. New York: The Psychological Cor-
        poration, 1941.
Leiter International Performance Scale
    Leiter, R. G. *Leiter International Performance Scale*. Washington, D. C.: The Psychological Service Center
        Press, 1948.
    Arthur, G. *Arthur adaptation of the Leiter international performance scale*. Washington, D. C.: The
        Psychological Service Center Press, 1952.
McCarthy Scales of Children's Abilities
    McCarthy, D. *McCarthy Scales of Children's Abilities*. New York: Psychological Corporation, 1972.
    Kaufman, A. S., & Kaufman, N. L. *Clinical evaluation of young children with the McCarthy scales*. New
        York: Grune & Stratton, 1977.
Merrill–Palmer Scale of Mental Tests*
    Stutsman, R. *Mental measurement of preschool children*. Yonkers-on-Hudson, NY: World Book, 1931.
Nonverbal Test of Cognitive Skills
    Johnson, G. O., & Boyd, H. F. *Nonverbal Test of Cognitive Skills*. Columbus, OH: Merrill, 1981.
Pictorial Test of Intelligence*
    French, J. L. *Pictorial Test of Intelligence*. Boston: Houghton-Mifflin, 1960.
Raven Progressive Matrices
    Raven, J. *Guide to the standard progressive matrices: Sets A, B, C, D, E*. London: H. K. Lewis, 1960.
    Raven, J. *Advanced Progressive Matrices: Sets I and II*. London: H. K. Lewis, 1965.
    Coloured Progressive Matrices
        Raven, J. *Guide to using the Coloured Progressive Matrices*. London: H. K. Lewis, 1963.
Slosson Intelligence Test
    Slosson, R. L. *Slosson Intelligence Test*. East Aurora, NY: Slosson Educational Publications, 1981.
Stanford-Binet Intelligence Scale*
    Terman, L. M., & Merrill, M. A. *Stanford-Binet Intelligence Scale: Manual for the third revision*, Form
        L-M. Boston: Houghton Mifflin, 1960.
Test of Nonverbal Intelligence
    Brown, L., Sherbenou, R. J., & Dollar, S. J. *The Test of Nonverbal Intelligence: A language free measure
        of cognitive ability*. Austin, TX: Pro-ed, 1982.
Weschler Preschool and Primary Scale of Intelligence*
    Weschler, D. *Weschler Preschool and Primary Scale of Intelligence*. New York: The Psychological Corpora-
        tion, 1976.
Weschler Intelligence Scale for Children—Revised
    Weschler, D. *Manual for the Weschler Intelligence Scale for Children*. New York: The Psychological Cor-
        poration, 1974.
Weschler Adult Intelligence Scale
    Weschler, D. *Manual for the Weschler Adult Intelligence Scale*. New York: The Psychological Corporation, 1955.

---

*Denotes language items have been analyzed within the framework of an earlier version of the SLPM as reported in:
Aram, D. M., & Nation, J. E. Intelligence tests for children: A language analysis. *Ohio Journal of Speech and Hearing*, 1971, *6*, 22–43.

b. GENERAL DEVELOPMENT TOOLS

Developmental Potential of Preschool Children

Haeussermann, E. *Developmental Potential of Preschool Children.* New York: Grune & Stratton, 1958.

Denver Developmental Screening Test

Frankenburg, W. K., & Dodds, J. B. *Denver Developmental Screening Test.* Denver: University of Colorado Medical Center, 1967.

Frankenburg, W., Dodds, J., & Fandal, A. *Denver Developmental Screening Test.* Denver: University of Colorado Medical Center, 1970.

Preschool Attainment Record

Doll, E. A. *Preschool Attainment Record.* Circle Pines, MN: American Guidance Service, 1966.

Rockford Infant Developmental Evaluation Scales

Project RHISE/Outreach. *Rockford Infant Developmental Evaluation Scales.* Bensenville, IL: Scholastic Testing Service, 1979.

Vineland Social Maturity Scale

Doll, E. A. *Vineland Social Maturity Scale: Condensed manual of directions.* Circle Pines, MN: American Guidance Service, 1965.

c. SOCIAL AND PSYCHOLOGICAL ADJUSTMENT AND BEHAVIOR RATING TOOLS

Autism Screening Instrument for Educational Planning

Krag, D. A., Arick, J. R., & Almond, P. J. *Autism Screening Instrument for Educational Planning.* Portland, OR: ASIEP Ed., 1980.

California Test of Personality

Thorpe, L. P., Clark, W. W., & Tiegs, E. W. *California Test of Personality.* Monterey, CA: California Test Bureau, 1953.

Child Behavior Checklist

Achenbach, T. M. *Child Behavior Checklist.* Burlington, VT: University of Vermont, 1981.

Child Behavior Rating Scale

Cassell, R. *Child Behavior Rating Scale.* Los Angeles: Western Psychological Services, 1962.

Children's Apperception Test

Bellak, L., & Bellak, S. S. *Children's Apperception Test* (5th ed.). Los Angeles: Western Psychological Services, 1971.

Bellak, L. *The Thematic Apperception Test and the Children's Apperception Test in clinical use.* New York: Grune & Stratton, 1954.

Haworth, M. R. *The CAT: Facts about fantasy.* New York: Grune & Stratton, 1966.

Mother–Child Relationship Evaluation

Roth, R. M. *Mother–Child Relationship Evaluation.* Beverly Hills, CA: Western Psychological Services, 1961.

Thematic Apperception Test

Murray, H. A. *Thematic Apperception Test.* Cambridge, MA: Harvard University Press, 1943.

Bellak, L. The thematic apperception test and the children's apperception test in clinical use. New York: Grune & Stratton, 1954.

3. Production Segment

a. MOTOR PERFORMANCE TOOLS

Bruininks–Oseretsky Test of Motor Proficiency

Bruininks, R. H. *Bruininks–Oseretsky Test of Motor Proficiency: Examiner's manual.* Circle Pines, MN: American Guidance Service, 1978.

Oseretsky Test of Motor Proficiency

Doll, E. A. (Ed.) *Oseretsky Test of Motor Proficiency.* Circle Pines, MN: American Guidance Service, 1964.

Harris Tests of Lateral Dominance

Harris, A. J. *Harris Tests of Lateral Dominance.* New York: The Psychological Corporation, 1955.

Motor Problems Inventory

Riley, G. D. *Motor Problems Inventory: Manual.* Los Angeles: Western Psychological Services, 1972.

Purdue Pegboard

Tiffin, J. *Examiner manual for the Purdue Pegboard.* Chicago: Science Research Associates, 1948.

Purdue Perceptual–Motor Survey

Roach, E., & Kephart, N. *The Purdue Perceptual–Motor Survey.* Columbus, OH: Merrill, 1966.

Southern California Motor Accuracy Test
   Ayres, A. J. *Southern California Motor Accuracy Test.* Los Angeles: Western Psychological Services, 1964.
Southern California Perceptual–Motor Test
   Ayres, A. J. *Southern California Perceptual–Motor Test.* Los Angeles: Western Psychological Services, 1968.

C. Associated Problem Areas

Tools examining related problem areas are grouped as follows: Visual Perception Tools; Visual–Motor Coordination Tools; Academic Readiness Tools; Academic Achievement Tools; Reading Tools; Written Language Tools; and Learning Disabilities Screening Tools. Again, Salvia and Ysseldyke (1981) is an excellent resource for studying these tools.

1. VISUAL PERCEPTION TOOLS

Benton Revised Visual Retention Test
   Benton, A. *Benton Revised Visual Retention Test.* New York: The Psychological Corporation, 1974.
Developmental Test of Visual Perception
   Frostig, M., Lefever, D., Maslow, P., & Whittlesley, R. *Marianne Frostig Developmental Test of Visual Perception.* Palo Alto, CA: Consulting Psychologists Press, 1964.
Memory-for-Designs Test
   Graham, R., & Kendall, B. *Memory-for-Designs Test.* Missoula, MT: Psychological Test Specialists.
   Graham, F. K., & Kendall, B. S. Memory-for-Designs Test: Revised general manual. *Percept. Motor Skills,* 1960, *11,* 147–190.
Motor-Free Visual Perception Test
   Colarusso, R., & Hammill, D. *Motor-free Visual Perception Test.* San Rafael, CA: Academic Therapy Publications, 1972.
Primary Visual Motor Test
   Haworth, M. *The Primary Visual Motor Test.* New York: Grune & Stratton, 1970.
Southern California Figure–Ground Visual Perception Test
   Ayres, A. J. *Southern California Figure–Ground Visual Perception Test.* Los Angeles: Western Psychological Services, 1966.

2. VISUAL-MOTOR COORDINATION TOOLS

Ayres Space Test
   Ayres, A. J. *Ayres Space Test.* Los Angeles: Western Psychological Services, 1962.
Bender-Gestalt Test for Young Children
   Bender, L. A visual motor gestalt test and its clinical use. New York: *American Orthopsychiatric Association, Research Monogr. No. 3,* 1938.
   Koppitz, E. M. *Bender-Gestalt Test for young children.* New York: The Psychological Corporation, 1964.
Developmental Test of Visual Motor Integration
   Beery, K. E., & Buktenica, N. A. *Developmental Test of Visual Motor Integration: Administration and scoring manual.* Chicago: Follet, 1967.

3. ACADEMIC READINESS TOOLS

Anton Brenner Developmental Gestalt Test of School Readiness
   Brenner, A. *Anton Brenner Developmental Gestalt Test of School Readiness.* Los Angeles: Western Psychological Services, 1964.
Test of Early Reading Ability
   Reid, D. K., Hresko, W. D., & Hammill, D. D. *Test of Early Reading Ability.* Allen, TX: Developmental Learning Materials, 1981.
Clymer–Barrett Prereading Battery
   Clymer, T., & Barrett, T. C. *Prereading battery.* Princeton, NJ: Personnel Press, 1967.

4. ACADEMIC ACHIEVEMENT TOOLS

Metropolitan Achievement Tests
   Durost, W. N., Bixler, H. H., Hildreth, G. H., Lund, K. W., & Wrightstone, J. W. *Metropolitan Achievement Tests: Advanced battery.* New York: World Book, 1958.

Durost, W. N., Bixler, H. H., Wrightstone, J. W., Prescott, G. A., & Balow, I. H. *Metropolitan Achievement Tests: Primary II. Form F.* New York: Harcourt Brace Jovanovich, 1970.

Peabody Individual Achievement Tests
Dunn, L. M., & Markwardt, F. C. *Peabody Individual Achievement Tests.* Circle Pines, MN: American Guidance Service, 1970.

Wide Range Achievement Test
Jastak, J. F., Bijou, S. W., & Jastak, S. *Wide Range Achievement Test.* Wilmington, DE: Jastak Assoc., 1978.

Woodcock–Johnson Psycho-Educational Battery
Woodcock, R. W., & Johnson, M. B. *Woodcock–Johnson Psycho-Educational Battery.* Hingham, MA: Teaching Resources, 1977.

5. READING TOOLS

Botel Reading Inventory Word Opposites
Botel, M. *Botel Reading Inventory.* Chicago: Follett Educational Corp., 1970.

Durrell Analysis of Reading Difficulty
Durrell, D. D. *Manual of directions for Durrell Analysis of Reading Difficulty.* New York: Harcourt Brace Jovanovich, 1937.

Gates Advanced Primary Reading Test
Gates, A. Gates Advanced Primary Reading Test. New York: Columbia University, Teachers College Press, 1958.

Gates–McKillop Reading Diagnostic Test
Gates, A. I., & McKillop, A. S. *Gates–McKillop Reading Diagnostic Test.* New York: Teachers College Press, Columbia University, 1962.

Stanford Diagnostic Reading Test
Karlsen, B., Madden, R., & Gardner, E. F. *Stanford Diagnostic Reading Test.* New York: Harcourt Brace Jovanovich, 1966.

Test of Reading Comprehension
Brown, V. L., Hammill, D. D., & Wiederholt, J. L. *Test of reading comprehension.* Austin, TX: Pro-ed, 1978.

Woodcock Reading Mastery Tests
Woodcock, R. W. *Woodcock Reading Mastery Tests.* Circle Pines, MN: American Guidance Service, 1973.

6. WRITTEN LANGUAGE TOOLS

Picture Story Language Test
Myklebust, H. *Development and disorders of written language: Picture Story Language Test* (Vol. I). New York: Grune & Stratton, 1965.

Test of Written Language
Hammill, D. D., & Larsen, S. C. *Test of Written Language.* Allen, TX: Developmental Learning Materials, 1983.

Test of Written Spelling
Larsen, S. C., & Hammill, D. D. *Test of Written Spelling.* Allen, TX: Developmental Learning Materials, 1976.

7. LEARNING DISABILITIES SCREENING TOOLS

Meeting Street School Screening Test
Hainsworth, P. K., & Signeland, M. L. *Early identification of children with learning disabilities: The Meeting Street School Screening test.* Providence, RI: Crippled Children and Adults of Rhode Island, 1969.

Pupil Rating Scale: Screening for Learning Disabilities
Myklebust, H. R. *Pupil Rating Scale: Screening for Learning Disabilities.* New York: Grune & Stratton, 1971.

Screening Tests for Identifying Children with Specific Language Disability
Slingerland, B. H. *Screening Tests for Identifying Children with Specific Language Disability.* Cambridge, MA: Educators Publishing Service, 1967.

Speech mechanism examination form

SPEECH MECHANISM EXAMINATION

Name _____ Birth date _____ Age ____ Center No. ____
Examiner _____ Date _____

Adequacy for speech ratings
1 = Normal
2 = Slight deviation—probably no adverse effect on speech
3 = Moderate deviation—possible adverse effect on speech; remedial services may be required particularly if other structures of the speech mechanism are also deviant
4 = Extreme deviation—sufficient to prevent normal production of speech; modification of structure required if possible, either with or without clinical speech services, or speech services needed to compensate for the structural deviation

General physical appearance _____
_____
_____

General appearance of head and face

Symmetry, size and shape of head and face _____
_____

Scars _____
_____

Facial grimaces noted during speech _____
_____

Muscles of facial expression—ability to: Smile __ Wink __ Wrinkle forehead __
Eyes
Intraocular distance: Normal _____ Other _____
Ptosis: None _____ Right _____ Left _____ Bilateral _____

Nose

Structure

Deviated septum: No _____ To right _____ To left _____
Deviated columella: No _____ To right _____ To left _____

SPEECH MECHANISM EXAMINATION—Cont'd

Nose—Cont'd

Function

History of upper respiratory infections: No _____ Yes _____ Explain _____

_____

Nasal obstruction: No _____ Right _____ Left _____ Bilateral _____ Describe _____

_____

Mouth breathing: No _____ Yes _____ Chronic _____ Acute _____ Describe _____

_____

Adequacy for speech: 1 _____ 2 _____ 3 _____ 4 _____

Lips

Structure

   Upper lip length: Normal __ Short __ Markedly short __
   Symmetric: Yes_____No_____
   Do lips touch when teeth are in occlusion? Yes __ No __
   Other abnormalities _____

   _____

Function

   Describe instructions necessary to obtain performance (e.g., imitation, tactile
   stimulation, etc.) _____

   _____

   Protrude: Yes_____No_____Tense and press: Yes_____No_____Eversion:
   Yes _____ No _____
   Retraction: Right_____Left_____ Bilateral symmetry: Yes_____No_____

	Trials			Rating		
	1	*2*	*3*	*Above av.*	*Av.*	*Below av.*
Rounding and retraction of lips (o-ee-o-ee) in 10 sec (5 times in 15 sec)[1]						
Number of times can say /pʌ/ in 5 sec (range 3.0-5.5 per sec)[2,3,5]						

   Description of function _____

Adequacy for speech: 1 _____ 2 _____ 3 _____ 4 _____

Continued.

SPEECH MECHANISM EXAMINATION—Cont'd

Mandible

Structure

Size _____

_____

Shape _____

_____

Function

Ability to chew _____

Diadochokinesis (rate and rhythm) _____ /ja/

Adequacy for speech: 1 _____ 2 _____ 3 _____ 4 _____

Teeth

Occlusion: Normal _____ Neutroclusion _____Distoclusion _____Mesioclusion _____

Vertical relationship of anterior teeth: Normal ___ Open bite ___ Closed bite ___

Crossbite _____

Maxillary collapse: No_____Yes_____Right_____Left_____Bilateral_____

Anterior-posterior relation of incisors: Normal _____ Linguoversion _____ Labioversion _____ Mixed _____

Diastema: No_____Yes_____Mild_____Moderate_____Severe_____Which teeth_____

Missing teeth:	8 7	6 5 4 3 2 1	1 2 3 4 5 6	7 8
	8 7	6 5 4 3 2 1	1 2 3 4 5 6	7 8

(Circle)

Condition of dental hygiene: Excellent _____ Good _____ Poor _____

Dental prosthesis: No_____Yes_____Partial_____Complete_____

Adequacy for speech: 1 _____ 2 _____ 3 _____ 4 _____

Tongue

Structure

Size in relation to dental arches: Normal _____ Large _____ Small _____

Atrophy: No ___ Yes ___ Fissures: No ___ Yes ___ Frenum: Normal ___

Short _____

Function

Tremors or fasciculations at rest: Yes _____ No _____

Extension-retraction pattern present: Yes _____ No _____

Continued.

SPEECH MECHANISM EXAMINATION—Cont'd

Tongue—Cont'd

Function—Cont'd

Describe instructions needed to obtain performance (e.g., imitation, tactile stimulation, etc.) _____

_____

_____

_____

Protrude: Yes _____ No _____ Deviation: To right _____ To left

_____

Lateralize: Right _____ Left _____
Elevate

Tip: Yes ____ No ____ Back: Yes ____ No ____ Relationship of elevation to lingual frenum and extent of mouth opening_____

_____

	Trials			Rating		
	1	*2*	*3*	*Above av.*	*Av.*	*Below av.*
Number of times can say /t ʌ/ in 5 sec (range 3.0-5.5 per sec)[3,5]						
Number of times tongue can touch alveolar ridge without speech (range 3.5-6.0 per sec)[4]						
Number of times can move tongue tip from one corner of mouth to the other in 5 sec (can use above ranges for average)						
Number of times can say /kʌ/ in 5 sec (range 3.5-5.5 per sec)[2,3,5]						
Number of times can say /p ʌ t ʌ kʌ/ in 5 sec (range 1.0-1.75 per sec)[3,5]						

Description for possible tongue thrust pattern (swallowing)

Extreme tension in muscles of mastication and orbicularis oris: Yes _____ No _____

Lack of contraction of masseter muscle when swallowing: Yes _____ No _____

Tongue protrusion when labial seal is broken: Yes _____ No _____

Adequacy for speech: 1 _____ 2 _____ 3 _____ 4 _____

Continued.

SPEECH MECHANISM EXAMINATION—Cont'd

Hard palate

Width: Normal _____ Narrow _____ Wide _____ Height: Normal _____ Vaulted _____
Low _____
Symmetric: Yes _____ No _____ Explain _____

_____

_____

Color of tissue: Pink _____ Whitish _____ Mottled _____
Cleft: Repaired _____ Unrepaired _____ Submucous _____ Describe degree and condition

_____

_____

Adequacy for speech: 1 _____ 2 _____ 3 _____ 4 _____

Velopharyngeal port mechanism

Structure

Soft palate and uvula
　At rest: Deviation _____ Right _____ Left _____
　Length of soft palate in relation to depth of oropharynx: Adequate _____
　Inadequate _____ Describe _____

_____

　Cleft: Absent uvula ____ Bifid uvula ____ Repaired ____ Unrepaired ____
　Describe degree and condition_____

_____

Fauces
　Palatoglossus: Present _____ Absent _____ Scarred _____
　Palatopharyngeus: Present _____ Absent _____ Scarred _____
　Faucial isthmus: Average _____ Large _____ Restricted _____
　Tonsils: Normal _____ Atrophied _____ Enlarged _____ Inflamed
　_____ Absent _____

Function

Velopharyngeal closure: Blow out match _____ Drink from straw _____
Soft palate movement
　Prolonged /ɑ/: Elevation pronounced and maintained _____ Elevation pro-
　nounced and erratic _____ Moderate movement _____ Slight move-
　ment _____ No movement _____ Other _____

_____

　Levator dimples: Prominent _____ Slight _____ Absent _____
　Short rapid productions of /ɑ/: Elevation pronounced and maintained _____
　Elevation pronounced and erratic _____ Moderate movement _____
　Slight movement _____ No movement _____ Other _____

_____

_____

Continued.

SPEECH MECHANISM EXAMINATION—Cont'd

Velopharyngeal port mechanism—cont'd

Function—cont'd

Panting: Elevation pronounced and maintained _____ Elevation pronounced and erratic _____ Moderate movement _____ Slight movement _____ No movement _____ Other _____

_____

Gag reflex
Could not be elicited _____
Movement of palate and pharyngeal walls:
Vigorous _____ Moderate _____ Slight _____
Symmetric movement: Yes _____ No _____ Other observations

_____

Movement of posterior pharyngeal walls (noted under the above activities):
Mesially _____ Superiorly _____ Both_____
Pressure ratio: Instrument used _____

	Trials			Notes
	1	*2*	*3*	
Nostrils open				
Nostrils occluded				
Obtained ratio				

Comments regarding velopharyngeal closure for speech production_____

_____

Adequacy for speech: 1 _____ 2 _____ 3 _____ 4 _____

Breathing

"Clavicular breathing" noted: Yes _____ No _____
Voluntary control of breathing: Rhythm _____ Inhalation _____
Exhalation _____ Panting _____

Continued.

SPEECH MECHANISM EXAMINATION—Cont'd

Breathing—cont'd

	Trials			Rating		
	1	2	3	Above av.	Av.	Below av.
Ability to sustain steady exhalation (10 sec)[1]						
Length of time can sustain steady phonation of /ɑ/ or /m/ (10 sec)[1]						

References

1. Westlake, H. Suggested minimum physiological essentials for speech. In *A system for developing speech with cerebral palsied children*. Available from the National Society for Crippled Children and Adults.

2. Bloomquist, B. L. Diadochokinetic movements of nine-, ten-, and eleven-year-old children. *Journal of Speech and Hearing Disorders*, 1950, *15*, 159-164.

3. Sprague, A. L. The relationship between selected measures of expressive language and motor skill in eight-year-old boys. Doctoral dissertation, University of Iowa, 1961.

4. Fairbanks, G., and Spriestersback, D. C. A study of minor organic deviations in "functional" disorders of articulation: 1. Rate of movement of oral structures. *Journal of Speech and Hearing Disorders*, 1950, *15*, 60-69.

5. Fletcher, S. G. *The Fletcher Time-by-Count Test of Diadochokinetic Syllable Rate*. Tigard, Oregon: C. C. Publications, Inc., 1978.

Examples for writing clinical reports and parental (patient) report letters

THE CLINICAL REPORT

The following are *example* excerpts from reports demonstrating how the various sections of reports may be written. We have provided different types of information within each section. Following the excerpts is an entire example clinical report. The student should return to Chapter 10 for a discussion of what is included within each section, potential ways of ordering the information, and variations that might exist depending on the nature of the client and his problem.

I. Identification

As previously mentioned, this section is generally dictated by the work setting.

II. Statement of the problem

- Mrs. Sam Whaley, age 48 years, was referred to this clinic by Dr. Paul Keller after being diagnosed as having vocal nodules and periodic hoarseness during the 3 months prior to April 1, 1983. Mrs. Whaley reported that she seems to have a mild case of laryngitis and often loses her voice completely.

- James "Michael" Lund, 5 years, 0 months of age, was brought to the speech and hearing clinic by his mother for an evaluation of "unclear" speech. Miss Martha Moore, Director of Services for Exceptional Children in Cobb County, suggested that Mrs. Lund contact the speech and hearing clinic concerning the problem.

  During the interview, Mrs. Lund stated that Michael seemed to understand everything said to him but talked infrequently. She further reported that his speech is very hard to understand and he frequently "points" without using speech.

- Rodney McCoy, 7 years, 7 months old, was referred to the University Speech and Hearing Clinic by Mrs. Frances T. Horseman, Public Health Nurse of Clarke County. Since Rodney is not yet in school and has not been provided with a special educational program, Mrs. Horseman wanted further evaluation of speech, hearing, psychological, and educational needs.

III. Background history

- According to Mr. and Mrs. Jen, Herman babbled and cooed during his first 6 months and spoke his first word at 10 months. During the first year, he was not indifferent to sound and responded when he was spoken to. He had acquired some meaningful speech. At 13 months of age Herman contracted bacterial meningitis (see medical history).

Following this, Herman's vocalizations consisted of yelling and screeching to attract attention or express annoyance. He became markedly alert to gesture, facial expression, and movement.

Presently, Herman has little meaningful speech, but he does use the words "stop," "mama," and "daddy." He points to things he wants and babbles for objects. he is alert to gestures but does not respond to speech.

- Mrs. Lund stated that Michael babbled and cooed within the first 6 months. The date of Michael's first intelligible word could not be determined. Jargon was used in place of meaningful speech until the age of 2 years. Between the ages of 2 and 3 years single distorted words such as "mama," "boy," and "girl" were first spoken. Two-word sentences and short phrases have increased in frequency up to the present time.

Mrs. Lund first became concerned about Michael's speech in the summer of 1983. At that time Michael appeared to comprehend the speech of others but spoke very little. Gestures were used in situations where speech was more applicable. Speech was highly distorted and almost unintelligible when attempted. Hesitations and repetitions of single words and sounds were also noted by Mrs. Lund.

- According to a medical report received from Dr. Paul Keller, Mrs. Whaley was seen by him in April, 1983, at which time she complained of periodic hoarseness. On examination she was found to have "very small vocal nodules on the anterior third of her vocal cords bilaterally." She was therefore advised to use her voice as little as possible, and if the nodules persisted, voice retraining was recommended. Mrs. Whaley reported that she took a short vacation at the doctor's suggestion but had to return home sooner than planned because of a family problem. After returning to work, she found it difficult to follow the doctor's orders of vocal rest since she felt that her customers would not understand.

- When Herman was 10 months old, he had severe bronchial pneumonia with fevers up to 104°F. At 13 months of age, December, 1983, he had acute bacterial meningitis accompanied by high fevers (104°F) and convulsions. Herman had 3-day measles at 1 year and a head injury at 14 months of age; both of these conditions were reported to be mild.

- Mrs. Nat had a normal pregnancy with Steve. The length of labor was 23 hours, and instruments were used in delivery. There was so supplementary oxygen required and no evidence of jaundice at birth. Birth weight was 7 pounds, 9½ ounces. No health or feeding problems occurred during the first 2 weeks of life.

- Mrs. Lund reported that labor was induced by drugs because she was 3 weeks overdue. It was feared that serious complications might result if the child was carried for a longer period. Labor lasted 3 hours. No instruments were used, but anesthesia was administered. Birth weight was 9 pounds, 2 ounces, and was regained during the first week. No postnatal problems were reported for the first 2 weeks of life.

Mrs. Lund stated that Michael held his head erect while lying on his stomach at an age comparable to his siblings. Michael sat alone unsupported at 6 months, crawled at 9 months, walked unaided at 16 months, was fed with a spoon at 2 weeks, and was toilet trained while awake at 2 years and while sleeping at 3 years.

- Jeffrey entered Mrs. Richards' kindergarten class in Lapham School on November 12, 1983. Mrs. Richard indicated the following: "Our readiness activities do not spark his interest, and he has shown he needs help with many primary concepts such as color recognition, counting and number recognition, knowledge of shapes, etc."

- During the interview with Mrs. Lund, she reported that Michael is rejected by playmates his age due to "his speech problem." As a result, he tends to play with children younger than himself or alone.

  According to Mrs. Lund, Michael is easily frustrated when others fail to understand his speech. It appears to irritate Michael that he cannot talk as well as his 2-year-old brother Billy. Michael becomes very "stubborn" and hard to discipline when such frustrations occur. During these periods Michael chews his fingernails and toenails.

- Mrs. Ober described Jeffrey as a happy child "who likes school and his teacher but is very conscious of talking." Mrs. Richard indicated that Jeffrey has shown "immaturity in social and emotional growth." According to her, "Jeffrey needs firm control because he is impulsive in his actions. He becomes very restless and disturbs other children." She also mentioned that he fidgets, daydreams, and is irresponsible.

- Larry has been seen at the Psycho-Educational Clinic in regard to his learning and behavior difficulties. A report dated January 2, 1983, from Robert Birch stated that Larry obtained an intelligence score of 94 on the Stanford-Binet Intelligence Scale (Form L-M). His performance on the Bender–Gestalt Test for Young Children and the Graham–Kendall Memory-for-Design Test shows "immature, but adequate, perceptual abilities." The report also states that Larry is an anxious child whose anxiety is "manifest in rapid speech, motor hyperactivity, short attention span, and inability to concentrate for extended periods of time." It is felt that his excessive anxiety underlies Larry's learning difficulties. Larry has been referred to the Dane County Guidance Center for further evaluation and therapy.

IV. Testing and observation

- Rodney went willingly with the examiners. He was responsive to visual stimuli and movement. He attended visually to people moving about the room as well as objects that were new to him. He also responded readily to touch by turning in the appropriate direction and smiling. It was evident throughout this examination that Rodney responded very favorably to human contact, concern, and approval.

- Eleanor separated easily from her parents. Testing was begun with a spontaneous speech sample talking about toys to be unwrapped. The majority of her language consisted of one-word responses, consonant-vowel syllables, or vowel sounds. Approximately 10% of her spontaneous speech consisted of nine two-word phrases: no more, more toy, no toy, big ball, big baby, bye bunny, my book, two eye, and more pow, in descending order of frequency. Total vocabulary output was less than 25 words. Intonation was appropriate and used to indicate a question or a statement.

  The Peabody Picture Vocabulary Test (PPVT), Form B, was administered. Without a basal being established, Eleanor received a vocabulary comprehension age of 2 years, 1 month (chronological age of 3 years, 0 months). The reliability of this test is questionable for Eleanor's responses were erratic.

  The Utah Test of Language Development yielded a language-age equivalent of 2 years, 2 months. She could follow simple instructions, recognize body parts, recognize the names of common objects, and identify common pictures when named. Expressively, she named two common pictures and used some two-word combinations spontaneously. She did not respond to simple commands, name colors, or identify action in pictures.

- Mrs. Smith was very cooperative and said that she understood the purpose of testing and was willing to do her best. The Language Modalities Test for Aphasia designed by Wepman and Jones was administered and the entire test completed. The only errors on the screening section were spelling and articulation; the response for "cat" was "C-A... oh, oh, C-A-C," with no response ("I don't know") to spelling and writing "give." The repetition of words on the screening test was characterized by the production of incorrect phonemes with the exception of the correct production of "seven." Matching of both visual and auditory stimuli to pictures presented few problems for Mrs. Smith; one error was pointing to a picture of two tops instead of one (visual sentence); the second error was pointing to one plant growing rather than to several (visual sentence); the third error was pointing to "these bells ring" for "three bells ring" (auditory sentence). Oral responses showed mainly errors consisting of using an incorrect phoneme usually, but not exclusively, in the initial syllable of a word. Once she got past the first syllable, a sequence of syllables could usually be produced without the pauses that characterized the initiation of the sentence. Graphic responses were either correctly done, not attempted, or not completed after a correct attempt was begun. When Mrs. Smith wrote, she did it slowly, had to use her nonpreferred left hand, and often paused after writing one or more letters. The tell-a-story items evoked responses that were mainly content words containing incorrect phonemes, some phrases that were ended by hesitation, and a few sentences. In general, the stories told by Mrs. Smith were short, did not describe all aspects of the picture, contained many pauses and interjections, and were usually ended by "I don't know" after being urged by the examiner to tell more. According to Wepman and Jones' scoring, the patient exhibited syntactic and some semantic language problems on the tell-a-story items, phonemic and semantic errors on oral responses to visual and auditory stimuli, and correct or "no response" errors on graphic responses to visual and auditory stimuli. In cycles 1 and 2 of the Language Modalities Test for Aphasia, about 50% of the oral and graphic responses were correct and only 3 out of 60 matching items were missed.

- Tim went willingly with the examiner and adjusted quickly to the testing situation. He understood all the tasks and worked steadily for over 1½ hours. The following testing procedures were used:

    1. Peabody Picture Vocabulary Test (PPVT), Form B
    2. Vocabulary Usage Test (VUT)
    3. Wepman's Auditory Discrimination Test
    4. Templin-Darley Screening Articulation Test
    5. Hejna's Developmental Articulation Test
    6. Speech mechanism examination
    7. Pure tone air conduction audiometric screening
    8. Stimulability testing as well as informal measures for auditory comprehension and retention span, cognitive behavior, and sentence structure

The primary finding was inadequate phonologic development. On the Templin-Darley Articulation Screening Test he had one correct response out of 50. Children his age and sex should have approximately 35 correct responses. An analysis of his errors on the sounds tested on both the Templin-Darley and Hejna tests revealed a rather consistent use of the /t/ and /d/ phonemes or these phonemes in combination with another distorted phoneme for most all of the consonant singles and blends. Other phonemes he used correctly with some consistency were /p, b, m, n, k, g/ and occasionally /f and v/. The vowels used were almost always distorted. Another phoneme problem that revealed itself was a pattern of unvoicing a final voiced consonant as in the word "bed." This phoneme pattern resulted in speech that was unintelligible unless the examiner knew the subject matter. (See articulation tests for detailed articulation results.)

- The 50-item screening test and the 43-item Iowa Pressure Test from the Templin-Darley Tests of Articulation were administered. Donna produced nine correct responses on the screening test. By 12 years of age a perfect score should be obtained. On the Iowa Pressure Test Donna produced three correct responses. The Iowa Pressure Test includes items selected to assess the adequacy of intra-oral pressure for speech production and thus, inferentially, the adequacy of velopharyngeal closure.

  Donna generally produced bilabial plosives in all positions. A velar or pharyngeal fricative was sustained for the linguoalveolar and linguovelar plosives in most positions, while a glottal stop was substituted for medial /k and g/; /t/ was transcribed as correct in the medial position by two examiners, but apparently it was an acoustic approximation. Most fricatives were either omitted or substituted by the velar fricative. /z/ was transcribed in the word 'crayons' by both examiners. /f/ was never produced, although Donna sometimes put her lower lip in contact with the upper central incisors but no sound was produced. Affricates always had the velar substitution. All nasals were produced as were the glides /r/ and /l/ as singles. In the final position the r-colored vowel occasionally had no coloring. Glides were generally produced in two- and three-item consonant clusters; two-item clusters involving any fricative or plosive were always substituted by the velar fricative.

  Varying amounts of nasal emission and nasality accompanied the phonemes that were produced.

  Modfiability was attempted on all plosives, fricatives, and affricates. Even with intensive stimulation involving manipulation of the articulators, /t, d, k, g, / were always substituted by the velar fricative; there was no anterior approximation at all. A fairly good /s and z/ could be produced in isolation; in syllables the tendency was toward a more posterior production. An anterior approximation was achieved on /ʃ, θ, ð, ʒ, tʃ/; /dʒ/ was still produced with a velar substitution.

- Observations of Mrs. Whaley's voice quality were made for different types of vocalizations such as production of isolated vowels /ɑ, i/, reading of words and sentences, and conversational speech. Speaking situations differed in the following ways: the voice was high, then low; the muscles were tensed, then relaxed; the head was bent forward, then backwards. In general, her voice quality was hoarse; however, it was much clearer when producing isolated sounds and reading than in conversational speech. Mrs. Whaley was unable to increase the loudness of her voice to any noticeable degree, and when attempts were made, pitch breaks were evident. When speaking softly, she used a "loud whisper," and her voice was as strained as in habitual use.

- A speech mechanism examination revealed a postoperative left unilateral complete cleft of the primary and secondary palates. Some asymmetry of the vermilion border of the lip and depression of the left nares are evident. Asymmetry of the palate is also evident; the left half of the soft palate is more elongated than the right. Two potential fistulas were noted; one in the medial portion of the hard palate, and the second in the posterior aspect of the soft palate. It is not known if these fistulas are complete. The premaxilla is partially collapsed, resulting in a mesiocclusion. The low attachment of the superior labial frenulum is restricting the mobility of the upper lip. The tonsils are present and do not appear inflamed. On phonation of "ah" only slight movement of the soft palate on the left was noted and no lateral wall movement was noted. The oral manometer readings, indicating Maury's ability to build intraoral breath pressure, revealed an average of 3.6 ounces with the nostrils unoccluded and 4.5 ounces with the nostrils occluded. The measure was not considered reliable because of a weak labial closure that allowed air to escape out of the mouth. It does indicate, however, that velopharyngeal closure is probably not complete. Tongue protrusion, lateralization, and elevation were adequate.

V. Clinical evaluation

- From all indications, Mrs. Whaley's voice problem is a manifestation of her difficulties in coping with day-to-day problems. The vocal nodules have apparently resulted from excessive strain and tension brought on by increased responsibilities and greater use of a voice that even in its normal function was not a good speaking voice.

    Throughout the interview she displayed signs of general tension, particularly in speech musculature, which probably has some relationship to her voice disorder. Although Mrs. Whaley is aware that she has tensions, she evidently does not understand the possibility of casual relationships between these tensions, her voice abuse, and resulting vocal nodules.

- A review of the case history and evaluation of present speech and language abilities suggests the possibility of brain injury, resulting in both an aphasic disorder and retarded mental development.

    The case history gives evidence of the possible occurrence of brain injury. The umbilical rupture and necessity for induced labor serve as possible causal factors. Michael's expressive language problems, reduced attention span, retarded language development, distractibility, difficulties in visual discrimination and relationships, and intense preoccupation with very fine detail are behavioral characteristics indicative of possible central nervous system dysfunction.

    Mental retardation was also indicated by many of Michael's behaviors. The Leiter International Performance Scale and Peabody Picture Vocabulary Test results indicated slow mental development. However, due to the language problems, these test results should be interpreted with caution.

    It is therefore believed that Michael should presently be considered as having aphasic problems with an accompanying delay in mental development.

- Donna has a severe articulation-resonation disorder, the main component being production of a velar fricative as a substitution for most plosives, fricatives, and affricates. Her articulation scores on both tests were extremely low and were commensurate with the performance of a normal child 3 years of age and below. Although both parents stated that Donna was easy to understand, this examiner does not concur. Even when the subject was known, intelligibility was below 50%.

    The nature and severity of Donna's disorder are the product of many variables. It is generally believed that children cannot improve phonemic production unless they are able to practice and experiment with their articulators. Donna was confined to bed because of her heart problem for the first 4 years. She had major illnesses and surgery throughout her life, significantly the laryngeal operations at 8, 9, and 10 years of age with varying lengths of forced vocal rest. When Donna did learn to speak, she did so with an incompetent mechanism, that is, inadequate velopharyngeal closure. The paralysis of the palate was not discovered until she was 10 years old, and corrective surgery was not performed until the following year. Therefore the patterns of speech that were first developed were perpetuated; that is, the sounds that require a buildup of intraoral pressure could not be produced, so Donna compensated by producing a velar fricative or glottal stop as substitutions. At the present time it seems possible that Donna has *potential* velopharyngeal closure as evidenced by the pressure ratios, her ability to modify some of the speech sounds, and the Iowa Pressure Test, which showed that an increase in the number of items in consonant clusters did not affect production.

VI. Diagnosis

- Mrs. Janes has a severe aphasia resulting from a cerebrovascular accident.
- Gary's speech and language problem is very complex. The case history, previous speech therapy, and the present speech and language evaluation suggest the possibility of an aphasic language disorder and slow mental development stemming from brain injury.
- Grady has a mild articulation disorder associated with tongue thrust.
- Karyn has a severe speech production problem affecting all speech production subprocesses resulting in disordered voice, resonance, prosody, and phonetic structure. This major disorder is associated with the neurologic damage sustained in an automobile accident.
- Jess is delayed in all language abilities; this is apparently related to both intellectual and emotional factors.
- It is felt that Robert's major problem is one of general retardation. However, language comprehension and formulation appear to be poorer than would be expected from the retardation.
- Mr. Natjen has an extremely hoarse voice quality due to ventricular phonation.

VII. Recommendations

- Intensive language stimulation and articulation therapy should be initiated in an effort to prepare Ramon for entrance into school. A group situation with children his age might be especially helpful in preparing him to interact socially in kindergarten.

    Referral for psychological testing is recommended and would best be presented to the parent as an aid in determining Ramon's readiness for school.

    Referral for a dental evaluation would be helpful in planning articulation therapy and in helping the child to have a better facial appearance.

    Parent counseling with Mrs. Jablonski should be continued to help in parental attitudes toward the speech problem and reduce tendencies toward overprotection.

- Voice therapy to begin in the Fall of 1983 and designed to relax muscular tension in the laryngeal area, establish adequate breathing patterns, and alter vocal usage.

    Counseling in regard to the many pressures present in her life that may be affecting vocal use.

    Periodic examinations by an otolaryngologist.

    Periodic audiometric examinations.

    The following recommendations were given to Mrs. Whaley in regard to use of the speech mechanism until therapy can be arranged:

    1. Reduce the amount of coughing and clearing of the throat
    2. Vocal rest
    3. Use soft vocal attacks and breathy voice
    4. Eliminate speaking on residual air

- Because Larry's behavior at this time limits any improvement that could result from speech therapy, a program of speech therapy is not recommended at the present time. It is recommended that Larry be seen by the Dane County Guidance Center for an evaluation of his behavioral problems and recommendations for treatment.

Following this evaluation and the recommendations made by the Center, further plans for speech therapy can be made. In accordance with their advice a choice can be made between the following possibilities.

1. If it is felt that treatment of Larry's underlying difficulties will allow him to modify his behavior, speech therapy can be delayed until such modifications have taken place.

2. If Larry's behavior problems are not felt to be symptomatic of underlying emotional difficulties but are felt to exist independently from such difficulties, speech therapy can begin immediately. If this is the case, attempts will be made during therapy to deal with Larry's behavior as it exists.

3. Speech therapy for Larry must be directed to correction of articulation errors, elimination of word and sound omissions, and establishment of an appropriate rate of speech. Control must then be developed so that these techniques can be carried over into conversational speech.

CLINICAL REPORT EXAMPLE

November 22, 1983

I. IDENTIFICATION

Name:	James Richards
Birth date:	October 19, 1973
Parents' name:	Mr. and Mrs. James W. Richards
	1322 Glen Street
	Belton, Wisconsin
Examined at:	United Speech and Hearing Services
	Belton General Hospital
	Belton, Wisconsin
Date of examination:	October 22, 1983
From:	Dr. James Edwards

II. STATEMENT OF THE PROBLEM

James Richards (Ricky) was seen at the United Speech and Hearing Services Clinic (USHS) for speech evaluations and therapy. The present consultation was to determine how much speech progress might be expected with the existing speech mechanism. At this time, Ricky is 10 years of age.

III. HISTORY

A. Medical and surgical history

Ricky was born on October 19, 1973, following a normal pregnancy. The length of labor was approximately 6 hours and no instruments were used in delivery. Birth

---

Continued.

CLINICAL REPORT EXAMPLE—Cont'd

III. HISTORY—Cont'd

A. Medical and surgical history—Cont'd

weight was 6 pounds, 8 ounces. Apparent at birth was an extensive cleft lip and palate. At 1 month of age Ricky was referred to the Cleft Lip and Palate Clinic and has been followed by them since. The original diagnosis of the cleft condition at that time by Dr. Jackson, pediatrician, stated: "Bears a severe cleft on the left side that involves a large portion of the palate. There is some rotation of the dental ridge on the right side of the cleft. The lip and nose are involved in the process."

Ricky's surgical history reveals a cleft lip repair on December 2, 1973, and a cleft palate repair on August 2, 1975. A clinic visit on January 13, 1976 revealed that the palate and lip were closed. Dr. Thompson suggested that "in a few years he will need narrowing of the left nares."

From 1976 to the present, Ricky has been followed by the Cleft Lip and Palate Clinic. Dental treatment has been carried out, but no orthodontic work has been recommended by Dr. Wells. No further surgical procedures have been done although the possibility of narrowing the left nares (Dr. Thompson, 1976), an Abbe Estlander flap (Dr. Thompson, 1979), and work on the upper lip and narrowed "arphis" (Dr. Grimball, 1982) were considered.

In October, 1982, Mr. Poolwall, speech pathologist, indicated limited improvement in speech apparently related to inadequate velopharyngeal closure. (See speech history.) He felt that pharyngeal flap surgery should be considered. In October, 1982, Dr. Grimball concurred. The possibility of pharyngeal flap surgery will be discussed by Dr. Thompson with Dr. Nelson in Madison, Wisconsin.

B. History of speech development and hearing

According to Mr. and Mrs. Richards, Ricky began to say single words at 20 months of age and began using simple sentences at age 22 months. The parents talked baby talk to the child but felt that he received much speech stimulation. At times they would anticipate his wants before he could communicate his need. They believe that Ricky's present vocabulary is average but his speech is inferior. They do not feel that Ricky's cleft palate condition interferes with his amount of communication.

On March 14, 1978, Ricky was first seen by a speech pathologist (Mr. Obers, United Speech and Hearing Services). He was unable to get an adequate speech sample, but from the sounds that were heard and the parent's report of speech, he felt that a marked nasality and articulatory involvement were present. Speech therapy was recommended but was not initiated. A reevaluation (Mr. Obers) on May 5, 1979 revealed adequate vowel production but severe sibilant distortions. Speech therapy was again recommended.

Ricky has received periodic speech therapy from June, 1979, to the present time. Therapy has been concentrated around improving articulatory skills by increasing Ricky's ability to direct and control the breath stream. Some nasality and nasal emission have been decreased as a result of this therapy. On June 28, 1983, Mr. Poolwall,

Continued.

CLINICAL REPORT EXAMPLE—Cont'd

III. HISTORY—Cont'd

B. History of speech development and hearing—Cont'd

speech pathologist (USHS), believed that with Ricky's present inadequate velopharyngeal closure as much speech compensation as possible had taken place. He suggested the possibility of pharyngeal flap surgery. (See medical history.)

Mr. and Mrs. Richards do not believe that Ricky has heard adequately during his development. Previous otologic and audiometric examinations bear this out. A series of air conduction audiograms taken from 1979 to 1981 reveal a mild bilateral hearing loss. An otologic report to the speech clinic in 1979 indicated "fluid in the ears," scarring of the tympanic membrane, and inflammation of the tonsils and adenoids, which were removed at age 5 according to the parents.

C. Educational history

Ricky's parents report that he makes average grades in the fourth grade at Central Grammar School where Mrs. Wicker is his teacher. He attended Marshall School during the first three grades, failing the first grade. He likes school.

D. Personality adjustment

Ricky has many playmates with whom he usually gets along well. He prefers outdoor activities and likes to participate in activities involving others. He belongs to the Cub Scouts. He is taken care of by his grandmother when his mother is away. His parents stated that Ricky is concerned about the "bump on his mouth and he wants to have lips." He doesn't seem shy about it and will talk to other children about this problem when they ask him what is wrong. However, children tease him sometimes and he does mind this.

The other children in the family don't say anything to him about his problem, and they all understand his speech.

E. Family history

Ricky is the oldest of five children. He has three sisters, ages 7, 5, and 3, and a brother who is 20 months old. No speech, hearing, or physical problem is reported for any of the other children. Ricky's mother, who is 27 years old, completed the ninth grade and is a textile worker. His father, who is 30 years of age, also completed the ninth grade. They are both employed at the Belton Yarn Plant where Mr. Richards is a textile supervisor. They own their six and a half room home, which is located within the city limits.

IV. TESTING AND OBSERVATION

Selected parts of the Templin-Darley Test of Articulation were adminstered to assess adequacy of articulation.

One of Ricky's primary substitution errors in the initial position was using the nasal/m or n/ sound in place of a sound requiring buildup of oral breath pressure,

Continued.

CLINICAL REPORT EXAMPLE—Cont'd

IV. TESTING AND OBSERVATION—Cont'd

for example, /m/b, m/s, m/st, m/sm, s̃m/sp, mp̃/spl, mp̃/spr, n/sn, and nl/sl. This nasal sound substitution error was used primarily in words containing an /s/ sound.

Other errors of substitution in blends in the initial position included: /w/sw, w/kw, w/tw, l/sl, l/kl, r/dr, r/pr, r/kr, r/fr, r/tr, and r/ʃr/. The common error here generally is one of omitting the aspect of the blend that required buildup of oral breath pressure. The /l, r, and w/ are produced correctly according to articulatory position but at times are nasal.

Errors of omission occurred on /p, k, t, d, s, and ʃ/ in the initial position, /k, t, s, and ʃ/ in the medial position, and /t and s/ in final position. Many of the sounds tested were distorted by nasality and nasal emission.

The errors of omission and distortion reveal that certain sounds are inconsistently produced. The plosives, fricatives, and affricates are at times omitted but when produced are almost always characterized by nasality (~) or nasal emission (≫). All vowels were at times produced nasally. Ricky's best consonant production requiring oral breath pressure was the production of /g/. Whenever Ricky was instructed to try very hard when producing consonant sounds, greater nasality and nasal emission were noted.

In spontaneous speech the above errors tended to make Ricky's speech highly unintelligible unless the context was known. His sentences contained many nasalized vowels, glottals, and some weak consonants.

Integral stimulation revealed that Ricky had only limited ability to modify his production of speech sounds in isolation. Most modifications still resulted in the sound being nasally emitted.

A. Oral examination

Examination of the peripheral speech mechanism revealed a repaired cleft lip and palate with the upper lip being extremely tight. This seems to interfere with protrusion and eversion of the upper lip as Ricky was observed to speak primarily out of the left side of the mouth. Scar tissue is present on both the hard and soft palate. The nasality and nasal emission noted in his speech indicated that he is not attaining proper velopharyngeal closure. Very little movement of the palate was noted on phonation of "ah." The oral manometer was used to obtain an indication of intraoral breath pressure. The average breath pressure with the nostrils open was 10 ounces. The average with the nostrils occluded was 15. This indicates that velopharyngeal closure is not adequate.

B. Hearing examination

An audiometric pure tone air conduction test was administered bilaterally for the frequencies from 250 to 8,000 Hz. The results indicated acuity within the normal range (approximately 10 to 15 dB over the speech frequencies).

Continued.

CLINICAL REPORT EXAMPLE—Cont'd

V. CLINICAL EVALUATION

Ricky has a severe articulation-resonation problem including errors of substitution, distortion, and omission accompanied by excess nasality and nasal emission. The examination indicates that the problem is primarily related to his inability to obtain the adequate velopharyngeal closure needed to produce speech sounds requiring intraoral breath pressure.

The history of limited success in speech therapy, the present oral manometer readings, the limited palatal movement seen, and his inability to reduce the nasality and nasal emission on sounds under stimulation indicate that his present mechanism is not adequate. It is therefore not expected that much improvement is to be gained with a speech therapy program alone.

Richard was cooperative throughout the testing, and it would seem that his motivation for speech would be high. During the examination, he not only answered questions readily, but conversed easily.

VI. DIAGNOSIS

Ricky has a severe articulation-resonation problem accompanied by excessive nasality and nasal emission resulting from inadequate velopharyngeal closure.

VII. RECOMMENDATIONS

1. Consideration for further surgical or prosthetic procedures to obtain better velopharyngeal closure.
2. Consideration for further surgical procedures to gain better flexibility of the upper lip.
3. Continued audiometric and otologic examinations. Any further hearing loss must be prevented.
4. Speech therapy after the completion of any procedure utilized for obtaining better closure. (NOTE: Ricky should be evaluated carefully after the procedures for closure have been completed. His ability to produce each sound must be noted as well as his ability to modify any incorrect sounds.

James Edwards, Ph.D.
Speech Pathologist

THE PARENTAL (PATIENT) REPORT LETTER

This report is generally a brief letter to the parents or the patient and should be worded so that they understand most of the terms used. Remember, however, that these reports follow your discussion with the parents or patient during the interpretive conference. They should not include information that has not been previously discussed, unless you indicated during the interpretive conference that it would be provided.

These reports in some way should incorporate the following:

1. Identification of the patient
2. When and where the patient was examined
3. The results of the examination
4. The diagnosis
5. Possible causal and related factors
6. The recommendations
7. The action being taken

Dear Mr. and Mrs. Rostar:

As you know, Leon was seen in our clinic on November 19, 1983. At this time we tried to find out what Leon's problem might be. At present we feel that it may be related to a hearing loss; however, we are not certain. We need to see Leon for regular observations and testing. We would like to start this as soon as possible beginning in December. Before that time you can help us a great deal by finding out as much as you can about his hearing. We would like for you to tell us such things as what he does when you tell him to do something such as "Look for your shirt," or whether or not you have to point to things you want him to get, and how much attention he pays to your face when you talk, etc. Thank you very much for your help, which will aid us in helping Leon.

We will let you know when we can begin seeing Leon on a regular basis.

If you have any questions or need help with Leon, please call Miss Josephine.

Dear Mrs. Whaley:

As you know, our voice examination results revealed that your voice has a hoarse quality that is a result of the vocal nodules and related to the increased amount of tension present in your life.

We feel that voice therapy beginning in 2 months when you return from vacation will be helpful in teaching you a better voice quality and reducing the amount of vocal misuse resulting from the increased muscular tension. Until then, however, we would like to remind you of the following recommendations in regard to the use of your voice:

1. Reduce the amount of coughing and clearing of the throat.
2. Talk as little as possible, especially under strained conditions.
3. Begin your words with a breathy voice and continue talking with this breathy quality.
4. Remember to take another breath of air rather than to talk when you are out of breath.

We will notify you in September to schedule voice therapy.

If we fail to contact you or if you have any questions concerning your problem, please feel free to call us.

Dear Mr. and Mrs. Whitney:

As you know, Scott was seen in our clinic on February 11, 1983. At that time we found that he has a problem of delayed use of sounds characterized by sound substitutions, omissions, and distortions. We found that his vocabulary comprehension is adequate for a child of his age. As you have pointed out, he is using his tongue inappropriately during conversation.

We also noted that Scott had some negative reactions to speech as evidenced by his responding with "I don't know" and I don't want to." He also asked the examiner to name a number of objects that probably were familiar to him rather than having to name them himself. We believe that he may feel that his speech is inadequate or not understandable to the listener; thus the negative reactions on his part.

We recommend speech therapy and are placing Scott's name on the waiting list. In the meantime, we would suggest that you reinforce his speech with correct words rather than repeating his errors; for example, if he says, "Where's my 'woo' (for shoe)?" respond with the word in a sentence such as "Let's look for your shoe, Scott," etc. It is recommended that he never be forced to say a word correctly. At his age he probably is not ready to produce some of the more difficult sounds such as (ch) and (sh). Also, he should not be given directions as to tongue placement for certain sounds with which he is having difficulty.

Attention to Scott's speech can be given indirectly through certain activities such as looking at pictures and books together and letting him make responses when he wishes. Spontaneous response, without pressure, should be acceptable in every situation.

We feel that maturation, along with reducing any pressures regarding speech, and a therapy program would indicate a favorable prognosis for Scott.

We will contact you concerning a therapy schedule for him.

If you have any questions, please do not hesitate to call or write.

Dear Mr. Herber:

As you know, your daughter Donna Kay was brought to the Speech and Hearing Clinic on November 5, 1983, by her grandmother Mrs. Hart for a speech evaluation. Results of our examination indicated that Kay has a severe articulation problem accompanied by excessive nasality. A test of hearing also indicated a moderate hearing loss in both ears. Kay was found to be below average for her age in vocabulary comprehension; she does not understand as many words as she should for a child her age.

Our main concern at the time of the evaluation was to try to find a reason for Kay's excessive nasality. An examination of her speech mechanism indicated that Kay has a very immobile soft palate. This makes it difficult, if not impossible, for Kay to get enough closure in the back part of her mouth to keep sounds from coming out of her nose. It is our belief that this lack of movement of the palate may be caused by a physical abnormality in that area. We want Dr. George Erwin to see Kay again to help us determine any physical problems she may have. Dr. Erwin will advise you concerning further medical examinations for Kay. In the meantime, we will arrange for Kay to be seen in our clinic for more extensive hearing tests and for tests to determine any special educational needs.

We will advise you as to a time that Kay can be scheduled for the two examinations in our clinic. We do feel that Kay's speech can be improved and that we will be better able to help her after the other examinations have been made.

Dear Mr. and Mrs. Bobkoff:

As you know, Juan was seen in our clinic on July 20, 1983, for a speech evaluation. At that time, a test was administered to assess Juan's use of speech sounds. Certain sounds were found to be in error; however, we are not overly concerned about the errors at this time because Juan is just about 3 years old, and his sound system will still be developing for several more years. With maturation the sounds should be correctly incorporated into his sound system.

Since you were most concerned about Juan's "stuttering" behavior, the major portion of the evaluation time was spent in evaluating Juan's spontaneous speech. Before discussing the results obtained from this speech sample, we would like to review in a general way, the development of speech in children. Rather than using the term "stuttering," we will refer to the behavior of hesitating on words or repeating words or sounds as "disfluent" speech. All normal children in the process of acquiring speech and language hesitate and repeat on words. Young children must, within the space of several years, acquire a complex language system. From the one-word level of a 1-year-old, they progress through several stages until they are speaking in complex sentences. During their second year, children learn simple and compound sentences. Their speech rhythm is often broken. Many children use gestures and other substitutive behavior while they are developing a growing vocabulary. During the third and fourth years, the length of sentences increases, and parts of speech such as pronouns, prepositions, and conjunctions are added. Many children of 3 and 4 years of age do not have the vocabulary, the articulation skills, or the facility with grammar to keep their fluency or speech rhythm up to adult standards. Children may try to master the adult patterns of speech too quickly and their attempts may be marked with disfluencies. It is similar to children tripping themselves when they try to run when they are just learning to walk.

Juan is still at the age of acquiring a language system. If one compared him to an adult speaker, his disfluent behavior might seem excessive. However, it is important to remember that he is not an adult speaker. Children lack both the fine muscular ability and the knowledge of a complete language system that adults have. It is also important to remember that all children acquire this ability at different rates, while still being within normal limits.

There are some conditions that have been thought to increase the amount of disfluent speech. Examples are a lowered physical vitality or sickness, lack of sufficient sleep and rest, competition with another child, a feeling of not being loved or wanted by one or both parents or a teacher, overprotection by a parent or another person, an aggressive or domineering person in the home or school, and the expectation of too much from a child either at home or at school. It is known, too, that disfluent speech varies with situations of emotional stress. It may increase at times when the speaker feels fear, insecurity, or excitement.

When Juan was playing with the examiner, his spontaneous speech had very few disfluencies. Later, he seemed excited to be with you again, and when he talked to you, we did hear the repetitions that you had described to us. Your telling us that Juan is most disfluent when he is tired, excited, or talking at the same time as his brother was also helpful to our assessment of Juan's speech. Because of his young age and because so much of Juan's speech does run smoothly, his disfluencies cannot be classified as excessive at the present time. We feel, however, that you were very wise to bring him in for an evaluation because at a later time, should this behavior continue, it might be significant. Although Juan's disfluencies are not a serious problem, we do have several suggestions for you that may help his speech develop normally without excessive repetitions.

It has been found that disfluent speakers are often very fluent when they feel secure and relaxed. You have already noted this, for Juan speaks smoothly when playing quietly. By your appearing calm and relaxed about Juan's speech, you can set an atmosphere that will help him to also feel calm and relaxed about his own speech. It is important to avoid giving undue attention to any periods of disfluent speech. Therefore it would be helpful to avoid discussing his speech with anyone in Juan's presence and also to avoid saying directly to him such statements as, "Stop and begin again" or "don't talk so fast." (Many 3- and 4-year-old children speak very fast because they want to say so much at one time.) Similarly, do not try to speak for him or supply him with a word or phrase. Just wait until he finishes what he is saying. Honest, sincere praise for tasks well accomplished will help a disfluent child feel more competent and important and help bolster his feelings of security and accomplishment.

The most important thing is that Juan continue to enjoy talking and to have the opportunity to share his feelings and experiences with those who are important to him. Always listen to Juan and allow him to talk when he wants to without pressuring him to talk by asking excessive questions. Your practice of preventing competition between your two sons by giving each a turn to speak when they begin talking together is a good one, so keep it up.

Because disfluencies are less frequent when Juan is relaxed and calm, it would be a good idea to set aside a short period of time during the day when Juan could be alone with you just to talk together. Early in the morning, after lunch, or perhaps right before bedtime might be suitable for this "quiet talking time." You can just chat, or talk about pictures, or play a quiet game together. You did this very naturally at the center when we asked you to play with Juan. It will give Juan a chance to talk when calm and relaxed, a break from the normal excitement of a little boy's day. Both of you could spend this time with Juan if you have time or perhaps you could take turns.

We hope that these suggestions will assist you in working with Juan. The center will contact you in 6 months to schedule a reevaluation time so that we can see how Juan is progressing. If, before then, you notice that Juan's disfluencies are becoming much more frequent, you can call the center and the appointment can be set up at an earlier time. Should you have any questions, please do not hesitate to get in touch with us.

REFERENCES*

Abbs, J. H., & Kennedy, J. G. III. Neurophysiological processes of speech movement control. In N.J. Lass, L. V. McReynolds, J. L. Northern, & D. E. Yoder (Eds), *Speech, language, and hearing: Normal processes* (Vol. 1). Philadelphia: Saunders, 1982.

Adams, M., & Reis, R. The influence of the onset of phonation on the frequency of stuttering. *Journal of Speech and Hearing Research,* 1971, *14,* 639–644.

American Speech–Language–Hearing Association. *1982 directory.* Washington, D.C.: American Speech–Language–Hearing Association, 1982.

Anderson, R. M., Miles, M., & Matheny, P. A. *Communicative evaluation chart from infancy to five years.* Cambridge, MA: Educators Publishing Service, 1963.

Andrews, G., & Harris, M. *The syndrome of stuttering.* London: Heinemann, 1964.

Aram, D. M., Ekelman, B. L., & Nation, J. E. *Preschool language disorders: Ten years later.* (In press).

Aram, D. M., & Nation, J. E. Intelligence tests for children: A language analysis. *Ohio Journal of Speech and Hearing,* 1971, *6,* 22–43.

Aram, D. M., & Nation, J. E. Patterns of language behavior in children with developmental language disorders. *Journal of Speech and Hearing Research,* 1975, *18,* 229–241.

Aram, D. M., & Nation, J. E. Preschool language disorders and subsequent language and academic difficulties. *Journal of Communication Disorders,* 1980, *13,* 159–170.

Aram, D. M., & Nation, J. E. *Child language disorders.* St. Louis: Mosby, 1982.

Aronson, A. E. *Clinical voice disorders.* New York: Theime–Stratton, 1980.

Aronson, A. E. Early motor unit disease masquerading as psychogenic breathy dysphonia: A clinical case presentation. *Journal of Speech and Hearing Disorders,* 1971, *36,* 115–123.

Aronson, A. E., Peterson, H. W., & Litin, E. M. Voice symptomatology in functional dysphonia and aphonia. *Journal of Speech and Hearing Disorders,* 1964, *29,* 367–380.

Aronson, A. E., Peterson, H. W., & Litin, E. M. Psychiatric symptomatology in functional dysphonia and aphonia. *Journal of Speech and Hearing Disorders,* 1966, *31,* 115–127.

Asha Committee on Audiometric Evaluation. Guidelines for identification audiometry. *Asha,* 1975, *17,* 94–99.

Austin, J. *How to do things with words.* Cambridge: Harvard University Press, 1962.

Baker, H. J., & Leland, B. *Detroit Test of Learning Aptitude: Examiner's handbook.* Indianapolis: Bobbs-Merrill, 1967.

Bangs, T. E. *Language and learning disorders of the preacademic child with curriculum guide* (2nd ed.). Englewood Cliffs, NJ: Prentice-Hall, 1982.

Bar, A. Decreasing the no-show rate in an urban speech and hearing clinic *Asha,* 1975, *17,* 455–456.

Barsch, R. H. *The parent of the handicapped child.* Springfield, IL: Thomas, 1968.

Bates, E. *Language and context: The acquisition of pragmatics.* New York: Academic Press, 1976.

Bayles, K. A., & Boone, D. R. The potential of language tasks for identifying senile dementia. *Journal of Speech and Hearing Disorders,* 1982, *47,* 204–210.

Bentin, S., Silverberg, R., & Gordon, H. W. Asymmetrical cognitive deterioration in demented and Parkinson patients. *Cortex,* 1981, *17,* 533–544.

Bernstein, B. A sociolinguistic approach to socialization: With some reference to educability. In F. Williams (Ed.), *Language and poverty: Perspectives on a theme.* Chicago: Markham Press, 1970.

Berry, M. F. Developmental history of stuttering children. *Journal of Pediatrics,* 1938, *12,* 209–217.

Berry, M. F. *Language disorders of children: The bases and diagnosis.* New York: Appleton–Century–Crofts, 1969.

Berry, W. R. (Ed.) *Clinical dysarthria.* San Diego: College-Hill Press, 1983.

Bess, F. H., & McConnell, F. E. *Audiology, education, and the hearing impaired child.* St. Louis: Mosby, 1981.

Bingham, W. V., & Moore, B. V. *How to interview.* New York: Harper & Row, 1941.

Blalock, H. M. *Causal models in the social sciences.* Chicago: Aldine, 1971.

Blank, M., Rose, S. A., & Berlin, L. *The language of learning: The preschool years.* New York: Grune & Stratton, 1978.

Bloodstein, O. A rating scale of conditions under which stuttering is reduced or absent. *Journal of Speech and Hearing Disorders,* 1950, *15,* 29–36.

Bloodstein, O. The anticipatory struggle hopothesis: Implications of research on the variability of stuttering. *Journal of Speech and Hearing Research,* 1972, *15,* 487–499.

---

* Bibliographic information for tests and other diagnostic procedures are included in Tool Retrieval Tables: Appendix III.

Bloodstein, O. The rules of early stuttering. *Journal of Speech and Hearing Disorders,* 1974, *39,* 379–394.

Bloodstein, O. *A handbook on stuttering* (3rd ed.). Chicago: National Easter Seal Society for Crippled Children and Adults, 1981.

Bloom, L. *Language development: Form and function in emerging grammars.* Cambridge, MA: MIT Press, 1970.

Bloom, L. Talking, understanding, and thinking. In R. L. Schiefelbusch & L. L. Lloyd (Eds.), *Language perspectives—Acquisition, retardation, and intervention.* Baltimore: University Park Press, 1974.

Bloom, L., & Lahey, M. *Language development and language disorders.* New York: Wiley, 1978.

Boller, F., Kim, Y., & Mack, J. L. Auditory comprehension in aphasia. In H. Whitaker, & H. A. Whitaker (Eds.), *Studies in neurolinguistics* (Vol. 3). New York: Academic Press, 1977.

Boone, D. R. *The voice and voice therapy* (2nd ed.). Englewood Cliffs, NJ: Prentice–Hall, 1977.

Bowerman, M. *Early syntactic development: A cross-linguistic study with special reference to Finnish.* Cambridge: Cambridge University Press, 1973.

Brady, J. P. Studies on the metronome effect on stuttering. *Behavior Research and Therapy,* 1969, *7,* 197–204.

Brenner, N. C., Perkins, W. H. & Soderberg, G. A. The effect of rehearsal on frequency of stuttering. *Journal of Speech and Hearing Research,* 1972, *15,* 483–486.

Bright, K. E., & Matkin, N. D. *Psychometric review of selected central auditory tests for children.* Paper presented at the Arizona Speech–Language–Hearing Association Convention, Tucson, AZ, 1983.

Broca, P. Nouvelle observation d'aphémie produite par une lésion de la mortié posterieure des deuxième et troisième circonvolutions frontales. *Bull. Soc. Anat. Paris,* 1861, 398–407. (a)

Broca, P. Remarques sur le siegè de la faculté du langage articulé, suivés d'une obseration d'aphémie. *Bull. Soc. Anat. Paris,* 1861, 330–357. (b)

Brodbeck, A. J. & Irwin, O. C. The speech behavior of infants without families. *Child Development,* 1946, *17,* 145–156.

Brodnitz, F. S. Contact ulcer of the larynx. *Arch. Otolaryng.,* 1961, *74,* 70-80.

Brodnitz, F. S. Letter to the editor. *Asha,* 1983, *25,* (1), 5.

Brookshire, R. H. Effects of task difficulty on naming performance of aphasic subjects. *Journal of Speech and Hearing Research,* 1972, *15,* 551–558.

Brookshire, R. H. *An introduction to aphasia.* Minneapolis: BRK, 1973.

Brown, C. W., & Ghiselli, E. E. *Scientific method in psychology.* New York: McGraw–Hill, 1955.

Brown, R. Development of the first language in the human species. *American Psychologist,* 1973, *28,* 9–106. (a)

Brown, R. *A first language: The early stages.* Cambridge, MA: Harvard University Press, 1973 (b)

Brutten, G. J., & Shoemaker, D. J. *The modification of stuttering.* Englewood Cliffs, NJ: Prentice–Hall, 1967.

Buckingham, H. W., Jr. Neuropsychological models of language. In N. J. Lass, L. V. McReynolds, J. L. Northern, & D. E. Yoder (Eds.), *Speech, language, and hearing: Normal processes.* (Vol. 1). Philadelphia: Saunders, 1982.

Burt, M. K., Dulay, H. C., & Hernández-Chávez, E. Evaluation of linguistic proficiency in bilingual children. In S. Singh, & J. Lynch (Eds.), *Diagnostic procedures in hearing, language, and speech.* Baltimore: University Park Press, 1978.

Byrne, M. C., & Shervanian, C. C. *Introduction to communicative disorders.* New York: Harper & Row, 1977.

Bzoch, K. R. (Ed.) *Communicative disorders related to cleft lip and palate* (2nd ed.). Boston: Little, Brown, 1979.

Caplan, D. *Biological studies of mental processes.* Cambridge, MA: MIT Press, 1980.

Carrow, M.A. The development of auditory comprehension of language structure in children. *Journal of Speech and Hearing Disorders,* 1968, *33,* 99–111.

Chalfant, J., & Scheffelin, M. *Central processing dysfunctions in children: A review of research.* NINDS Monograph No. 9. Bethesda, MD: U.S Department of Health, Education and Welfare, 1969.

Chapman, D. C., & Nation, J. E. Patterns of language performance in educable mentally retarded children. *Journal of Communication Disorders,* 1981, *14,* 245–254.

Chapman, R. S. Discussion summary: The developmental relationship between receptive and expressive language. In R. L. Schiefelbusch & L. Lloyd (Eds.), *Language perspectives—Acquisition, retardation and intervention.* Baltimore: University Park Press, 1974.

Chapman, R. S. Comprehension strategies in children. In J. F. Kavanagh & W. Strange (Eds.), *Speech and language in the laboratory, school and clinic.* Cambridge, MA: MIT Press, 1978.

Chapman, R. S., & Miller, J. F. Word order in early two- and three-word utterances: Does production precede comprehension? *Journal of Speech and Hearing Research,* 1975, *18,* 355–371.

Chapman, R. S., & Miller, J. F. Analyzing language and communication in the child. In R. L. Schiefelbush (Ed.), *Nonspeech language intervention.* Baltimore: University Park Press, 1980.

Chase, R. A. Neurological aspects of language disorders in children. In J. V. Irwin & M. Marge (Eds.), *Principles of childhood language disabilities.* New York: Appleton–Century–Crofts, 1972.

Cherry, E. C., & Sayers, B. M. Experiments upon the total inhibition of stammering by external control, and some clinical results. *Journal of Psychosomatic Research,* 1956, *1,* 233–246.

Chesson, A. L., Jr. Aphasia following a right thalamic hemorrhage. *Brain and Language,* 1983, *19,* 306–316.

Chomsky, C. S. *The acquisition of syntax in children from five to ten.* Cambridge, MA: MIT Press, 1969.

Chomsky, N. *Syntactic structures.* The Hague: Mouton, 1957.

Chomsky, N. *Aspects of the theory of syntax.* Cambridge, MA: MIT Press, 1965.

Chomsky, N., & Halle, M. *The sound patterns of English.* New York: Harper & Row, 1968.

Church, J., & Stone, L. *Childhood and adolescence: A psychology of the growing person.* New York: Random House, 1973.

Chusid, J. G. *Correlative neuroanatomy and functional neurology* (14th ed.). Los Altos, CA: Lange Med. Pub., 1970.

Clark, E. What's in a word? On the child's acquisition of semantics in his first language. In T. E. Moore (Ed.), *Cognitive development and the acquisition of language.* New York: Academic Press, 1973.

Compton, A. J., & Hutton, J. S. *Compton–Hutton phonological assessment.* San Francisco: Carousel House, 1978.

Conture, E. *Stuttering.* Englewood Cliffs, NJ: Prentice–Hall, 1982.

Cooper, H. K., Harding, R. L., Krogman, W. M., Mazaheri, M., & Millard, R. T. (Eds.), *Cleft palate and cleft lip: A team approach to clinical management and rehabilitation of the patient.* Philadelphia: Saunders, 1979.

Cooper, M., & Cooper, M. (Eds.) *Approaches to vocal rehabilitation.* Springfield, IL: Thomas, 1977.

Corlew, M. M., & Nation, J. E. Characteristics of visual stimuli and naming performance in aphasic adults. *Cortex,* 1975, *11,* 186–191.

Counihan, D. T. Oral and nasal airflow and air pressure measures. In W. C. Grabb, S. W. Rosenstein, & D. R. Bzoch (Eds.), *Cleft lip and palate: Surgical, dental and speech aspects.* Boston: Little, Brown, 1971. (a)

Counihan, D. T. Oral and nasal airflow and sound pressure measures. In W. C. Grabb, S. W. Rosenstein, & D. R. Bzoch (Eds.), *Cleft lip and palate: Surgical, dental, and speech aspects.* Boston: Little, Brown, 1971. (b)

Crane, S. L., & Cooper, E. B. Speech–language clinician personality variables and clinical effectiveness. *Journal of Speech and Hearing Disorders,* 1983, *48,* 140–145.

Crystal, D., Fletcher, P., & Garman, M. *The grammatical analysis of language disability.* New York: Elsevier, 1976.

Curtiss, S., Prutting, C. A., & Lowell, E. L. Pragmatic and semantic development in young children with impaired hearing. *Journal of Speech and Hearing Research,* 1979, *22,* 534–552.

Dale, P. S. *Language development: Structure and function.* Hinsdale, IL: Dryden Press, 1972.

Dalton, P., & Hardcastle, W. J. *Disorders of fluency.* New York: Elsevier, 1977.

Daniloff, R. G. Normal articulation processes. In F. D. Minifie, T. J. Hixon, & F. Williams (Eds.), *Normal aspects of speech, hearing and language.* Englewood Cliffs, NJ: Prentice–Hall, 1973.

Darby, J. K., Jr. *Speech evaluation in medicine.* New York: Grune & Stratton, 1981.

Darley, F. L. *Diagnosis and appraisal of communication disorders.* Englewood Cliffs, NJ: Prentice–Hall, 1964.

Darley, F. L. *Evaluation and management of neurogenic speech and language disorders: Interaction between neurology and speech pathology.* Paper presented at the Annual Convention of the American Speech and Hearing Association, Detroit, 1973.

Darley, F. L. (Ed.) *Evaluation of appraisal techniques in speech and language pathology.* Reading, MA: Addison–Wesley, 1979.

Darley, F. L. *Aphasia.* Philadelphia: Saunders, 1982.

Darley, F. L., Aronson, A. E., & Brown, J. R. Differential diagnostic patterns of dysarthria. *Journal of Speech and Hearing Research,* 1969, *12,* 246–269. (a)

Darley, F. L., Aronson, A. E., & Brown, J. R. Clusters of deviant speech dimensions in the dysarthrias. *Journal of Speech and Hearing Research,* 1969, *12,* 462–496. (b)

Darley, F. L., Aronson, A. E., & Brown, J. R. *Motor speech disorders.* Philadelphia: Saunders, 1975. (a)

Darley, F. L., Aronson, A. E., & Brown, J. R. *Motor speech disorders: Audio seminars in speech pathology.* Philadelphia: Saunders, 1975. (b)

Darley, F. L., & Spriestersbach, D. C. *Diagnostic methods in speech pathology* (2nd ed.). New York: Harper & Row, 1978.

Davis, J., & Blasdell, R. Perceptual strategies employed by normal-hearing and hearing-impaired children in the comprehension of sentences containing relative clauses. *Journal of Speech and Hearing Research,* 1975, *18,* 281–295.

De Hirsch, K. Differential diagnosis between aphasic and schizophrenic language in children. *Journal of Speech and Hearing Disorders,* 1967, *32,* 3–10.

Demetras, M. J., Matkin, A. M., & Swisher, L. *Speech and language behaviors of preschool children: A clinical review of tests.* Paper presented at the annual convention of the American Speech–Language–Hearing Association, Toronto, Canada, 1982.

DeRenzi, E., & Vignolo, L. A. The token test: A sensitive test to detect receptive disturbances in aphasia. *Brain,* 1962, *85,* 665–678.

Derman, S., & Manaster, A. Family counseling with relatives of aphasic patients at Schwab Rehabilitation Hospital. *Asha,* 1967, *9,* 175–177.

deVilliers, J. G., & deVilliers, P. A. *Language acquisition.* Cambridge: Harvard University Press, 1978.

Dickson, S. Incipient stuttering and spontaneous remission of stuttered speech. *Journal of Communication Disorders,* 1971, *4,* 99–110.

Dickson, S., & Jann, G. R. Diagnostic principles and procedures. In S. Dickson (Ed.), *Communication disorders: Remedial principles and practices.* Glenview, IL: Scott, Foresman, 1974.

Dore, J. A pragmatic description of early language development. *Journal of Psycholinguistic Research,* 1974, *3,* 343–350.

Dore, J. Holophrases, speech acts and language universals. *Journal of Child Language,* 1975, *2,* 21–40.

Dreher, B. B., & Baltes, L. Bibliotherapy for the communication disordered: Rationale and materials. *Asha,* 1973, *15,* 528–534.

Duchan, J. F. Language processing and geodesic domes. In T. M. Gallagher & C. A. Prutting (Eds.), *Pragmatic assessment and intervention issues in language.* San Diego: College-Hill Press, 1983.

Duffy, J. R., Watt, J., & Duffy, R. J. Path analysis: A strategy for investigating multivariate causal relationships in communication disorders. *Journal of Speech and Hearing Research,* 1981, *24,* 474–490.

Dulay, H. C., Hernández-Chávez, E. & Burt, M. K. The process of becoming bilingual. In S. Singh, & J. Lynch (Eds.), *Diagnostic procedures in hearing, language, and speech.* Baltimore: University Park Press, 1978.

Dworkin, J. P. II. Differential diagnosis of motor speech disorders: The clinical examination of the speech mechanism. *Journal of National Student Speech and Hearing Association,* 1978, *8,* 37–62.

Dworkin, J. P., & Culatta, R. A. *Dworkin–Culatta oral mechanism examination.* Nicholasville, KN: Edgewood Press, 1980.

Edwards, M., & Watson, A. C. H. (Eds.) *Advances in the management of cleft palate.* New York: Churchill Livingstone, 1980.

Edwards, M. L., & Shriberg, L. D. *Phonology Applications in communicative disorders.* San Diego: College-Hill Press, 1983.

Eisenson, J. *Aphasia in children.* New York: Harper & Row Publishers, 1972.

Eisenson, J. *Adult aphasia: Assessment and treatment.* New York: Appleton–Century–Crofts, 1973.

Elliot, L. L., & Vegely, A. B. Notes on clinical record-keeping systems. *Asha,* 1971, *13,* 444–446.

Elliott, L. L., Vegely, A. B., & Falvey, N. J. Description of a computer-oriented record-keeping system. *Asha,* 1971, *13,* 435–443.

Emerick, L. L. *The parent interview.* Danville, IL: Interstate Printers & Publishers, 1969.

Emerick, L. L., & Hatten, J. T. *Diagnosis and evaluation in speech pathology* (2nd ed.). Englewood Cliffs, NJ: Prentice–Hall, 1979.

Erickson, R., & Van Riper, C. Demonstration therapy in a university training center. *Asha,* 1967, *9,* 33–35.

Ervin-Tripp, S., & Mitchell-Kernan, C. (Eds) *Child discourse.* New York: Academic Press, 1977.

Faircloth, M. A., & Faircloth, S. R. An analysis of the articulatory behavior of a speech-defective child in connected speech and in isolated-word responses. *Journal of Speech and Hearing Disorders,* 1970, *35,* 51–61.

Fenlason, A. F. *Essentials in interviewing: For the interviewer offering professional services.* New York: Harper & Row, 1952.

Fillmore, C. J. The case for case. In E. Bach & R. J. Harms (Eds.), *Universals in linguistic theory.* New York: Holt, Rinehart & Winston, 1968.

Fisher, H. B. *Improving voice and articulation.* Boston: Houghton Mifflin, 1966.

Fisher, H. B., & Logemann, J. A. Objective evaluation of therapy for vocal nodules: A case report. *Journal of Speech and Hearing Disorders,* 1970, *35,* 277–285.

Fluharty, N. B. The design and standardization of a speech and language screening test for use with preschool children. *Journal of Speech and Hearing Disorders,* 1974, *39,* 75–88.

Folkins, J. W., & Kuehn, D. P. Speech production. In N.J. Lass, L. V. McReynolds, J. L. Northern, & D. E. Yoder (Eds.), *Speech, language, and hearing,* Vol. 1, *Normal processes.* Philadelphia: Saunders, 1982.

Forscher, B. K., & Wertz, R. Organizing the scientific paper. *Asha,* 1970, *12,* 494–497.

Fox, D., Lynch, J., & Brookshire, B. Selected developmental factors of cleft palate children between two and thirty-three months of age. *Cleft Palate Journal,* 1978, *15,* 239–245.

Francis, W. N. *The structure of American English.* New York: Ronald Press, 1958.

Fransella, F., & Beech, H. R. An experimental analysis of the effect of rhythm on the speech of stutterers. *Behavior Research and Therapy,* 1965, *3,* 195–201.

Freeman, F. J. Prosody in perception, production, and pathologies. In N. J. Lass, L. V. McReynolds, J. L. Northern, & D. E. Yoder (Eds.), *Speech, language, and hearing: Pathologies of speech and language* (Vol. 2). Philadelphia: Saunders 1982.

Froeschels, E. New viewpoints on stuttering. *Folia Phoniatrica,* 1961, *13,* 187–201.

Gallagher, T. M. Pre-assessment: A procedure for accommodating language use variability. In T. M. Gallagher & C. A. Prutting (Eds.), *Pragmatic assessment and intervention issues in language.* San Diego: College-Hill Press, 1983.

Gallagher, T. M., & Prutting, C. A. (Eds.) *Pragmatic assessment and intervention issues in language.* San Diego: College-Hill Press, 1983.

Garrett, A. *Interviewing: Its principles and methods* (2nd ed., Revised by E. P. Zaki & M. M. Mangold). New York: Family Service Association of America, 1972.

Garstecki, D. C., Borton, T. E., Stark, E. W., & Kennedy, B. T. Speech, language, and hearing problems in the Laurence–Moon–Biedl syndrome. *Journal of Speech and Hearing Disorders,* 1972, *37,* 407–413.

Gleason, H. A. *An introduction to descriptive linguistics* (rev. ed.). New York: Holt, Rinehart & Winston, 1961.

Goldfarb, W. Effects of psychological deprivation in infancy and subsequent stimulation. *American Journal of Psychiatry,* 1945–1946, *102,* 18–33.

Goldstein, R. Neurophysiology of hearing. In N. J. Lass, L. V. McReynolds, J. L. Northern, & D. E. Yoder (Eds.), *Speech, language, and hearing: Normal processes* (Vol. 1). Philadelphia: Saunders, 1982.

Golper, L. A. C., Nutt, J. G., Rau, M. T., & Coleman, R. O. Focal cranial dystonia. *Journal of Speech and Hearing Disorders,* 1983, *48,* 128-134.

Goodglass, H. Studies on the grammar of aphasics. In S. Rosenberg & J. H. Koplin (Eds.), *Developments in applied psycholinguistics research.* New York: Macmillan, 1968.

Goodglass, J., & Kaplan, E. *The assessment of aphasia and related disorders.* Philadelphia: Lea & Febiger, 1972.

Goodglass, H., Klein, B., Carey, P., & Jones, K. J. Specific semantic word categories in aphasia. *Cortex,* 1966, *2,* 74–89.

Goodstein, L. D. Psychosocial aspects of cleft palate. In D. C. Spriestersbach & D. Sherman (Eds.), *Cleft palate and communication.* New York: Academic Press, 1968.

Gregory, H. *Controversies about stuttering therapy.* Baltimore: University Park Press, 1979.

Guyette, T. W., & Diedrich, W. M. A critical review of developmental apraxia of speech. In N. Lass & (Ed.), *Speech and language: Advances in basic research and practice* (Vol.5). New York: Academic Press, 1981.

Hall, P. The occurrence of disfluencies in language-disordered school-age children. *Journal of Speech and Hearing Disorders,* 1977, *42,* 364–370.

Halliday, M. A. K. *Explorations in the functions of language.* New York: Elsevier/North-Holland, 1977. (a)

Halliday, M. A. K. *Learning how to mean: Explorations in the development of language.* New York: Elsevier/North-Holland, 1977. (b)

Hammond, K. R., & Allen, J. M. *Writing clinical reports.* New York: Prentice–Hall, 1953.

Hanley, T. O., & Peters, R. The speech and hearing laboratory. In L. E. Travis (Ed.), *Handbook of speech pathology and audiology.* New York: Appleton–Century–Crofts, 1971.

Hannah, J. E., & Sheeley, E. C. The audiologist's model for test selection. *Asha,* 1975, *17,* 83–89.

Hayes, C. S. Audiological problems associated with cleft palate. *Asha Monograph,* 1965, *1,* 83–90.

Haynes, W. O., & Oratio, A. R. A study of clients' perceptions of therapeutic effectiveness. *Journal of Speech and Hearing Disorders,* 1978, *43,* 21–33.

Hirano, M. *Clinical examination of the voice.* New York: Springer-Verlag, 1981.

Hixon, T. J., & Hardy, J. C. Restricted motility of the speech articulators in cerebral palsy. *Journal of Speech and Hearing Disorders,* 1964, *29,* 293–306.

Hixon, T. J., Shriberg, L. D., & Saxman, J. H. (Eds.) *Introduction to communication disorders.* Englewood Cliffs, NJ: Prentice–Hall, 1980.

Hodson, B. W., & Paden, E. P. *Targeting intelligible speech: A phonological approach to remediation.* San Diego: College-Hill Press, 1983.

Hollien, H., & Shipp, T. Speaking fundamental frequency and chronologic age in males. *Journal of Speech and Hearing Research,* 1972, *15,* 155–159.

Hood, S. B. The assessment of fluency disorders. In S. Singh, & J. Lynch (Eds.), *Diagnostic procedures in hearing, language, and speech.* Baltimore: University Park Press, 1978.

Hopper, R., & Naremore, R. *Children's speech: A practical introduction to communication development.* New York: Harper & Row, 1973.

Horwitz, S. J. Neurological findings with children with developmental verbal apraxia. In D. M. Aram (Ed.), *Seminars in speech and language: Developmental verbal apraxia.* (Projected 1984).

Hubbell, R. D. *Children's language disorders: An integrated approach.* Englewood Cliffs, NJ: Prentice–Hall, 1981.

Ingram, D. The relationship between comprehension and production. In R. L. Schiefelbusch & L. L. Lloyd (Eds.), *Language perspectives—Acquisition, retardation, and intervention.* Baltimore: University Park Press, 1974.

Ingram, D. *Phonological disability in children.* New York: Elsevier/North-Holland, 1976.

Irwin, J., & Marge, M. (Eds.) *Principles of childhood language disabilities*. Englewood Cliffs, NJ: Prentice–Hall, 1972.

Jacobs, R. J., Philips, B. J., & Harrison, R. J. A stimulability test for cleft-palate children. *Journal of Speech and Hearing Disorders*, 1970, *35*, 354–360.

Jakobson, R., Fant, C. G. M., & Halle, M. *Preliminaries to speech analysis*. Cambridge, MA: MIT Press, 1963.

Jenkins, J. L., Jimenez-Pabon, E., Shaw, R. E., & Safter, J. D. *Schuell's aphasia in adults: Diagnosis, prognosis, and treatment* (2nd ed.). New York: Harper & Row, 1975.

Jerger, J. Scientific writing can be readable. *Asha*, 1962, *4*, 101–104.

Johns, D. F. (Ed.) *Clinical management of neurogenic communicative disorders*. Boston: Little, Brown, 1978.

Johnson, D. J., & Myklebust, H. R. *Learning disabilities: Educational principles and practice*. New York: Grune & Stratton, 1967.

Johnson, M. R., & Tomblin, J. B. The reliability of developmental sentence scoring as a function of sample size. *Journal of Speech and Hearing Research*, 1975, *18*, 372–380.

Johnson, O. G. *Tests and measurements in child development: Handbook II* (2 Vols.). San Francisco: Jossey–Bass, 1976.

Johnson, W. A study of the onset and development of stuttering. *Journal of Speech Disorders*, 1942, *7*, 251–257.

Johnson, O. G., & Bommarito, J. W. *Tests and measurements in child development: A handbook*. San Francisco: Jossey–Bass, 1971.

Johnson, W., & Ainsworth, S. Studies in the psychology of stuttering: X, Constancy of loci of expectancy of stuttering. *Journal of Speech Disorders*, 1938, *3*, 101–104.

Johnson, W., Darley, F., & Spriestersbach, D. *Diagnostic methods in speech pathology*. New York: Harper & Row, 1963.

Johnston, J. R. The language disordered child. In N. J. Lass, L. V. McReynolds, J. L. Northern, & D. E. Yoder (Eds.), *Speech, language and hearing: Pathologies of speech and language* (Vol. II). Philadelphia: Saunders, 1982.

Kahane, J. C. Anatomy and physiology of the organs of the peripheral speech mechanism. In N. J. Lass, L. V. McReynolds, J. L. Northern, & D. E. Yoder (Eds.), *Speech, language, and hearing: Normal processes* (Vol. 1). Philadelphia: Saunders, 1982.

Kamhi, A. G. Problem solving in child language disorders: The clinician as clinical scientist. *Language, Speech, and Hearing Services in Schools*, in press.

Kamhi, A. G., & Johnston, J. R. Towards an understanding of retarded children's linguistic deficiencies. *Journal of Speech and Hearing Research*, 1982, *25*, 435–445.

Keith, R. *Central auditory dysfunction*. New York: Grune & Stratton, 1977.

Kenny, D. A. *Correlation and causality*. New York: Wiley, 1979.

Kent, R. D. *Is the seriation of speech movements governed by motor programs or feedback?* Paper presented at the Annual Convention of the American Speech and Hearing Association, Detroit, 1973.

Kent, R. D. Models of speech production. In N. J. Lass (Ed.), *Contemporary issues in experimental phonetics*. New York: Academic Press, 1976.

Kent, L. R., & Chabon, S. S. Problem-oriented record in a university speech and hearing clinic. *Asha*, 1980, *22*, 151–158.

Kent, R., & Netsell, R. A case study of an ataxic dysarthric: Cineradiographic and spectrographic observations. *Journal of Speech and Hearing Disorders*, 1975, *40*, 115–134.

Kertesz, A. (Ed.) *Localization in neuropsychology*. New York: Academic Press, 1983.

Kessler, J. W. *Psychopathology of childhood*. Englewood Cliff, NJ: Prentice–Hall, 1966.

Kessler, J. W. Nosology in child psychopathology. In H. E. Rie (Ed.), *Perspectives in child psychopathology*. Chicago: Aldine, 1971.

Kidd, K. K., Heimbuch, R. C., Records, M. A., Oehlert, G., & Webster, R. L. Familial stuttering patterns are not related to one measure of severity. *Journal of Speech and Hearing Research*, 1980, *23*, 539–545.

Kidd, K. K., Kidd, J. R., & Records, M. A. The possible causes of the sex ratio in stuttering and its implications. *Journal of Fluency Disorders*, 1978, *3*, 13–23.

Khan, L. M. L. A review of 16 major phonological processes. *Language, Speech, and Hearing Services in Schools*, 1982, *13*, 77–85.

Klatt, D. The duration of /s/ in English words. *Journal of Speech and Hearing Research*, 1974, *17*, 51–63.

Knepflar, K. J. *Report writing in the field of communication disorders*. Danville, IL: Interstate Printers & Publishers, 1976.

Knobloch, H., & Pasamanick, B. (Eds.) *Gessell and Amatruda's developmental diagnosis: The evaluation and management of normal and abnormal neuropsychologic development in infancy and early childhood* (3rd ed.). New York: Harper & Row, 1974.

Knott, J. R., Johnson, W., & Webster, M. Studies in the psychology of stuttering: I, A quantitative evaluation of expectation of stuttering in relation to the occurence of stuttering. *Journal of Speech Disorders*, 1937, *2*, 20–22.

Kuehn, D. P. Assessment of resonance disorders. In N. J. Lass, L. V. McReynolds, J. L. Northern, & D. E. Yoder (Eds.), *Speech, language, and hearing: Pathologies of speech and language* (Vol. II). Philadelphia: Saunders, 1982.

Kuhl, P. K. Speech perception: An overview of current issues. In N. J. Lass, L. V. McReynolds, J. L. Northern, & D. E. Yoder (Eds.), *Speech, language and hearing: Normal processes* (Vol. 1). Philadelphia: Saunders, 1982.

Lamb, S. M. *Outline of stratificational grammar*. Washington, D.C.: Georgetown University Press, 1966.

Lass, N. J., McReynolds, L. V., Northern, J. L., & Yoder, D. E. (Eds.)*Speech, language, and hearing* (Vols. I, II, & III). Philadelphia: Saunders, 1982.

Lee, L. L. Developmental sentence types: A method for comparing normal and deviant syntactic development. *Journal of Speech and Hearing Disorders*, 1966, *31*, 311–330.

Lee, L. L. A screening test for syntax development. *Journal of Speech and Hearing Disorders*, 1970, *35*, 103–112.

Lee, L. L. Developmental sentence analysis. Evanston, IL: Northwestern University Press, 1974.

Lee, L. L., & Canter, S. M. Developmental sentence scoring: A clinical procedure for estimating syntactic development in children's spontaneous speech. *Journal of Speech and Hearing Disorders*, 1971, *36*, 315–340.

Lemme, M. L., & Daves, N. H. Models of linguistic processing. In N. J. Lass, L. V. McReynolds, J. L. Northern, & D. E. Yoder (Eds.), *Speech, language, and hearing: Normal processes* (Vol. 1). Philadelphia: Saunders, 1982.

Lenneberg, E. H. *Biological foundations of language*. New York: Wiley, 1967.

Leonard, L. B. What is deviant language? *Journal of Speech and Hearing Disorders*, 1972, *37*, 427–446.

Leonard, L. B. *Meaning in child language: Issues in the study of early semantic development*. New York: Grune & Stratton, 1976.

Leonard, L. B. Language impairment in children. *Merrill–Palmer Quarterly*, 1979, *25*, 205–232.

Leonard, L. B., Camarata, S., Rowan, L. E., & Chapman, K. The communicative functions of lexical usage by language impaired children. *Applied Psycholinguistics*, 1982, *3*, 109–125.

Leonard, L. B., Prutting, C. A., Perozzi, J. A., & Berkley, R. K. Nonstandardized approaches to the assessment of language behaviors. *Asha*, 1978, *20*, 371–379.

Lesser, R. *Linguistic investigations of aphasia*. London: Arnold, 1978.

Lezak, M. D. *Neuropsychological assessment*. New York: Oxford University Press, 1976.

Lillywhite, H. S., & Bradley, D. P. *Communication problems in mental retardation: Diagnosis and management*. New York: Harper & Row, 1969.

Littlejohn, S. W. *Theories of human communication* (2nd ed.). Belmont, CA: Wadsworth, 1983.

Locke, J. L. The inference of speech perception in the phonologically disordered child. Part I: A rationale, some criteria, the conventional tests. *Journal of Speech and Hearing Disorders*, 1980, *45*, 431–444. (a)

Locke, J. L. The inference of speech perception in the phonologically disordered child. Part II: Some clinically novel procedures, their use, some findings. *Journal of Speech and Hearing Disorders*, 1980, *45*, 445–468. (b)

Luria, A. R. *Higher cortical functions in man*. New York: Basic Books, 1966.

MacDonald, J. D., & Blott, J. P. Environmental language intervention: The rationale for a diagnostic and training strategy through rules, context, and generalization. *Journal of Speech and Hearing Disorders*, 1974, *39*, 244–256.

Marshall, L. Auditory processing in aging listeners. *Journal of Speech and Hearing Disorders*, 1981, *46*, 226–240.

Marshall, N. R., & Goldstein, S. G. Imparting diagnostic information to mothers: A comparison of methodologies. *Journal of Speech and Hearing Research*, 1969, *12*, 65–72.

Marshall, N. R., & Goldstein, S. G. The maintenance of diagnostic information imparted by three methods: One year later. *Journal of Speech and Hearing Research*, 1970, *13*, 447–448.

Mason, R. M., & Grandstaff, H. L. Evaluating the velopharyngeal mechanism in hypernasal speakers. *Ohio Journal of Speech and Hearing*, 1970, *4*, 23–28. (Reprinted in *Language, Speech, Hearing Services in Schools*, 1971, *4*, 53–61.)

Massaro, D. W. *Understanding language*. New York: Academic Press, 1975.

Mayo Clinic. *Clinical examinations in neurology* (3rd ed.). Philadelphia: Saunders, 1971.

McCabe, P. A. A coding procedure for classification of cleft lip and cleft palate. *Cleft Palate Journal*, 1966, *3*, 383–391.

McCarthy, D. Language development in children. In L. Carmichael (Ed.), *Manual of child psychology*. New York: Wiley, 1954.

McCarthy, J. J., & McCarthy, J. F. *Learning disabilities*. Boston: Allyn & Bacon, 1973.

McCauley, R. J., & Swisher, L. *Psychometric review of language and articulation tests for preschool children*. *Journal of Speech and Hearing Disorders*, in press.

McLean, J. E., & Snyder-McLean, L. K. *A transactional approach to early language training.* Columbus, OH: Merrill, 1978.

McNeill, D. *The acquisition of language: The study of developmental psycholinguistics.* New York: Harper & Row, 1970.

McReynolds, L. V. Operant conditioning for investigating speech sound discrimination in aphasic children. *Journal of Speech and Hearing Research,* 1966, *7,* 519–528.

McReynolds, L. V., & Engmann, D. L. *Distinctive feature analysis of misarticulations.* Baltimore: University Park Press, 1975.

McReynolds, L. V., & Huston, K. A distinctive feature analysis of children's misarticulations. *Journal of Speech and Hearing Disorders,* 1971, *36,* 155–166.

McWilliams, B. J., Musgrave, R., & Crozier, P. The influence of head position upon velopharyngeal closure. *Cleft Palate Journal,* 1968, *5,* 117–124.

Menyuk, P. *Sentences children use.* Cambridge, MA: MIT Press, 1969.

Menyuk, P. Early development of receptive language: From babbling to words. In R. L. Schiefelbusch & L. L. Lloyd (Eds.), *Language perspectives—Acquisition, retardation, and intervention.* Baltimore: University Park Press, 1974.

Menyuk, P. *The acquisition and development of language.* Englewood Cliffs, NJ: Prentice–Hall, 1971.

Menyuk, P. *Language and maturation.* Cambridge: MIT Press, 1977.

Menyuk, P., & Looney, P. L. A problem of language disorder: Length versus structure. *Journal of Speech and Hearing Research,* 1972, *15,* 264–279.

Merits-Patterson, R., & Reed, C. G. Disfluencies in the speech of language-delayed children. *Journal of Speech and Hearing Research,* 1981, *46,* 55–58.

Messick, S. Test validity and the ethics of assessment. *American Psychologist.* 1980. *35.* 1012–1027.

Milisen, R. Methods of evaluation and diagnosis of speech disorders. In L. E. Travis (Ed.), *Handbook of speech pathology.* New York: Appleton–Century–Crofts, 1957.

Milisen, R. (Ed.) The disorder of articulation: A systematic clinical and experimental approach. *Journal of Speech and Hearing Disorders,* 1954, *4,* Monogr. Suppl.

Miller, G. A., & Nicely, P. E. An analysis of perceptual confusions among some English consonants. *Journal of the Acoustical Society of America,* 1955, *27,* 338–352.

Miller, J. F. Assessing children's language behavior: A developmental process approach. In R. L. Schiefelbusch (Ed.), *Bases of language intervention.* Baltimore: University Park Press, 1978.

Miller, J. F. *Assessing language production in children.* Baltimore: University Park Press, 1981.

Miller, J. F., & Chapman, R. S. The relation between age and mean length of utterance in morphemes. *Journal of Speech and Hearing Research,* 1981, *24,* 154–161.

Miller, J. F., & Yoder, D. E. An ontogenetic language teaching strategy for retarded children. In R. L. Schiefelbusch & L. L. Lloyd (Eds.), *Language perspectives—Acquisition, retardation and intervention.* Baltimore: University Park Press, 1974.

Miller, J., Yoder, D. E., & Schiefelbusch, R. (Eds.). Contemporary issues in language intervention. *ASHA Reports,* 12, 1983.

Mills, A. E. (Ed.) *Language acquisition in the blind child: Normal and deficient.* San Diego: College-Hill Press, 1983.

Miner, L. E. Scoring procedures for the length–complexity index: A preliminary report. *Journal of Communication Disorders,* 1969, *2,* 224–240.

Minifie, F. D., Darley, F. L., & Sherman, D. Temporal reliability of seven language measures. *Journal of Speech and Hearing Research,* 1963, *6,* 139–148.

Moll, K. L. A focus on our common goal: Presidential address—1974 National Convention, *Asha,* 1975, *17,* 3–8.

Molyneaux, D., & Lane, V. W. *Effective interviewing: Techniques and analysis.* Boston: Allyn & Bacon, 1982.

Moncur, J. P., & Brackett, I. P. *Modifying vocal behavior.* New York: Harper & Row, 1974.

Moore, G. P. *Organic voice disorders.* Englewood Cliffs, NJ: Prentice–Hall, 1971. (a)

Moore, G. P. Voice disorders organically based. In L. E. Travis (Ed.), *Handbook of speech pathology and audiology.* New York: Appleton–Century–Crofts, 1971. (b)

Moore, M. V. Pathological writing. *Asha,* 1969, *11,* 535–538.

Morehead, D. M., & Ingram, D. The development of base syntax in normal and linguistically deviant children. *Journal of Speech and Hearing Research,* 1973, *16,* 330–352.

Morley, M. E. *The development and disorders of speech in childhood* (3rd ed.). London: Churchill Livingstone, 1972.

Morris, H. D., Spriestersbach, D. C., & Darley, F. L. An articulation test for assessing competency for velopharyngeal closure. *Journal of Speech and Hearing Research,* 1961, *1,* 48–55.

Mortensen, C. D. *Communication: The study of human interaction.* New York: McGraw-Hill, 1972.

Muma, J. R. *Language handbook: Concepts, assessment, intervention*. Englewood Cliffs, NJ: Prentice–Hall, 1978.

Muma, J. R. *Language primer for the clinical fields*. Lubbock, TX: Natural Child, 1981.

Mussen, P. H., Conger, J. J., & Kagan, J. *Child development and personality* (3rd ed.). New York: Harper & Row, 1969.

Myklebust, H. R. *Auditory disorders in children: A manual for differential diagnosis*. New York: Grune & Stratton, 1954.

Mysak, E. D. *Speech pathology and feedback theory*. Springfield, IL: Thomas, 1966.

Mysak, E. D. Cerebral palsy speech habilitation. In L. Travis (Ed.), *Handbook of speech pathology and audiology*. New York: Appleton–Century–Crofts, 1971.

Mysak, E. D. *Pathologies of speech systems*. Baltimore: Williams & Wilkins, 1976.

Naremore, R. C., & Dever, R. B. Language performance of educable mentally retarded and normal children at five age levels. *Journal of Speech and Hearing Research*, 1975, *18*, 82–95.

Nation, J. E. Determinants of vocabulary development of preschool cleft palate children. *Cleft Palate Journal*, 1970, *7*, 645–651.

Nation, J. E. A vocabulary usage test. *Journal of Psycholinguistic Research*, 1972, *1*, 221–231.

Nation, J. E. Management of speech and language disorders. In N. J. Lass, L. V. McReynolds, J. L. Northern, & D. E. Yoder, *Speech, language and hearing: Pathologies of speech and language* (Vol. II). Philadelphia: Saunders, 1982.

Nation, J. E., & Aram, D. M. *Diagnosis of speech and language disorders*. St. Louis: Mosby, 1977.

Nation, J. E., & Corlew, M. M. Aphasia tests: Differences among naming tasks. *Archives of Physical Medicine and Rehabilitation*, 1974, *55*, 228–231.

Naylor, R. V. Letter to the editor. *Asha*, 1983, *25* (6), 4.

Needham, L. S., & Swisher, L. P. A comparison of three tests of auditory comprehension for adult aphasics. *Journal of Speech and Hearing Disorders*, 1972, *37*, 123–131.

Nelson, K. Some evidence for the cognitive primacy of categorization and its functional basis. *Merrill–Palmer Quarterly*, 1973, *19*, 21–39.

Nelson, K. *Children's language*. New York: Gardner Press, 1978.

Nelson, E. E., Hunter, N., & Walter, M. Stuttering in twin types. *Journal of Speech Disorders*, 1945, *10*, 335–343.

Netsell, R. Speech physiology. In F. D. Minifie, T. J. Hixon, & F. Williams (Eds.), *Normal aspects of speech, hearing, and language*. Englewood Cliffs, NJ: Prentice-Hall, 1973.

Noland, R. L. (Ed.) *Counseling parents of the ill and the handicapped*. Springfield, IL: Thomas, 1971.

Northern, J. L., & Downs, M. P. *Hearing in children* (2nd ed.). Baltimore: Williams & Wilkins, 1978.

Oller, D. K. Regularities in abnormal child phonology. *Journal of Speech and Hearing Disorders*, 1973, *38*, 36–47.

Owens, R. E., Haney, M. J., Giesow, V. E., Dooley, L. F., & Kelly, R. J. Language test content: A comparative study. *Language, Speech, and Hearing Services in the Schools*, 1983, *14*, 7–21.

Oyer, H. J., & Oyer, E. J. *Aging and communication*. Baltimore: University Park Press, 1976.

Palmer, J. O. *The psychological assessment of children*. New York: Wiley, 1970.

Pannbacker, M. Diagnostic report writing. *Journal of Speech and Hearing Disorders*, 1975, *40*, 367–379.

Peins, M. Adaptation effect and spontaneous recovery in stuttering expectancy. *Journal of Speech and Hearing Research*, 1961, *4*, 91–99.

Perkins, W. H. Vocal function: A behavioral analysis. In L. Travis (Ed.), *Handbook of speech pathology and audiology*. New York: Appleton–Century–Crofts, 1971. (a)

Perkins, W. H. Vocal function: Assessment and therapy. In L. Travis (Ed.), *Handbook of speech pathology and audiology*. New York: Appleton–Century–Crofts, 1971. (b)

Perkins, W. H. *Speech pathology: An applied behavioral science* (2nd ed.). St. Louis: Mosby, 1977.

Perkins, W. H., & Curlee, R. F. Causality in speech pathology. *Journal of Speech and Hearing Disorders*, 1969, *34*, 231–238.

Peterson, H. A., & Marquardt, T. P. *Appraisal and diagnosis of speech and language disorders*. Englewood Cliffs, NJ: Prentice–Hall, 1981.

Peterson-Falzone, S. J. Articulation disorders in orofacial anomalies. In N. J. Lass, L. V. McReynolds, J. L. Northern, & D. E. Yoder (Eds.), *Speech, language, and hearing: Pathologies of speech and language* (Vol. 2). Saunders, 1982.

Platt, L. J., Andrews, G., & Howie, P. M. Dysarthria of adult cerebral palsy: II. Phonemic analysis of articulation errors. *Journal of Speech and Hearing Research*, 1980, *23*, 41–55.

Platt, L. J., Andrews, G., Young, M., & Quinn, P. T. Dysarthria of adult cerebral palsy: I. Intelligibility and articulatory impairment. *Journal of Speech and Hearing Research*, 1980, *23*, 28–40.

Poole, I. Genetic development of articulation of consonant sounds in speech. *Elementary English Review*, 1934, *11*, 159–161.

Porch, B. E. *Porch Index of Communicative Ability: Administration, scoring and interpretation* (Vol. 2, rev. ed.). Palo Alto, CA: Consulting Psychologists Press, 1971.

Porter, H. V. K. Studies in the psychology of stuttering: XIV, Stuttering phenomena in relation to size and personnel of audience. *Journal of Speech Disorders,* 1939, *4,* 323–333.

Prather, E. M., Hedrick, D. L., & Kern, C. A. Articulation development in children aged two to four years. *Journal of Speech and Hearing Disorders,* 1975, *40,* 179–191.

Prins, D., & Lohr, F. Behavioral dimensions of stuttered speech. *Journal of Speech and Hearing Research,* 1972, *15,* 61–71.

Prutting, C. A. Process /pra/,ses/ n: The action of moving forward progressively from one point to another on the way to completion. *Journal of Speech and Hearing Disorders,* 1979, *44,* 3–30.

Prutting, C. *Observational protocol for pragmatic behaviors.* Manual developed for the University of California Speech and Hearing Clinic, 1982. (a)

Prutting, C. A. Pragmatics as social competence. *Journal of Speech and Hearing Disorders,*1982, *47,* 123–134. (b)

Prutting, C. A. Scientific inquiry and communicative disorders: An emerging paradigm across six decades. In T. M. Gallagher & C. A. Prutting (Eds.), *Pragmatic assessment and intervention issues in language.* San Diego: College-Hill Press, 1983.

Prutting, C. A., & Kirchner, D. M. Applied pragmatics. In T. M. Gallagher & C. A. Prutting (Eds.), *Pragmatic assessment and intervention issues in language.* San Diego, CA: College-Hill Press, 1983.

Ramer, A. L. H., & Rees, N. S. Selected aspects of the development of English morphology in black American children of low socioeconomic background. *Journal of Speech and Hearing Research,* 1973, *16,* 569–577.

Ramig, L. A., & Ringel, R. L. Effects of physiological aging on selected acoustic characteristics of voice. *Journal of Speech and Hearing Research,* 1983, *26,* 22–30.

Rapin, I. L., & Wilson, B. C. Children with developmental language disability: Neurological aspects and assessment. In M. Wyke (Ed.), *Developmental dysphasia.* New York: Academic Press, 1978.

Ratusnik, D. L., & Koeningsknecht, R. A. Internal consistency of the Northwestern Syntax Screening Test. *Journal of Speech and Hearing Disorders,* 1975, *40,* 59–68.

Rees, M., Herbert, E. L., & Coates, N. H. Development of a standard case record form. *Journal of Speech and Hearing Disorders,* 1969, *34,* 68–81.

Rees, N. S. Auditory processing factors in language disorders: The view from Procrustes' bed. *Journal of Speech and Hearing Disorders,* 1973, *38,* 304–315.

Rees, N. S. Art and science of diagnosis in hearing, language, and speech. In S. Singh & J. Lynch (Eds.), *Diagnostic procedures in hearing, language, and speech.* Baltimore: University Park Press, 1978.

Rees, N. S., & Shulman, M. I don't understand what you mean by comprehension. *Journal of Speech and Hearing Disorders,* 1978, *43,* 208–219.

Rheingold, H. L. Interpreting mental retardation to parents. *Journal of Consulting Psychologists,* 1945, *9,* 142–148.

Richardson, S., Dohrenwend, B. S., & Klein, D. *Interviewing: Its forms and functions.* New York: Basic Books, 1965.

Rieber, R. W., & Brubaker, R. S. *Speech pathology.* Philadelphia: Lippincott, 1966.

Ringel, R. L. The clinician and the researcher: An artificial dichotomy. *Asha,* 1972, *14,* 351–353.

Rogers, C. R. *Counseling and psychotherapy.* Boston: Houghton Mifflin, 1942.

Rosch, E. H. On the internal structure of perceptual and semantic categories. In T. E. Moore (Ed.), *Cognitive development and the acquisition of language.* New York: Academic Press, 1973.

Rosenbek, J. C., & LaPointe, L. L. The dysarthrias: Description, diagnosis, and treatment. In D. F. Johns (Ed.), *Clinical management of neurogenic communicative disorders.* Boston: Little, Brown, 1978.

Salvia, J., & Ysseldyke, J. E. *Assessment in special and remedial education* (2nd ed.). Boston: Houghton Mifflin, 1981.

Sameroff, A. J. Early influences on development: Fact or fancy? *Merrill–Palmer Quarterly,* 1975, *21,* 267–294.

Sander, E. K. Counseling parents of stuttering children. *Journal of Speech and Hearing Disorders,* 1959, *24,* 262–271.

Sander, E. When are speech sounds learned? *Journal of Speech and Hearing Disorders,* 1972, *37,* 55–63.

Sanders, D. A. A model for communication. In L.L. Lloyd (Ed.), *Communication assessment and intervention strategies.* Baltimore: University Park Press, 1976.

Sanders, L. J. *Procedure guides for evaluation of speech and language disorders in children* (4th ed.). Danville, IL: Interstate Printers and Publishers, 1979.

Sarno, M. T. (Ed.) *Acquired aphasia.* New York: Academic Press, 1981.

Schlesinger, I. M. Production of utterances and language acquisition. In D. I. Slobin (Ed.), *The ontogenesis of grammar.* New York: Academic Press, 1971.

Schultz, M. C. *An analysis of clinical behavior in speech and hearing.* Englewood Cliffs, NJ: Prentice–Hall, 1972.

Schultz, M. C. The bases of speech pathology and audiology: Evaluation as the resolution of uncertainty. *Journal of Speech and Hearing Disorders,* 1973, *38,* 147–155.

Schwartz, M. F. Acoustic measures of nasalization and nasality. In W. C. Grabb, S. W. Rosenstein, & K. R. Bzoch (Eds.), *Cleft lip and palate: Surgical, dental, and speech aspects.* Boston: Little, Brown, 1971.

Searle, J. *Speech acts: An essay in the philosophy of language.* Cambridge: Cambridge University Press, 1969.

Segalowitz, S. J. *Language functions and brain organization.* New York: Academic Press, 1983.

Shames, G. H., & Wiig, E. H. (Eds.) *Human communication disorders: An introduction.* Columbus, OH: Merrill, 1982.

Sharf, D. J. Some relationships between measures of early language development. *Journal of Speech and Hearing Disorders,* 1972, *37,* 64–74.

Sheehan, J. G., & Martyn, M. M. Stuttering and its disappearance. *Journal of Speech and Hearing Research,* 1970, *13,* 279–289.

Shewan, C. M., & Canter, G. J. Effects of vocabulary, syntax, and sentence length on auditory comprehension in aphasic patients. *Cortex,* 1971, *7,* 209–226.

Shriberg, L. D. The effect of examiner social behavior on children's articulation test performance. *Journal of Speech and Hearing Research,* 1971, *14,* 659–672.

Shriberg, L. D. Articulation judgments: Some perceptual considerations. *Journal of Speech and Hearing Research,* 1972, *15,* 876–882.

Shriberg, L., & Kwiatkowski, J. *Natural process analysis: (NPA): A procedure for phonological analysis of continuous speech samples.* New York: Wiley, 1980.

Shriberg, L. D., & Kwiatkowski, J. Phonological disorders I: A diagnostic classification system. *Journal of Speech and Hearing Disorders,* 1982, *47,* 226–241.

Shriberg, L. D., & Smith, A. J. Phonological correlates of middle-ear involvement in speech-delayed children: A methodological note. *Journal of Speech and Hearing Research,* 1983, *26,* 293–297.

Shriner, T. H. A comparison of selected measures with psychological scale values of language development. *Journal of Speech and Hearing Research,* 1967, *10,* 828–835.

Shriner, T. H. A review of mean length of response as a measure of expressive language development in children. *Journal of Speech and Language Disorders,* 1969, *34,* 61–68.

Shriner, T., & Sherman, D. An equation for assessing language development. *Journal of Speech and Hearing Research,* 1967, *10,* 41–48.

Shriner, T., Holloway, M., & Daniloff, R. The relationship between articulatory deficits and syntax in speech defective children. *Journal of Speech and Hearing Research,* 1969, *12,* 319–325.

Siegel-Sadewitz, V., & Shprintzen, R. J. The relationship of communication disorders to syndrome identification. *Journal of Speech and Hearing Disorders,* 1982, *47,* 338–354.

Silverman, E. M. Clustering: A characteristic of preschoolers' speech disfluency. *Journal of Speech and Hearing Research,* 1973, *16,* 578–583.

Singh, S., & Lynch, J. (Eds.) *Diagnostic procedures in hearing, language and speech.* Baltimore: University Park Press, 1978.

Slobin, D. I. Grammatical transformations in childhood and adulthood. *Journal of Verbal Learning and Verbal Behavior,* 1966, *5,* 219–227.

Slobin, D. I. Universals of grammatical development in children. In G. B. Flores D' Arcais & W. J. M. Levelt (Eds.), *Advances in psycholinguistics.* Amsterdam: North-Holland, 1970.

Smith, B. L., & Stoel-Gammon, C. A longitudinal study of the development of stop consonant production in normal and Down's syndrome children. *Journal of Speech and Hearing Disorders,* 1983, *48,* 114–118.

Smith, M. E. An investigation of the development of the sentence and the extent of vocabulary in young children. *University of Iowa studies in child welfare,* No. 3. Iowa City: University of Iowa, 1926.

Snow, C. E., & Ferguson, C. A. (Eds.) *Talking to children: Language imput and acquisition.* Cambridge: Cambridge University Press, 1977.

Soderberg, G. A. The relations of stuttering to word length and word frequency. *Journal of Speech and Hearing Research,* 1966, *9,* 584–589.

Spence, N. L. *The influence of stress, gesture, and speaker factors on auditory comprehension in aphasia.* Unpublished doctoral dissertation, Case Western Reserve University, 1983.

Starbuck, H., & Steer, M. D. The adaptation effect in stuttering speech behavior and normal speech. *Journal of Speech and Hearing Disorders,* 1953, *18,* 252–255.

Stark, R. E. (Ed.) *Language behavior in infancy and early childhood.* New York: Elsevier/North-Holland, 1981.

Stark, R. E., & Tallal, P. Selection of children with specific language deficits. *Journal of Speech and Hearing Disorders,* 1981, *46,* 114–122.

Starr, D. C. Dental and occlusal hazards to normal speech production. In W. C. Grabb, S. W. Rosenstein, & K. R. Bzoch (Eds.), *Cleft lip and palate: Surgical, dental, and speech aspects.* Boston: Little, Brown, 1971.

Steckol, K. F., & Leonard, L. B. Sensorimotor development and the use of prelinguistic performatives. *Journal of Speech and Hearing Research,* 1981, *24,* 262–268.

Steer, M. D. Symptomatologies of young stutterers. *Journal of Speech Disorders,* 1937, *2,* 3–16.

Stevenson, I. *The diagnostic interview* (2nd ed.). New York: Harper & Row, 1971.

Stoel-Gammon, C. Phonological analysis of four Down's syndrome children. *Applied Psycholinguistics,* 1980, *1,* 31–48.

Sullivan, H. S. *The psychiatric interview.* New York: Norton, 1954.

Tallent, N. *Report writing in special education.* Englewood Cliffs, NJ: Prentice–Hall, 1980.

Templin, M. C. *Certain language skills in children, their development and interrelationships.* Institute of Child Welfare, Monograph Series 26. Minneapolis: University of Minnesota Press, 1957. (a)

Templin, M. C. Templin Picture Sound Discrimination Test. In M. C. Templin, *Certain language skills in children.* Minneapolis: University of Minnesota Press, 1957. (b)

Terrell, S. L. (Ed.) Nonbiased assessment of language differences. *Topics in Language Disorders,* 1983, *3.*

Trantham, C. R., & Pederson, J. K. *Normal language development: The key to diagnosis and therapy for language-disordered children.* Baltimore: Williams & Wilkins, 1976.

Trost, J. E. Articulatory additions to the classical description of the speech of persons with cleft palate. *Cleft Palate Journal,* 1981, *18,* 193–203.

Tyack, D., & Gottsleben, R. *Language sampling, analysis and training: A handbook for teachers and clinicians.* Palo Alto, CA: Consulting Psychologists Press, 1974.

Uzgiris, I. C., & Hunt, J. McV. *Assessment in infancy.* Urbana, IL: University of Illinois Press, 1975.

Van Demark, D. R., Kuehn, D. P., & Tharp, R. F. Prediction of velopharyngeal competency. *Cleft Palate Journal,* 1975, *12,* 5–11.

Van Demark, D. R., & Tharp, R. A computer program for articulation tests. *Cleft Palate Journal,* 1973, *10,* 378–389.

Van Riper, C. *The nature of stuttering.* Englewood Cliffs, NJ: Prentice–Hall, 1971.

Van Riper, C. *Speech correction: Principles and methods* (5th ed.). Englewood Cliffs, NJ: Prentice–Hall, 1972.

Van Riper, C., & Irwin, J. V. *Voice and articulation.* Englewood Cliffs, NJ: Prentice–Hall, 1958.

Vaughan-Cooke, F. B. Improving language assessment in minority children. *Asha,* 1983, *25,* 9, 29–34.

Walker, V. G., Hardiman, C. J., Hedrick, D. L., & Holbrook, A. Speech and language characteristics of an aging population. In N. J. Lass (Ed.), *Speech and language: Advances in basic research and practice* (Vol. 6). New York: Academic Press, 1981.

Warner, W. L., Meeker, M., & Eells, K. *Social class in America.* New York: Harper & Row, 1960.

Waterson, N., & Snow, C. E. (Eds.) *The development of communication.* New York: Wiley, 1978.

Waryas, C., & Ruder, K. On the limitations of language comprehension procedures and an alternative. *Journal of Speech and Hearing Disorders,* 1974, *39,* 44–52.

Webster, E. J. *Counseling with parents of handicapped children: Guidelines for improving communication.* New York: Grune & Stratton, 1977.

Weed, L. L. *Medical records, medical education, and patient care.* Cleveland: Press of Case Western Reserve University, 1970.

Weinberg, B., Dexter, R., & Horii, Y. Selected speech and fundamental frequency characteristics of patients with acromegaly. *Journal of Speech and Hearing Disorders,* 1975, *40,* 253–259.

Weiner, F. F. *Phonological process analysis.* Baltimore: University Park Press, 1979.

Weiner, P. S. Stability and validity of two measures of intelligence used with children whose language development is delayed. *Journal of Speech and Hearing Research,* 1971, *14,* 254–261.

Weiner, P. S., & Hoock, W. C. The standardization of tests: Criteria and criticisms. *Journal of Speech and Hearing Research,* 1973, *16,* 616–626.

Wellman, B., Case, I., Mengert, I., & Bradbury, D. Speech sounds of young children. *University of Iowa Studies in Child Welfare,* 1931, *5,* 1–82.

Wells, C. *Cleft palate and its associated speech disorders.* New York: McGraw–Hill, 1971.

Wepman, J. M. Familial incidence in stammering. *Journal of Speech Disorders,* 1939, *4,* 199–204.

Whitaker, H. A. Neurolinguistics. In W. O. Dingwall (Ed.), *A survey of linguistic science.* College Park, MD: Linguistic program, University of Maryland, 1971.

Wiig, E. H., & Semel, E. M. Comprehension of linguistic concepts requiring logical operations by learning-disabled children. *Journal of Speech and Hearing Research,* 1973, *16,* 627–636.

Wiig, E. H., & Semel, E. M. *Language disabilities in children and adolescents.* Columbus, OH: Merrill, 1976.

Wiig, E. H., & Semel, E. M. *Language assessment and intervention for the learning disabled.* Columbus, OH: Merrill, 1980.

Wilcox, M. J., & Howse, P. Children's use of gestural and verbal behavior in communicative misunderstandings. *Applied Psycholinguistics,* 1982, *3,* 15–27.

Williams, D. E., Silverman, F. H., & Kools, J. A. Disfluency behavior of elementary school stutterers and non-stutterers: The adaptation effect. *Journal of Speech and Hearing Research,* 1968, *11,* 622–630.

Wilson, D. K. *Voice problems of children* (2nd ed.). Baltimore: Williams & Wilkins, 1979.

Wilson, M. E. A standardized method for obtaining a spoken language sample. *Journal of Speech and Hearing Research,* 1969, *12,* 95–102.

Wingate, M. Recovery from stuttering. *Journal of Speech and Hearing Disorders,* 1964, *29,* 312–321.

Wingate, M. Prosody in stuttering adaptation. *Journal of Speech and Hearing Research,* 1966, *9,* 550–556.

Wingate, M. Sound and pattern in "artificial" fluency. *Journal of Speech and Hearing Research,* 1969, *12,* 677–686.

Wingate, M. E. Stuttering and word length. *Journal of Speech and Hearing Research,* 1967, *10,* 146–152.

Winitz, H. *Articulatory acquisition and behavior.* New York: Appleton–Century–Crofts, 1969.

Winitz, H. (Ed.) *Treating language disorders: For clinicians by clinicians.* Baltimore: University Park Press, 1983.

Wischner, G. J. An experimental approach to expectancy and anxiety in stuttering behavior. *Journal of Speech and Hearing Disorders,* 1952, *17,* 139–154.

Wood, B. S. *Children and communication: Verbal and nonverbal language development.* Englewood Cliffs, NJ: Prentice–Hall, 1976.

Wood, K. S. The parent's role in the clinical program. *Journal of Speech and Hearing Disorders,* 1948, *13,* 209–210.

Wyke, M. A. (Ed.) *Developmental dysphasia.* New York: Academic Press, 1978.

Yoss, K. A., & Darley, F. L. Developmental apraxia of speech in children with defective articulation. *Journal of Speech and Hearing Research,* 1974, *17,* 399–416.

Young, M. A. Onset, prevalence, and recovery from stuttering. *Journal of Speech and Hearing Disorders,* 1975, *40,* 49–58.

Zimmerman, G. Articulatory behaviors associated with stuttering: A cinefluorographic analysis. *Journal of Speech and Hearing Research,* 1980, *23,* 108–121. (a)

Zimmerman, G. Articulatory dynamics of fluent utterances of stutterers and nonstutterers. *Journal of Speech and Hearing Research,* 1980, *23,* 73–94. (b)

Zimmerman, G. Stuttering: A disorder of movement. *Journal of Speech and Hearing Research,* 1980, *23,* 122–136. (c)

Zimmerman, G. N., Smith, A., & Hanley, J. M. Stuttering: In need of a unifying conceptual framework. *Journal of Speech and Hearing Research,* 1981, *46,* 25–31.

copy pg 32:

Author Index

A

Abbs, J. H., 36
Achenback, T. M., 213, 351
Adams, M., 241
Addicott, M. A., 347
Ainsworth, S., 242
Allen, D. V., 340
Allen, J. M., 270
Almond, P. J., 351
Ammons, H. S., 210, 327
Ammons, R., 330
Ammons, R. B., 210, 327
Anderson, M., 323
Andrews, G., 205, 240
Anthony, A., 325
Aram, D. M., 7, 9, 12, 32, 34, 50, 78, 111, 112, 114, 143, 144, 163, 165, 167, 169, 170, 236, 350
Arick, J. R., 351
Arlt, P. B., 328
Arthur, G., 168, 169, 350
Aten, J., 206, 324
Austin, J., 47
Ayres, A. J., 352

B

Baker, J. H., 148, 324
Balow, I. H., 353
Baltes, L., 274
Bangs, T., 321
Bangs, T. E., 114, 257, 260, 274, 345, 346
Bankson, N. W., 320
Bar, A., 74
Barrett, M., 213, 334, 347
Barrett, T. C., 352
Barsch, R. H., 114
Bates, E., 47
Bayles, K. A., 8
Bayley, N., 148, 350
Beech, H. R., 241
Beery, K. E., 352
Bellak, L., 351
Bellak, S. S., 351
Bender, L., 352
Benten, S., 247
Benton, A., 352
Benton, A. L., 333
Bernstein, A., 172
Berry, M., 213, 321
Berry, M. F., 111, 240

Berry, W. R., 114, 181
Bess, F. H., 114
Beukelman, D. R., 181, 318
Bijou, S. W., 353
Bingham, V., 321
Bingham, W. V., 155, 213
Bixler, H. S., 352, 353
Blagden, C. M., 329
Blakely, R. W., 340
Blalock, H. M., 82
Blank, M., 34, 148, 168, 213, 336
Blasdell, R., 247
Bliss, L. S., 340
Bloodstein, O., 10, 114, 181, 241
Bloom, L., 7, 46, 148
Bloomquist, B. L., 360
Blott, J. P., 157
Blum, L., 350
Boehm, A. E., 321
Boller, F., 148
Boone, D. R., 8, 42, 181, 204
Bommarito, J. W., 182
Borton, T. E., 247
Botel, M., 353
Bowan, M. L., 321
Bowerman, M., 46
Boyd, H. F., 350
Brackett, I. P., 50
Bradbury, D., 225
Bradley, D. P., 113
Brady, J. P., 241
Brassel, E., 317
Breecher, S. V. A., 340
Bremner, A., 352
Brenner, N. C., 242
Bright, K. E., 161, 163
Broca, P., 32
Brodbeck, A. J., 126
Brookshire, B., 124, 204
Brown, A. W., 350
Brown, C. W., 51, 75
Brown, J. R., 114, 181, 203, 234
Brown, L., 350
Brown, R., 7, 46
Brown, V. L., 343, 353
Brubaker, R. S., 81
Bruininks, G. H., 166, 170, 351
Brutten, E. J., 171, 181, 242
Bryant, B. R., 343
Bryant, D. L., 343
Buckingham, W. H., Jr., 19, 32

Lohr, F., 211
Looney, P. L., 230
Lorge, I., 350
Lowell, E. L., 247
Lund, 352
Luria, A. R., 31
Lynch, J., 15, 124

M

MacDonald, J. D., 157, 325, 326
Mack, J. L., 148
Madden, R., 353
Madison, C. L., 330
Mahoney, K. E., 325
Maldonado, A., 324
Manaster, A., 257
Marge, M., 111
Markwardt, F. C., 353
Marquardt, T. P., 15, 17
Marshall, L., 8
Marshall, N. R., 257
Martyn, M. M., 240, 253
Maslow, P., 352
Mason, R. M., 203
Massaro, D. W., 19, 32
Matheny, P., 323
Matkin, A. M., 163
Matkin, N. D., 161, 163
Mazaheri, M., 181
McCabe, P. A., 271
McCarthy, D., 7, 24, 111, 350
McCarthy, J., 158, 169, 175, 182, 202, 328
McCarthy, J. D., 111, 113
McCarthy, J. J., 111, 113
McCauley, R. L., 160, 161, 163, 182
McConnell, F., 319
McConnell, F. E., 114
McConnell, N. L., 329
McKillop, A. S., 353
McLean, J. E., 73
McNeill, D., 46
McNeill, M., 345
McReynolds, L. V., 18, 45, 112, 222
McWilliams, B. J., 203
Mecham, M., 340, 344, 346
Meeker, M., 103
Mengert, I., 225
Menyuk, P., 7, 46, 111, 148, 230
Merits-Patterson, R., 10
Merrill, M. A., 350
Messick, S., 160, 231, 237
Metraux, R. W., 323
Miles, M., 323
Milisen, R., 10, 88, 170
Millard, R. T., 181
Miller, G. A., 45

Miller, J. F., 5, 7, 46, 47, 148, 168, 182, 221, 230, 252, 318, 332
Mills, A. E., 7, 225
Miner, A., 347
Miner, L. E., 46, 221
Minifie, F. D., 221
Mitchell-Kernan, C., 47
Moll, K. L., 73
Molyneaux, D., 155, 184, 197, 213, 221
Moncur, J. P., 50
Moog, J. S., 328
Moore, B. V., 155, 213
Moore, G. P., 204
Moore, M. V., 270, 274
Morehead, D. M., 230
Morency, A., 182, 210, 213, 320
Morley, M. E., 19, 111, 113, 143, 144
Morris, H. D., 250
Morris, H. L., 329
Mortensen, C. D., 8
Muma, D. B., 333
Muma, J. R., 58, 333
Murray, H. A., 351
Musgrave, R., 203
Mussen, P. H., 113, 126
Myklebust, H. R., 113, 124, 143, 319, 353
Mysak, E. D., 19, 50, 63, 74, 203

N

Naremore, R. C., 111, 225
Nation, J. E., 7, 9, 10, 12, 32, 34, 50, 78, 111, 112, 114, 124, 143, 144, 157, 161, 163, 165, 167, 169, 170, 225, 236, 249, 252, 274, 346, 350
Needham, L. S., 161
Nelson, E. E., 240
Nelson, K., 46
Netsell, R., 43, 247
Newcomer, P. L., 344
Nicely, P. E., 45
Noland, R. L., 257
Northern, J. L., 18, 114
Nunnally, J. C., 341
Nutt, J. G., 247

O

Oliphant, G., 334
Oller, D. K., 45
Oratio, A. R., 189
Orzeck, A., 335
Owens, R. E., 165
Oyer, E. J., 8
Oyer, H. J., 8

Subject Index

A

Accident as causal factor affecting internal processing, 86

Acknowledgement
  letter, follow-up, 277
  of request for service, 276

Acoustic phonetics, 42

Administration, 67–72
  diagnostic session, 70–71
  flow chart, 68, 70–71
  follow-up, 71–72, 270–272
  intake procedures, 68–70
  & setting, 72

Administrative forms, 275–296

Allergies as causal factors affecting internal processing, 85–86

Analysis
  of clinical data, 53, 59–60, 219–227
  constituent, 75–115

Anatomy
  of auditory reception segment of internal speech & language processing component, 30
  of central language-thought segment of internal speech & language processing component, 33
  of speech production segment of internal speech & language processing component, 37

Angular gyrus, in auditory-verbal system, 33

Appointment letter, 295

Appraisal, definition of, 17

Arcuate fasciculus, in auditory-verbal system, 35

Assessment, definition of, 17

Audiologic chart, example of, 314

Audiologic tools, table, 348–349

Auditory acceptance-transduction, in auditory reception of internal speech & language processing component, 29–31

Auditory analysis-transmission, in auditory reception segment of internal speech & language processing component, 29–31

Auditory association areas in auditory-verbal system, 33

Auditory cortex, primary, in auditory reception-analysis, 30–31

Auditory programming
  in auditory reception segment of internal speech & language processing component, 29–30
  in central language-thought segment of internal speech & language processing component, 32–33

Auditory reception segment of processing model, 29–32

Authorization
  to obtain information, form for, 292
  to release information, form for, 296

B

Behavior section of children's history questionnaire, 99–100, 283

Behavioral correlates
  in categorizing effect constituents, 79–80
  in speech & language processing model, internal processing component, 27–28
    in auditory reception segment, 29–32
    in central language segment, 32–36
    in speech production segment, 36–38

Biological makeup, as causal factor, 84–85

Broca's area
  in central language-thought segment of internal speech & language processing component, 32–33
  in speech production, 37
  in speech programming, 35

C

Causal factor(s)
  basis for classification, 81–82
  chains of cause-effect interactions, 125
  directness perspective, 125–126
  impact on speech & language behavior, 130–133
  interactive view, 10–12
  multiple nature of, 124
  reporting in interpretive conference, 259–260
  scanning mechanism for, 82–86
  schematic of interactions, 131
  timing perspective, 126–129
  understanding, as goal of diagnosis, 2–3

Cause-effect relationships
  clinical hypothesis stated as, 135–137
  in development of hypothesis, 57–58
  identifying, 11
  schema for categorizing constituents, 78–86
  as viewed from speech & language processing model, 115

Central language-thought segment of processing model, 32–36
  comprehension, 32, 34
  formulation, 35
  integration, 34–35